W9-CTR-869

Lose your Gut Now!

Lose your Gut Now!

A Man's Plan for Shedding Pounds and Getting in Shape

Edited by Kenneth Winston Caine

A **Men'sHealth**® Book

RODALE®

Notice

This book is intended as a reference volume only, not as a medical manual. The information given here is designed to help you make informed decisions about your health. It is not intended as a substitute for any treatment that may have been prescribed by your doctor. If you suspect that you have a medical problem, we urge you to seek competent medical help.

© 2000 by Rodale Inc.

Feature cover photograph © by Blake Little
Inset cover photographs © by Rodale Images
Illustrations © by Mark Matcho

All rights reserved. No part of this publication may be reproduced or transmitted in any form or by any means, electronic or mechanical, including photocopying, recording, or any other information storage and retrieval system, without the written permission of the publisher.

Men's Health is a registered trademark of Rodale Inc.

Printed in the United States of America on acid-free 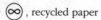 , recycled paper

"Mentally Fit" on page 110 has been reprinted with consent from Rod K. Dishman, Ph.D., professor of exercise science, the University of Georgia, Athens, Georgia 30602-6554. © 1978 by Rod K. Dishman. All rights reserved. No part of this publication may be reproduced, stored in a retrieval system, or transmitted in any form by any means, electronic, mechanical, photocopy, recording, or otherwise, without the prior written consent of Rod K. Dishman.

Library of Congress Cataloging-in-Publication Data

Lose your gut now! : a man's plan for shedding pounds and getting in shape / edited by
   Kenneth Winston Caine.
        p.   cm.
   Includes index.
   ISBN 1–57954–277–8 hardcover
   1. Weight loss.   2. Physical fitness for men.   3. Men—Health and hygiene.   I. Caine, K.
Winston.
   RM222.2 .L58   2000
   613.7'0449—dc21   00–023906

Distributed to the book trade by St. Martin's Press

2 4 6 8 10 9 7 5 3 1 hardcover

Visit us on the Web at www.menshealthbooks.com, or call us toll-free at (800) 848-4735.

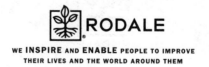

RODALE

WE **INSPIRE** AND **ENABLE** PEOPLE TO IMPROVE
THEIR LIVES AND THE WORLD AROUND THEM

Photo Credits
All interior photos are by Mitch Mandel/Rodale Images except:

page 25: Pulak Viscardi
page 28: © Clive Brunskill/Allsport
page 31: Courtesy of the U.S. Olympic Committee
page 60: Will Cofnuk
page 98: Tim Hancock/Sports File
page 100: Carey Frame/Joe Lewis Karate Systems
page 103: Courtesy of the National Basketball Association
page 118: Courtesy of NASA
page 120: Michael Ahearn
page 138: Jim Block
page 141: John Huet/Red Cat Productions
page 144: Doug Foreman
page 177: Courtesy of Robyn Rodgers
page 180: Photo courtesy of BEFIT Enterprises
page 183: Ron Kauk/© Galen Rowell/Mountain Light Photography
pages 219 (bottom) and 226: Anna Palma
page 278: Courtesy of Skyglass Inc.
page 281: Courtesy of Northwestern University
page 284: J. W. McDonnough/*Sports Illustrated*
page 313: Bill Lyle/Courtesy of Jacques Pépin
page 316: SportsChrom East/West
page 356: © Joni Palmer Photography

Lose Your Gut Now! Staff

MANAGING EDITOR: Kenneth Winston Caine

EDITORS: Jack Croft, Matthew Hoffman

WRITERS: Matthew Hoffman, Kenton Robinson, Deborah Pedron, Doug Hill, Brian Chichester, Kenneth Winston Caine, Jeff Bredenberg, Stephen C. George, Alisa Bauman, Brian Paul Kaufman, Perry Garfinkel, Jack Croft, Joely Johnson, Kathryn Piff, Selene Yeager

ART DIRECTOR: Charles Beasley

COVER DESIGNER: Joanna Williams

INTERIOR DESIGNER: Stephanie M. Tarone

PHOTO EDITOR: James A. Gallucci

COVER PHOTOGRAPHERS: John P. Hamel, Blake Little, Mitch Mandel, Kurt Wilson

ILLUSTRATOR: Mark Matcho

ASSISTANT RESEARCH MANAGER: Leah Flickinger

LEAD RESEARCHER: Mary S. Mesaros

PERMISSIONS: Lois Guarino Hazel

SENIOR COPY EDITOR: Susannah Hogendorn

COPY EDITOR: Kathryn C. LeSage

EDITORIAL PRODUCTION MANAGER: Marilyn Hauptly

LAYOUT DESIGNER: Jennifer M. Holgate

STUDIO MANAGER: Leslie M. Keefe

MANUFACTURING COORDINATORS: Brenda Miller, Jodi Schaffer, Patrick Smith

Rodale Active Living Books

VICE PRESIDENT AND PUBLISHER: Neil Wertheimer

EXECUTIVE EDITOR: Susan Clarey

EDITORIAL DIRECTOR: Michael Ward

MARKETING DIRECTOR: Janine Slaughter

PRODUCT MARKETING MANAGER: Kris Siessmayer

BOOK MANUFACTURING DIRECTOR: Helen Clogston

MANUFACTURING MANAGERS: Eileen Bauder, Mark Krahforst

RESEARCH MANAGER: Ann Gossy Yermish

COPY MANAGER: Lisa D. Andruscavage

PRODUCTION MANAGER: Robert V. Anderson Jr.

OFFICE MANAGER: Jacqueline Dornblaser

OFFICE STAFF: Julie Kehs, Mary Lou Stephen, Catherine E. Strouse

Contents

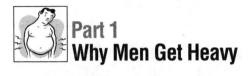

Part 5
How to Burn Calories Every Day

Part 6
The Aerobic Plan

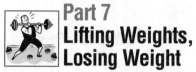

Part 7
Lifting Weights, Losing Weight

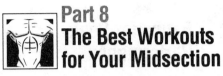

Part 1
WHY MEN GET HEAVY

How to Bust a Gut

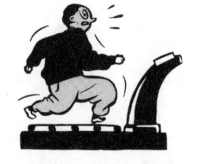

I t just sneaks up on us—the *gut*.
First, just a modicum of flab pushes over the belt. Yeah, it bothers us, but we know that it won't be there for long. It will burn off tomorrow. Or the next day. Or next week. Or sometime in the next couple of months.

Then it doesn't.

Instead, we let out our belts a notch. And then another. And then we shop for new (and bigger) trousers. It's okay, we tell ourselves; we needed new pants anyway.

This is a real-world scenario. It really happens to men. It happened to this author.

Soon, we have guts, spare tires. They're there. There's no denying it. So we go into denial. We try to forget about it. But we can't entirely. We don't want to take our shirts off anymore in public or in front of attractive women or in front of younger guys who we think look up to us. We have this secret shame. We wear it around our waists.

Then the mirror tells us there is more to this than just our guts. Something not so cool is happening to our chests and to our backs below our shoulders. To our necks. Our shirts are tighter. We've had to go up in neck size. And we've noticed that our faces are a little rounder, our jawlines no longer so jutting and defined. We don't like this. We don't know what to do about it.

Here's what to do about it.

Decide and declare that this problem will soon be over forever. Decide and declare that you will make simple, comfortable, significant, permanent changes in your lifestyle. Decide and declare that you want to be happy, healthy, and fit, and that you want to look it.

And you know what? You will. Follow this *Men's Health* program and you will be there in virtually no time at all.

No time at all means 3 to 4 short months if you are trying to trying to lose 20 to 25 pounds. All you have to make are little, significant changes. And soon you will look and feel healthy, alive, and more youthful than you have in perhaps years.

We're not going to ask you to do the impossible. We're going to show you how good health, good looks, and good shape are incredibly achievable. You're going to find what works for you. You're going to do it. And you're going to get into shape so much more quickly than you ever thought was possible. We know. We've done it. And so have thousands and thousands of other men. For inspiration, check out the Follow the Best chapters, profiles of guys who have made their efforts to stay in shape integral parts of their busy lives.

This is a design-your-own program. We give you literally hundreds and hundreds of tools you can use, systems you can follow, changes you can make, and you get to mix and match, pick and choose. Do that and you will get results.

We won't ask you to sacrifice and we won't ask you to suffer. We'll tease you, we'll coach you, we'll encourage you, we'll teach you.

You've taken a huge first step by purchasing this book with the slightly embarrassing title. You've admitted that there is a problem and you have committed time and money to solving it.

We're not going to waste your time and money; we're going to get right on with the program. First, we'll look at exactly what causes men to develop unattractive, unneeded, unseemly, unwanted flab around the midsection. Just what is fat, anyway?

What Is Fat?

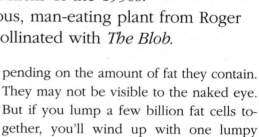

If you were to train a high-powered microscope on the inside of the belly of the typical overweight male, you'd probably be reminded of those low-budget sci-fi flicks of the 1950s. Seen up close, it resembles the voracious, man-eating plant from Roger Corman's *Little Shop of Horrors* cross-pollinated with *The Blob.*

Only Steve McQueen isn't around anymore to save the day.

Behind the belt of every man are billions of tiny blobs, each one emitting the same primal plea as Corman's campy carnivore.

"They're saying, 'Feed me. Feed me,'" says John P. Foreyt, Ph.D., director of the Nutrition Research Clinic at Baylor College of Medicine in Houston and author of *Living without Dieting.* "They're waiting to be filled."

They probably won't have to wait long. These blobs are fat cells, aptly described by Phillip M. Sinaikin, M.D., a Longwood, Florida, psychiatrist who specializes in the treatment of obesity, and the author of *Fat Madness: How to Stop the Diet Cycle and Achieve Permanent Well-Being,* as "kind of like a Baggie filled with oil."

It's not a pretty picture.

THE INCREDIBLE MR. LIPID

The average man has about 30 billion fat cells that can fluctuate wildly in size, de-pending on the amount of fat they contain. They may not be visible to the naked eye. But if you lump a few billion fat cells together, you'll wind up with one lumpy naked guy eyeing you contemptuously from the bathroom mirror.

The oily substances stored in fat cells are called lipids. But don't get confused. The term comes from the Greek word *lipos,* which means—you guessed it—fat.

We get fats from two sources: our bodies and our diets. "They're an integral part of all living systems," says Paul Saltman, Ph.D., professor of biology at the University of California, San Diego, and coauthor of *The University of California San Diego Nutrition Book.* "All creatures have fats. They're naturally produced and they're naturally a part of all the membranes and cells of our bodies."

Each of us seems to be born with a genetically determined capacity to make fat cells, which answer to the scientific name of adipose tissue. Despite how it may seem, they were not created solely to embarrass us with middle-age paunches. "The primary purpose for which God or nature put fat cells in our bodies was to be a reservoir for energy," says R. Paul Abernathy, Ph.D., professor in the department of foods and nutrition at Purdue University in West Lafayette, Indiana. "They're a place to put the energy until we need it. And when we need it, we get it out."

The problem is that most of us deposit far more than we withdraw. That's a great idea if you're talking about banking. But not with fat. Like the big-screen Blob, individual fat cells can expand to frightening proportions. "They can increase a thousandfold in volume," says Dr. Sinaikin.

They can also multiply. When fat cells expand to their outer limits—something Dr. Foreyt says occurs after a significant weight gain—they divide, forming new fat cells. And once a new fat cell is created, you have it for life. That is one of the primary reasons that it's so difficult to lose weight once you've ballooned up.

"A person with more fat cells has greater difficulty maintaining a lower body weight than a person with fewer fat cells," Dr. Foreyt says. "So you don't want to gain more fat cells. That's the bottom line. If you've got them, you can't get rid of them."

TROUBLE IN THE CELL BLOCK

Although a fat cell's main function is storing energy for future use, it also serves as a

LIPID LINGO

Cholesterol must have a great agent. In the world of fat and fatlike substances, it always gets star billing. So it may surprise you to learn that other forms of fat account for most of the fats, or lipids, in your body. Here's a quick guide to the three major classes of lipids.

Triglycerides. Found in both animal and plant foods, this is the form in which almost all of the fat in your body is stored. About 95 percent of lipids in fat cells are triglycerides, which occur when three fatty acids glom on to a molecule of glycerol. Your triglyceride level should register under 200 on a fasting test. If it's higher than that, you may be at risk for heart disease.

Phospholipids. These compounds mix fat with water, making them key players in the structures of cell membranes. They're similar to triglycerides, with one notable exception: One of the three fatty acids is traded for a molecule containing phosphorus. The best-known member of the phospholipid family is lecithin, which can be found in oatmeal, soybeans, cauliflower, peanuts, eggs, milk, and chocolate, among other foods. Proponents say that phospholipids may have health benefits ranging from improving memory to preventing liver damage from alcohol. But the jury is still out, and dietary supplements cannot be recommended.

Sterols. The most famous—and infamous—member of this lipid clan is cholesterol, which is found in animal tissues but not in plants. It serves many essential functions in your body. Too much cholesterol in your blood, however, increases your risk of heart disease. A level below 200 is considered desirable. Eggs and organ meats are particularly rich in cholesterol.

buffer that keeps excess blood sugar (glucose) and wayward globs of fat out of your bloodstream. But when fat cells are filled, they become less efficient. This means that they no longer can adequately keep harmful substances out of circulation. "The problems come not only from the fat cells but also from the things that the fat cells can't do," Dr. Abernathy says.

He likens the situation to overcrowded prisons. "It's not who's in the prison that's causing the damage. It's who's out on the streets."

In society, we have two choices: Either we can take steps to prevent crimes from being committed or we can build new cells to hold criminals. Your body is faced with the same choice when exposed to a high-fat diet. If you won't take preventive steps to cut down the amount of fat circulating through your system, your body will build new cells to store it.

By continuing to take in more energy than you can use, you'll soon fill up the new fat cells and then return even more fat and sugar to your bloodstream. This causes more insulin to be produced, which signals your body to make additional fat cells. At the same time, the excess fat and sugar in your bloodstream can eventually put you at greater risk for a raft of serious, often fatal health problems, such as heart disease, high blood pressure, and stroke.

The Beginning of a Belly

When excess dietary fat hits your system, it acts like an out-of-town conventioneer at an overbooked hotel, except without the funny hat. Instead of doing the sensible thing and leaving town, the fat lurches off in search of a room for the night. Chances are, it will wind up in Fat City—that section of the body known as the abdomen.

And there's always a neon sign out front, blinking "Vacancy."

But unlike obnoxious conventioneers, who eventually sober up and go home, the fat you eat tends to stick around. Once it's stored as body fat, it will establish permanent residency in your gut unless you forcibly evict it.

THE FIRST SHALL BE LAST

Most men consider fat to be simply abominable. But the real problem is that it's mainly abdominal.

Experts aren't sure why, but men tend to store fat in the abdominal region first. "Most men store their fat between the nipples and the navel. And most women store it between the navel and the knees," says Morton H. Shaevitz, Ph.D., associate clinical professor of psychiatry at the University of California, San Diego, School of Medicine and author of *Lean and Mean: The No Hassle Life-Extending Weight Loss Program for Men.*

And when it comes to getting rid of unwanted fat, your body is strictly a union shop: first hired, last fired. In other words, the fat in your abdomen is often the last fat to go since it's the first fat put on, says Phillip M. Sinaikin, M.D., a Longwood, Florida, psychiatrist who specializes in the treatment of obesity, and the author of *Fat Madness: How to Stop the Diet Cycle and Achieve Permanent Well-Being.*

Fat settles on your body in two patterns. Fat collecting in your abdomen and lower chest is known as apple-type distribution. Fat congregating in your hips, butt, and thighs is called the pear type.

"Men mostly fall into the apple type, which is the most dangerous," says John Erdman, Ph.D., professor of food science and director of the division of nutritional

HIDDEN DANGER

Jean-Pierre Despres, Ph.D., isn't overweight, but inside his abdominal cavity is a store of fat that increases his risk of heart disease and diabetes.

It's called visceral fat, and Dr. Despres, professor of exercise and physiology at the Laval University Lipid Research Center in Quebec, says that what you can't see can harm you. "Some normal-weight individuals will not show an obvious accumulation of abdominal fat, but they might have too much of this internal, visceral fat."

This may help explain why Old St. Nick has been around for so long. Having a belly that shakes like a bowl full of jelly is far less of a risk than having hidden abdominal fat and a hard belly, Dr. Despres says.

If you can grab the flab, that means that it's subcutaneous fat, located just underneath the skin, he says. "If it's a hard belly and you pinch the skin with your fingers and measure very little accumulation of subcutaneous fat, this individual is at very high risk because all the fat is in the abdominal cavity," explains Dr. Despres.

Men who are susceptible to this type of intra-abdominal fat storage need to be particularly vigilant about exercising regularly and avoiding excessive fat in their diets.

sciences at the University of Illinois at Urbana.

FORBIDDEN FRUIT

Maybe it goes back to the Garden of Eden. Man bit the apple; now, whenever he eats too much, he starts to look like one. Who said that God doesn't have a sense of humor?

But the health risks associated with apple-type fat storage are anything but funny. According to a review published by the President's Council on Physical Fitness and Sports, this fat pattern is "a risk factor for heart disease, high blood pressure, stroke, elevated blood lipids, and diabetes."

In fact, where fat accumulates may pose a greater health risk than how much fat you have, says Jack H. Wilmore, Ph.D., pro-

fessor in the department of kinesiology and health education at the University of Texas at Austin.

By contrast, the Widettes—those grotesquely wide-bottomed misfits portrayed by Dan Aykroyd, Jane Curtin, and John Belushi in the early years of *Saturday Night Live*—apparently would be in no great danger. "People could probably weigh more if most of that fat was in their behinds," says John P. Foreyt, Ph.D., director of the Nutrition Research Clinic at Baylor College of Medicine in Houston and author of *Living without Dieting*. That isn't to say that there's no risk at all, he adds. But research suggests that fat stored above the waist is far more dangerous than that stored below.

Experts aren't sure why abdominal fat is more dangerous. Perhaps it's because people with large amounts of belly fat have large concentrations of fat near vital organs and the hepatic portal circulatory system—the network of blood vessels that directly links the intestines to the liver.

"More recent evidence indicates that high levels of visceral fat—fat stored within the abdominal cavity—puts you at the highest risk," Dr. Wilmore says. "Not the fat that's directly under the skin, but the deep fat."

THE GATEKEEPER

How does excess dietary fat know where to go? Fat cells in certain areas are pro-grammed for storing fat, Dr. Wilmore says. More specifically, an enzyme called lipoprotein lipase is thought to serve as a "gatekeeper enzyme" that steers fat into waiting fat cells.

"It's sort of like a traffic cop. It sees fat and says, 'Stop, come in here,'" Dr. Wilmore says.

In men, the enzyme waves fat into adipose tissue in the abdomen, experts believe. "Why do you get big beer bellies in men? I suppose that's just where the fat is laid down," Dr. Foreyt says. "That's normal."

How We Eat

fig. 1

How does it feel to be wealthy?
Okay, maybe you're more a Rocky Balboa than a Rockefeller. But it's likely that to some degree you're wallowing in the astounding economic success that Americans have enjoyed over most of the past century.

Compared with the rest of the world, our food is less expensive—particularly meats, restaurant meals, and processed foods. At dinner, we can afford to give star billing to meat and cheese as opposed to, say, the rice commonly found on Asian tables. We've made dessert an indelible finale to the appetizer-salad-entrée progression. Elsewhere, it's different. Even the famed pastry chefs of Europe are only trotted out for special occasions. Day in and day out, those poor mopes overseas have only fruit to top off their meals.

Americans also revel in labor-saving machinery, such as power tools, vacuum cleaners, salad spinners, and riding lawn mowers. Driving a car is cheap in the United States, and our cities are designed to accommodate swarms of autos—unlike the claustrophobic lanes of Old World cities, which are more suited to foot traffic and bicycles.

But before you pat yourself on the back, pat yourself on the belly. What do you feel? A tractor-tread array of rippling abs? Or a balloon tire?

Chances are, it's the latter. Three-quarters of American men age 25 and over are above their recommended weight ranges, according to the Prevention Index, which tracks healthful behavior. And being overweight is a factor in a number of the nation's top killer diseases, such as cancer, heart disease, and stroke. In fact, these diseases account for 75 percent of the deaths in the United States each year. And each of them, scientists say, is directly related to how you eat.

In that light, our steak-and-leisure legacy seems more like a curse.

THE BALANCING ACT

Although most Americans actually do know a thing or two about nutrition, a study by CDB Research and Consulting in New York City found that 69 percent of men say that they find it very hard to eat a balanced diet. Two-thirds of Americans—more of them men than women—say that they're confused by news reports about what foods to avoid.

Saturated fat in the diet has been the topic of thousands of headlines. Red meat is the biggest source of saturated fat in an American man's diet. That's the stuff that stops up your arteries. What's more, eating a diet heavy on red meat and light on vegetables and fruits puts you at greater risk of developing colon and prostate cancer, which, after lung cancer, are the two cancers that kill the most men. If you have red meat five times a week, you're four times more likely to get colon cancer than if you eat it just once a month.

The FDA's Daily Values recommend that you take in no more than 30 percent of your calories from fat. (Some experts suggest that 20 percent or less would be better.) The Daily Values are based on 10 percent of your calories coming from protein and 60 percent from carbohydrates.

On average, we fall on the dangerous side of those recommendations. Men between the ages of 20 and 60 take in about 34 percent of their calories from fat, 47 percent from carbohydrates, around 15 percent from protein, and 4 percent from alcohol.

Grasping the dietary numbers is no picnic, but for many men, the hardest part of eating well is overcoming deeply ingrained attitudes about food. "People hold up ideals, which are socially and culturally set standards of what is a good meal," says Jeffery Sobal, Ph.D., a medical sociologist who specializes in nutrition research at Cornell University in Ithaca, New York. "These are root orientations that people use in deciding what to eat—and how to rationalize why they didn't choose something else."

Another confounding part of the equation is that men don't have a good handle on *how much* of certain foods they're eating.

A MATTER OF TASTE

Why do we decide to eat the foods that we do? The reasons are complex. Among the influences:

Personal preference. Maybe you just love garlicky Indian food.

Tradition. Lasagna has been on the family table since Grandpa came over on the boat.

Social interaction. Let's invite Sam over, order a pizza, and turn on the football game.

Convenience. Half a bagel, a quick slurp of coffee, and you're out the door in the morning.

Habit. What? I *always* eat peanut butter and jelly for lunch.

Belief. I'm giving up meat for Lent.

What's missing? Oh, yeah—nutrition. Certain foods will keep us healthy and lean.

All of the above reasons understandably influence what you eat, but nutrition needs to play a major role no matter what your mood or situation.

A survey commissioned by the Livestock and Meat Board showed that most guys believe that their eating closely follows the recommendations of the government's Food Guide Pyramid. While men, on average, think that they're getting 2.3 servings a day of dairy foods, they actually get 1.2. (Two to 3 servings are recommended.) And while they think that they're getting 2.1 servings of fruit per day, they're actually getting only 1. (Two to 4 servings are best.) Let's give credit where credit is due, though: Men think that they're getting 2.4 servings of vegetables a day, and that's accurate (although 3 to 5 servings are recommended).

A note about those ranges of servings: When health officials say that adults should eat 5 to 9 servings of fruits and vegetables,
they intend for men to gravitate toward the higher end because they eat more food than women. So the average man's total of 3 or 4 servings a day of fruits and vegetables falls far short of the ideal of 9.

Enough of the finger-wagging. There are also bright spots. A survey by the Calorie Control Council shows these trends.

- Seventy-four percent of American men say that they're eating more healthful diets than they were 3 years ago.
- Fifty-seven percent of men say that they always try to check nutrition labels for fat content.
- Fifty-two percent of men say that they always try to check nutrition labels for calorie content.

Alcohol and Weight

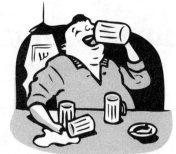

If you like to drink, you're going to have a tough time losing weight. The reason is simple, although health experts have only discovered it recently: Drinking alcohol has essentially the same effect on your weight that eating fatty foods does.

"We used to consider it liquid bread," says John P. Foreyt, Ph.D., director of the Nutrition Research Clinic at Baylor College of Medicine in Houston and author of *Living without Dieting.* "In other words, it was counted as a carbohydrate when doing food groups."

Although alcohol comes from fermented grains and fruits, chemically it's closer to fat. "Alcohol may not show itself as a layer of oil on top of a glass, but metabolically it's more like fat than like sugar," says J. P. Flatt, Ph.D., professor of biochemistry at the University of Massachusetts Medical School in Worcester.

And, like fat, alcohol has a high calorie content: about 7 calories per gram. A gram of fat has 9 calories, while carbohydrates and protein have about 4 calories per gram. In addition, when alcohol is consumed at the same time as food, the body tends to burn the alcohol first, sparing the fat.

"That helps explain why people get beer bellies," says Dr. Foreyt. "And it helps explain why you really have trouble losing or maintaining weight if you do a lot of drinking."

LIQUID FAT

The bottom line, when you're trying to cut back on fat, is to factor in the alcohol you drink. Suppose, for example, that you cut your calories from fat down to the 25 to 30 percent level recommended by experts. If you continue to consume 10 percent of your daily calories—which is about two drinks for most people—from booze, it's as though your diet contained 40 percent fat.

"If your dietary approach is to go to a very low fat diet, it won't work if you drink too much alcohol," Dr. Flatt says.

This isn't to say that you have to cut out alcohol entirely. It does mean that if you're going to drink and not gain weight, you had better cut a little more fat from your diet than you otherwise would.

But there's a catch. Even if you cut back on fat and drink alcohol in moderation, your weight-loss efforts may prove futile. First, there's the calorie issue: Drinking two 12-ounce cans of beer each day for a month is about the same as eating 550 grams of fat—or about 65 filets mignons. Then

LIQUID CALORIES

Here are the alcohol and calorie contents of a 12-ounce serving of some popular beers.

Brand	Calories	% Alcohol (By Volume)
Bud Dry	130	4.8
Bud Light	110	4.2
Budweiser	142	4.8
Busch	153	4.8
Busch Light	117	3.9
Coors Light	103	4.2
Coors Premium	141	4.7
Guinness Foreign Extra Stout	181	5.8
Killian's	172	5.4
Miller Genuine Draft	147	4.7
Miller Genuine Draft Light	98	4.2
Pete's Wicked Ale	170	5.0
Pilsner Urquell	150	5.5
Samuel Adams Boston Lager	160	4.9
Schmidt's	142	4.6

there's the small—or not so small—matter of appetite. "The circumstances under which you might enjoy alcohol are also conducive to eating more," Dr. Flatt says.

Although some experts advocate giving up drinking, at least during the initial stages of trying to lose weight, Dr. Foreyt warns that abstinence could make the heart grow fonder. "If you like a glass of wine at dinner, the worst thing you can do is give that up," he says. "You'll start thinking about it more. And psychologically, you're just setting yourself up for failure.

"If you do drink, you may have to cut back; that's true," he says. "If you're drinking a six-pack a day, you're not going to lose weight. You're going to have to gradually cut

back to one beer every other night or cut it back to weekends or something like that. But you don't want to cut beer out completely or wine out completely if you like it."

THE ALCOHOL BONUS

In countless bars over many generations, patrons have cheerily toasted, "To your health," before raising their glasses to their lips. Issues of weight aside, there's some truth to this—provided that you're only raising a glass or two. A number of studies have shown that moderate drinkers—men who have one to two drinks a day—are less likely to die from coronary disease than nondrinkers. Drinking raises the high-density lipoprotein (HDL) called the "good" cholesterol—that scoops away the artery-clogging "bad" cholesterol known as low-density lipoprotein (LDL), says Arthur Klatsky, M.D., senior consultant in cardiology at Kaiser Permanente Medical Center in Oakland, California. It may also hamper clot formation in the arteries by making blood less sticky, he says.

But physicians won't tell you to take two beers and call in the morning. Some people can't stop at two drinks, Dr. Klatsky says. Once you have six or more a day, you have a higher risk of dying from coronary heart disease than teetotalers or moderate drinkers. You're also at risk for a number of other diseases, including cirrhosis of the liver.

If you already drink an average of two a day—whether that's 24 ounces of beer, 10 ounces of wine, or 1¼ ounces of an 80-proof stiff one—there's no reason to stop, Dr. Klatsky says.

WEIGHING YOUR CHOICES

Back to the issue of drinking and weight. One study did show a correlation between beer drinking and overweight. Specifically, it suggested that given the choice between a glass of wine or a bottle of beer, men who choose the beer will gain more weight. The study, which looked at more than 12,000 men and women, found that those who drank more than six beers or other non-wine alcoholic drinks a week were 1.4 times more likely to have large guts than those who drank fewer than one. Meanwhile, those who drank more than six glasses of wine a week actually had leaner middles than those who didn't drink at all.

The researchers who did this study, however, admitted that the differences in weight between wine and beer drinkers could, in fact, be due to factors other than the booze, such as different eating habits.

THE BOTTOM LINE

When you consider the fact that there is virtually no nutritional value in alcohol, a man could possibly lose quite a bit of weight simply by giving up his nightly bottle of beer. If you're in the habit of drinking a beer every night after work, for example, you could—at least in theory—lose about 15 pounds a year just by cutting it out.

You could. But you would be depriving yourself of one of life's little pleasures. And since life gets pretty dull without its pleasures, there's not much point in that.

Clearly, what's needed is a comfortable middle zone. Here's what experts recommend.

Drink with measure. Every man needs to pay attention to how much he's drinking. A big tumblerful of bourbon is not a drink; it's two or three drinks. If you're in the habit of tipping a bottle of Scotch over the rocks each night, you should use a shot glass to measure it, just so you know how much you're actually drinking.

Switch to wine. "As far as weight loss is concerned, wine is probably the lowest-calorie beverage per standard drink," says Dr. Klatsky. "So you could make more of a case for wine in that regard."

Drink better. If you're not pouring down a six-pack every night, you can afford to buy something better. Savor one richly flavored microbrew instead of swilling several cans of cheap, mass-produced beer. Same goes for wine or Scotch. Buy the stuff you really like—just have less of it.

Dieting, Calorie Counting, and Other Lies

At any given time, the Institute of Medicine says, "tens of millions of people in this country are dieting." Americans shed pounds the way Madonna sheds clothes. There's only one big difference: Madonna's clothes tend to stay off.

According to the institute, which is part of the National Academy of Sciences in Washington, D.C., those who complete weight-loss programs will lose about 10 percent of their body weight, "only to regain two-thirds of it within 1 year and almost all of it within 5 years."

LOSING WEIGHT: IT'S A WAY OF LIFE

Most men view losing weight the same way college students approach studying for exams: Rather than working at it a little each night, they try to cram it all in at the last minute.

Taking a short-term approach to weight loss is shortsighted. And any results will almost certainly be short-lived, says Paul R. Thomas, R.D., Ed.D., a staff scientist with the Food and Nutrition Board of the National Academy of Sciences. "You do what

needs to be done to lose the weight, then you slowly go back to the old habits of eating and activity that got you into the problem in the first place," he points out.

Dieting can never be a quick fix, says Dale L. Anderson, M.D., head of the complementary medicine department at Park Nicollet Medical Center in Minneapolis. Indeed, the word *diet* hails from the Greek word for "mode of life." And that, experts say, is what we have to work on: not a temporary goal of losing 30 pounds for an upcoming high school reunion, for example, but keeping weight off for the long haul.

According to Morton H. Shaevitz, Ph.D., associate clinical professor of psychiatry at the University of California, San Diego, School of Medicine and author of *Lean and Mean: The No Hassle Life-Extending Weight Loss Program for Men*, when men come to him for help, they usually ask, "Doc, how much weight can I lose in the next 3 months?"

It's the wrong question. "The issue is, how much are you going to weigh in the next 3 years? The next 30 years? The next 50 years? That's very difficult for people to get a hold of," Dr. Shaevitz says.

DIETING IS DEAD

The problem with most diets is that they are based on deprivation, experts say. You may be able to deny yourself certain favorite foods for a short period of time, but sooner or later you're going to crave those foods again.

Another major problem is that most books, videos, and weight-loss products dictate exactly what you can and cannot eat. They don't leave a lot of room for flexibility and creativity.

"I call it no-brain dieting," says Martin Yadrick, R.D., a Los Angeles dietitian and spokesman for the American Dietetic Association. "You follow the orders and lose weight, but then when you're out in the real world, you don't know what to do and you gain it all back because you didn't learn anything."

If a basketball player who shoots 90 percent from the foul line stops practicing, his free-throw percentage will plummet. That's the way it is with dieters who regain weight, Dr. Shaevitz says. "You stop the behavior that was consistent with your success," he says.

THE MYTH OF CALORIE COUNTING

You would think that Dr. Thomas would be a nut for fine print. But when it comes to actually reading the nutrition labels he helped create, Dr. Thomas is like most men. "I'll admit I rarely look at nutrition labels outside of my professional life," he says.

It's not that Dr. Thomas doesn't care what's in his food. Just the opposite. But he knows that if he follows a few basic rules, he doesn't have to get caught up in calorie counting or complicated nutritional analyses. His diet will still be healthy.

You can do the same.

COUNTER INTELLIGENCE

When you talk about losing weight or cutting down on fat, the first thing people think of is calorie counting. That's all wrong. You can think about Count Dracula or Counting Crows or even counteroffensives, but do not—repeat, *do not*—think about counting calories.

Studies show that it's far more important to cut fat than calories. Eating fat, as you know, will make you fat. Researchers at Cornell University in Ithaca, New York, found that cutting fat intake can make people lose weight no matter how much food or how many calories they consume.

In one study, all subjects ate the same kinds of foods, but people in the low-fat group went without mayo on their turkey sandwiches, for example, or had low-fat yogurt instead of regular yogurt. After 11 weeks, the low-fat eaters had lost twice as much weight as people who ate more fat, even though the low-fat eaters had no calorie restrictions while the high-fat eaters were limited to 2,000 calories a day.

So, rather than trying to keep track of the calories you eat each day and the specific nutrient content of every item you buy, focus on the big picture. This means cutting back on fat generally by selecting mainly low-fat, minimally processed foods, and not getting hung up on minutiae.

"Nutrition labels are primarily useful in the beginning stages of making changes, particularly if you're going to be making changes by using low-fat or lower-fat alternatives to common products," Dr. Thomas says. "But once you establish your overall dietary pattern—the kinds of foods you're going to buy—it's no problem."

"I never count calories," says Paul Saltman, Ph.D., professor of biology at the University of California, San Diego, and coauthor of *The University of California San Diego Nutrition Book*. "And I tell people not to. It's compulsive-neurotic, and they'll lose track and eat too many."

In stressing calorie counting, Dr. Thomas says, some health experts have been guilty of promoting a strategy that can't possibly work. "The nutrition profession, by being so focused on the components of foods rather than the foods themselves, has led to unanticipated problems in how the general public thinks about eating," he notes. "When you're focusing on these individual parts, it does two things. Number one, it tends to take focus away from the whole. And second of all, it makes eating right seem incredibly complicated to do. And it's not."

WHAT YOU NEED TO KNOW

All your life you've been told to eat a balanced diet. But if you're like most American men, you probably need to tip the balance away from calorie-dense fats to carbohydrates, to avoid tipping the scales.

It's important to stress, though, that when it comes to your favorite foods, we're talking about cutting back, not cutting out.

"Think about a panorama of foods that gives you pleasure and a diversity that gives you nutrients," says Dr. Saltman. "Don't think of a single food, a single meal, or a single day in your life. Think of a 4- to 6-day integrated dietary program."

Here's what that diet should include.

Be a complex eater. If you're a meat-and-potatoes kind of guy—and let's face it, a lot of us still are—the last thing you want to hear is someone telling you to cut out the meat. But you probably need to think about eating more potatoes—and hold the sour cream, butter, or bacon bits—and less meat.

Carbohydrates can fill you up so that you crave less fat. At the same time, they burn fastest of all the body's energy sources and aren't easily converted into fat.

Nutrition experts recommend that at least 55 percent of your calories come from carbohydrates. The average U.S. male, however, gets only about 46 percent of his calories from carbohydrates.

One important distinction needs to be made, though: Not all carbohydrates are created equal. If you're looking to cut fat and increase carbohydrate consumption, the emphasis should be on eating more complex carbohydrates such as fruits and vegetables, which are also rich in fiber. Eating simple carbohydrates such as sugar can make losing weight harder.

Experts are well-aware, however, that men are especially resistant to making changes when meat is on the table for discussion.

"What I try to do is have them visualize a plate of food," explains Sandra Mowry, an applied clinical nutritionist in Wayne, Pennsylvania, who counsels individuals and corporate clients. "Where we used to think about having a big piece of steak and then a little bit of rice and a little bit of vegetables, I try to have them visualize a lot of rice and vegetables instead, with pieces of meat throughout."

Cut back on fat. Just as we eat too few carbohydrates, we generally consume too much fat. Although the government sets 30 percent as the target, many health experts say that we should aim to get 25 percent or fewer of our total calories from fat for maximum health benefits. The average man still gets about 34 percent of his calories from fat.

If men will follow four simple steps, they can easily keep their fat consumption within those guidelines, says Wayne C. Miller, Ph.D., assistant professor of kinesiology at Indiana University in Bloomington

and director of the university's weight-loss clinic. As part of a diet he helped develop, Dr. Miller offers the following tips.

- Don't cook in oil or fry in grease.
- Don't add butter or oil-based products to your foods.
- Eat and drink only low-fat dairy products.
- Eat only lean red meat, or fish and poultry without the skin.

"I'm not counting fat grams. I'm not weighing this, that, and the other," Dr. Miller says. "I'm not going to charts and tables and food exchanges. I'm just making some simple changes."

Don't be too pro-protein. High-protein foods, especially meats, are often rich in calories and loaded with fat. If you eat excessive amounts of protein, what your body doesn't burn for fuel it will store as fat.

Experts say that you should limit your protein consumption to less than 15 percent of your total calories. It probably won't be too hard, since several surveys have shown that the average man is already in that ballpark.

The Force of Genetics, the Counterforce of Choice

Talk about the American dream. When researchers announced that they'd identified and cloned a "fat gene" in mice, there was immediate speculation that someday scientists might come up with a pill to cure obesity.

Sorry, but there's a fat chance of that happening. Experts say that you'd be better off holding the mayo and going for a jog.

Although it seems clear that genetics plays a role in the amount of body fat we carry around with us, don't blame your parents if you have too much. Ultimately, tight jeans aren't the fault of your genes.

BIOLOGY OR BEHAVIOR?

The discovery of the obesity gene in mice revived a debate that has raged in scientific circles for decades. Does biology determine how fat we are, or does behavior? The answer, experts say, is both.

The role genetics plays in determining weight seems to vary greatly from individual to individual. But even if you are born with a genetic predisposition to overweight, the way you live is what will ultimately determine whether you get fat.

If you're living large, odds are that you'll be large.

"Clearly, the genes play a major role," says John P. Foreyt, Ph.D., director of the Nutrition Research Clinic at Baylor College of Medicine in Houston and author of *Living without Dieting.* "The genes, however, do not determine what you're going to have for dinner tonight or how much you're going to exercise."

OUT OF THE FEEDBACK LOOP

The discovery of what was dubbed the ob gene by a team of researchers from the Howard Hughes Medical Institute at Rockefeller University in New York City significantly bolsters the long-held theory that there is a feedback loop between fat cells and the brain.

Researchers believe that the ob gene makes fat cells secrete a protein that tells the brain when the body has had enough fat. Theoretically, once the brain receives that signal, it attempts to maintain constant body weight by suppressing appetite or speeding the rate at which your body burns calories.

In some cases, however, this feedback loop appears to short-circuit. In mice, for example, researchers found that those with a defective copy of the ob gene do not produce the signal-sending protein and so eat themselves into obesity. Experts believe that a similar pattern may occur in humans.

Genetics does more than tell us how much to eat. It controls our metabolisms as well. In mouse studies, for example, researchers have found that some animals that don't overeat still have a tendency to gain weight.

PUTTING FAT IN THE FIRE

Some guys can eat more and exercise less than others and not gain weight. To those others who complain that they got dealt a bad hand, Morton H. Shaevitz, Ph.D., associate clinical professor of psychiatry at the University of California, San Diego, School of Medicine and author of *Lean and Mean: The No Hassle Life-Extending Weight Loss Program for Men*, agrees. "You did. You got dealt bad genes. So in order to not get fat, you may have to watch what you eat more and exercise more than the other guy. So you either play your hand or ignore it."

THE BEST AND WORST FATS

Not all fats are created equal. While all are calorie-dense and can make you gain weight, some are better for you than others. Here's a quick primer.

Monounsaturated. Found mainly in vegetable and nut oils, such as olive and canola, these are often referred to as good fats. They help reduce blood cholesterol levels and protect against heart disease.

Polyunsaturated. These contain the essential nutrient linoleic acid and are found in fats that come from plants, such as safflower and corn oils. Like the monounsaturated variety, these also tend to reduce blood cholesterol levels.

Hydrogenated. These are liquid oils that have been chemically altered to a semisolid state. Margarine and vegetable shortening are prime examples. Hydrogenated fats are thought to clog coronary arteries, which places them in the "bad" category.

Saturated. These fats are found in all foods that come from animal sources, including meats and dairy products (milk, butter, cheese, cream, and so on). They are also found in oils such as coconut and palm-kernel oils. Saturated fats pose the highest risk for heart disease and some types of cancer. They are also found in nondairy dessert toppings and creamers.

FEEDING FRENZY:
IS IT HUNGER OR APPETITE?

Scientists believe that there's a circuit between fat cells and the brain. When the cells are full, they signal the brain, which says, "No more, thanks."

But humans are not automatons. There is a big difference between *hunger* and *appetite*. Hunger is what goes on in your belly, the physiological need to eat. Appetite refers to what goes on in your head, the psychological desire to eat.

For animals, at least in the laboratory, hunger is the key issue. "Mice, when you give them a cafeteria diet where they can pick and choose, will gorge for a while on one type of thing and then go back to eating a balanced diet over the period of a week," says Douglas L. Coleman, Ph.D., a biochemist and senior staff scientist emeritus at the Jackson Laboratory in Bar Harbor, Maine.

But people eat for reasons that have nothing to do with hunger. We eat when we're bored. We eat when we're depressed or under stress. Or we eat food for the same reason that some people strive to conquer a mountain: because it's there.

Appetite can also be driven by cravings—overpowering, not-to-be-denied yearnings for a special, usually high-fat food, says Marcia Levin Pelchat, Ph.D., a food-cravings expert at the Monell Chemical Senses Center in Philadelphia.

Although hunger and appetite roar full throttle for most of our lives, cravings appear to diminish. "One thing men can look forward to is that as they get older, they get fewer cravings and can resist them better," Dr. Pelchat says.

THE POWER OF CHOICE

In what is perhaps the most widely quoted line from the movie *Forrest Gump*, the lovable main character remarks, "Life is like a box of chocolates. You never know what you're going to get."

That's not entirely true. If you eat that box of chocolates, you know exactly what you're going to get—fat. Genetics may increase the risk that you'll put on weight, but it doesn't guarantee it. How you live your life does.

Men who are overweight invariably eat way too much fat in the form of steaks, candy bars, and corn dogs. Dietary fat in turn breeds body fat. The reason is simple: Fat is more than twice as, well, fattening as carbohydrates and protein. Specifically, 1 gram of fat packs a whopping 9 calories, while a gram of carbohydrates or protein carries only about 4 calories. A study that looked at 23 lean men and 23 obese men found little difference in their total sugar intake or the number of calories they consumed. But the overweight men took in an average of 33 percent of their total calories from fat, compared with 29 percent for their lean counterparts.

The study, led by Wayne C. Miller, Ph.D., assistant professor of kinesiology at Indiana University in Bloomington and director of the univer sity's weight-loss clinic, adds more credence to the message that health experts have preached for years: No more than 25 to 30 percent of your total daily calories should come from fat—ideally with less than 10 percent of calories coming from saturated fat, the most dangerous form.

"The real curse of fat, when push comes to shove, is that fat makes food taste good," says Paul Saltman, Ph.D., professor of biology at the University of California, San Diego, and coauthor of *The University of California San Diego Nutrition Book.* "When food tastes good, you eat more and you get more calories."

BEATING THE ODDS

Unless you're lucky enough to have been born with the metabolic intensity of a hummingbird, it doesn't matter all that much whether or not you're genetically predisposed to gain weight. The choice is yours. With a combination of smart eating and exercise, every man can lose all the weight he wants—and keep it off for good. Here's how.

Exercise late. It's every man's dream workout—literally. Researchers at the Human Energy Laboratory at Colorado State University in Fort Collins have found a way to burn more calories while you sleep. The key is exercising in the evening. Men who performed a 90-minute strength-training session in the evening woke up the next morning—15 hours after working out—with

their metabolisms still as much as 10 percent above normal.

Eat early. "Most people with weight problems eat 60 to 70 percent of their food between 6:00 P.M. and midnight and eat very little during the day," says Dr. Shaevitz. You need most of your calories during the day while you're active, so you should eat 70 percent of your day's food during daytime hours, he says.

Spice up your life. Spicy condiments such as hot peppers, horseradish, and chili powder serve double duty in the fight against fat. They fill you up more quickly and they speed up your metabolic rate. So if you're looking for something quick and easy to spice up that drab grilled chicken breast, forget the salt and try this: Stir a small amount of chili powder, cumin, chopped cucumber, and green onions into fat-free sour cream or plain yogurt. *Olé:* an instant Mexican topping.

Build up your bulk. When you get pumped up, you also pump up your metabolism. Studies have shown that for each extra pound of muscle you put on, you'll burn as many as 30 to 50 more calories a day because it takes more energy to sustain lean body mass than it does to sustain fat.

Buy foods with 3 grams of fat or less. "If you're looking at food labels, one rule of thumb is that if it has 3 grams of fat or less per serving, that would be acceptable," Dr. Miller says. "Not that you're not *ever* going to have anything that has more than that in it, but that's a good rule to follow."

Size matters. Even if you're strict about following the 3-gram rule, "you can get into trouble with quantities," says Paul R. Thomas, R.D., Ed.D., a staff scientist with the Food and Nutrition Board of the National Academy of Sciences in Washington, D.C. Suppose you're eating low-fat ice cream and the single-serving size is ½ cup. Don't routinely scarf down a pint in one sitting and then wonder why you haven't lost weight.

Keep on top of toppings. Even if you normally eat a lot of low-fat foods—potatoes, pasta, and bread, for example—you can lob a dietary bomb into the menu by piling on add-ons such as butter and sour cream. By all means, have a baked potato—but hold the butter and maybe substitute salsa.

Trim the fat. When shopping for red meat, look for cuts with the least fat. "Well-marbled meat with thick white streaks is going to be fattier than many other cuts," Dr. Thomas says.

In general, cuts with *loin* or *round* in the name are among the least fatty. And once you get the meat home, take a minute to trim away visible fat. Better to leave it on your plate than to see it on your waist.

Eat low-fat dairy foods. Most cheeses derive more than 70 percent of their calories from fat. So a 1-ounce chunk of Cheddar cheese contains more fat than a 3-ounce cut of T-bone steak.

White cheeses, such as Parmesan and mozzarella, are usually lower in fat than their yellow counterparts, such as Cheddar and American. Reduced-fat versions of the white cheeses can make an even bigger difference in any cheese lover's diet. And switching from whole milk to 1% or fat-free can also cut your fat intake substantially.

Ashrita Furman, Guinness Record Holder

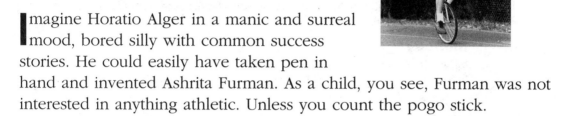

Imagine Horatio Alger in a manic and surreal mood, bored silly with common success stories. He could easily have taken pen in hand and invented Ashrita Furman. As a child, you see, Furman was not interested in anything athletic. Unless you count the pogo stick.

And darned if Furman didn't grow up to be one of the world's most prominent pogo-stickers, kachunking his way through the piranha-infested waters of the Amazon River and up and down 16 miles of Mount Fuji's foothills, breaking world records all the way.

This isn't whimsical fiction. Furman, the fiftyish manager of a health food store in Jamaica, New York, has made a career of gathering number-one citations in the *Guinness Book of Records*. At any one time, his name can usually be found next to *10 or 11* titles for sporting pursuits that we'll bet you've never tried.

Furman has broken Guinness records more than 50 times; he has broken some records several times over. But there's one event he will not be revisiting: underwater pogo-sticking.

"That was in the book for a couple of years, but they took it out," says Furman. "They said it was too dangerous. I pogo-sticked in the Amazon River, underwater. That was a thing that I invented. The piranhas were about 30 feet away. I had a rope tied around me in case of attack, although people tell me now that it would have been too late. I did that for 3 hours and 40 minutes. It was scary, but fun."

At one time or another, Furman has held the Guinness records for:

- Backward unicycling: 53 miles
- Basketball dribbling in 24 hours: 83 miles
- Brick carrying (9-pound brick in a one-handed pincer grip, palm down, walking): 64 miles
- Hopscotch (most games in 24 hours): 307

- Joggling (juggling and running at the same time) 50 miles: 8 hours, 52 minutes
- Joggling marathon: 3 hours, 22 minutes
- Milk-bottle balancing (glass bottle full of milk on the head): 70 miles
- Pogo-sticking: 15 miles
- Somersaults: 12¼ miles
- Squats, or deep knee bends, in an hour: 4,495
- Stepups (on and off a 15-inch exercise bench) in an hour: 2,229

RECORD TRAINING

Here's the training plan that Ashrita Furman followed as he prepared to break the Guinness records for brick carrying and stepups.

Monday
6:00–7:00 A.M.	Meditation
8:00 A.M.	3-mi run

Tuesday
6:00–7:00 A.M.	Meditation
8:00–8:30 A.M.	Jumping rope
3:00–3:45 P.M.	Weight lifting

Wednesday
6:00–7:00 A.M.	Meditation
8:00–8:40 A.M.	Jumping rope with high-speed intervals
3:00 P.M.	500 stepups

Thursday
6:00–7:00 A.M.	Meditation
8:00 A.M.	3-mi run
3:00–3:45 P.M.	Weight lifting

Friday
6:00–7:00 A.M.	Meditation
8:00–8:30 A.M.	Jumping rope

Saturday
6:00–7:00 A.M.	Meditation
10:00 A.M.–2:00 P.M.	Brick carrying

Sunday
6:00–7:00 A.M.	Meditation
8:00–10:00 A.M.	Brick carrying

THE INTUITIVE WORKOUT

To keep in shape for these stunts, Furman exercises almost daily, but he has no formal training schedule. "I'm very intuitive," he says. "My workouts revolve around whatever I'm training for. If I'm training for hopscotch, when I start getting into practices that last 7, 8, or 9 hours, then it takes me quite a long time to recover. So I have to work around that. I might work out with weights twice a week, run twice a week, and jump rope. I also like rowing on a rowing machine."

Furman works toward a record with a slow but sure buildup, adding more repetitions each time he practices. "You look at that deep-knee-bend record and do 500," he says. "'Wow, 500!' And the next time you do 600. It's progress you can see from day to day and week to week. The great thing is that the world is progressing, so you have to progress along with it. It would have been inconceivable for me to do 4,000 in an hour back in those days when the record was 1,800."

Furman has a flair for the exotic. The Guinness folks encourage sensational staging of events on the theory that it's hard to fake a record if there are thousands of witnesses and media coverage. Furman broke a knee-bend record in a hot-air balloon. He broke the walking-with-a-milk-bottle-on-your-head record in Indonesia and Switzerland. He broke the basketball-dribbling record in Fiji. And in Massachusetts, he somersaulted the entire length of Paul Revere's ride.

"The actual ride was Charlestown to Lexington," Furman says. "But I went the reverse because my friend told me that the hills were more in my favor. It turns out that they weren't. It was very hilly, and I got just as nauseated going down as going up."

NO LIMITS

Furman wasn't always such a dynamo. He grew up with the name *Keith* and was the class nerd. In the 1970s, he began studying Eastern philosophy and meditation under spiritual leader Sri Chinmoy, who gave him the name Ashrita, which means "protected by God."

In 1978, Furman decided to join friends in a 24-hour bicycle race in Central Park. Using meditation techniques that he had learned from Sri Chinmoy, he placed third out of thousands of participants, having ridden 405 miles.

"That was a major change, a major revelation for me—that anything is possible," he says. "If you can connect with your inner self, you can do anything. There are no limits."

Michael Chang, Tennis Ace

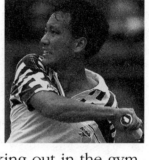

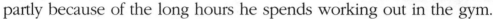

When Michael Chang makes short work of an opponent on the tennis court, it's partly because of the long hours he spends working out in the gym.

Chang lifts weights for up to 2 hours three times a week, working on the muscles most critical to tennis.

"Weight training gave me a more powerful serve," Chang says. "In the pros, everybody has a big serve. Everybody's acing each other 10 times a match. If you're weak, you have to strengthen and try to turn your serve into an asset. Make it a weapon, so it can help you end your game and save you a lot of energy."

To improve his volleys, Chang builds his forearms with wrist curls and by squeezing a tennis ball. To add pop to his serve, he strengthens his shoulders with military presses and bent-over flys. To put more power behind *all* of his shots, Chang exercises his midsection with crunches, seated barbell twists, and dumbbell sidebends. "Weight transfer plays a part in generating power, which is why the midsection is so important," Chang says. "It helps you get more power behind the ball."

To work his obliques (the muscles that run down the sides of the stomach), Chang plays catch with a trainer using a 15-pound medicine ball and rotating just his upper body. "All shots require twisting," says Chang, "so I do more abdominal work than anything else."

In 1989, at age 17, he became the youngest man ever to snare the French Open title. On the court, his preparation, speed, and guile have helped him reel in bigger, stronger opponents. His training plan turned one of the smallest players on the men's tour into one of the most feared.

That year, just as he burst onto the world scene, Chang fractured his hip. The diagnosis: too much pounding, aggravated by weak, inflexible hip muscles. Since then, he's become a devout stretcher. He keeps his back, butt, and hamstrings limber, but the primary focus is on his hips.

His exercise of choice is admittedly bizarre, but it gets the job done. He gets down on all fours and rotates his hips in a circular motion—to the right side, back, to the left, then forward—for a few minutes at

TOUGH DISCIPLINE

When he's in serious training, Michael Chang supplements his court time with weights and occasional running and swimming.

To stave off boredom, Chang varies his training schedule. In general, he spends 4 hours a day on the tennis court—2 hours in the morning and 2 in the afternoon. He lifts weights for up to 2 hours 3 days a week, focusing on the muscles crucial to tennis: shoulders, obliques (for twisting the midsection), abdominals, back, and forearms. He runs or does footwork drills 2 days a week.

a time. "I'm probably the only guy who does this exercise, because it looks so weird," he says. "But I do more running than just about anyone else on the tour, so I need more flexibility in my hips."

DIFFERENT STROKES

Chang has climbed to the top of the tennis rankings the old-fashioned way: through hard work and perseverance. There is no one secret to improving your game, he says.

"It's tricky. It varies," Chang says. "Take serving, for example. Goren Ivanisevic has a deceptive and effective serve. Great timing, but he tosses the ball low and serves on the rise. Pete Sampras doesn't snap his serve, but he's fluid, with a good rhythm, gets the ball high and out in front. Other guys aren't real accurate but have a lot of power. And then there's John McEnroe, who didn't serve hard but placed his shots so well that you weren't able to get them back. And if you did, it would just be an easy put-away for him.

"It's really a matter of what works for you, and practicing it enough to get yourself into a rhythm. Then add strength so you can add some pop to your serve. You can loosen the tension on your racket to give you more power on your serve. You can try to get more spin, for control and accuracy."

GONE FISHING

Endurance, concentration, patience, stealth. Michael Chang brings these traits to his favorite sport: fishing.

"It takes so much preparation and technique to fish," he says. "First, you decide what to fish for; then it's what type of boat; the hook; whether to use plastic worms, spinners, flies, or live bait like wigglers, crayfish, lizards, mealworms, or water dogs. It's such a big challenge."

NEVER GIVE UP

It's generally accepted in the tennis world that facing Chang is a losing proposition one way or the other. Even if you beat him, you'll be left with little energy to play the next match. Chang never gives up games or sets to conserve energy. He empties his tank every time. It's a strategy that pays a psychological dividend. "When you're out there, never stopping, that can be enough to beat someone," he says.

During play, which sometimes goes on for hours, he concentrates on each point and nothing else. He knows from experience that if he waits long enough, his opponent—Pete Sampras, Andre Agassi, the fish, it doesn't matter—might drop his guard and mess up. Says Chang, "Points turn into games. Games into sets. Sets into matches. Matches into tournaments. Tournaments into becoming number one."

Chang is a tireless scrambler who uses his speed to nullify the hard servers of the game. Part of his swiftness comes from his low center of gravity (he's 5 foot 9), but being speedy requires work. Each day, during 2-hour morning and afternoon practices, Chang does precision footwork drills with his brother-turned-coach, Carl. First, he does a series of sideways sprints, moving back and forth across the court as many as 20 times, keeping low and on his toes.

Then, he runs backward and forward from the net to the baseline. "I try to be really efficient with my movements," he says.

To keep his reflexes sharp, Chang has two trainers at the net fire tennis balls at him as he stands at the baseline, a mere 13 yards away, and works to return them. "They'll take turns and hit them high, low, and all over the place," he says. Thirty minutes is about all he can take.

Chang admits to having a weak spot for cheeseburgers, pizza, and most of the menu at Taco Bell, but his resolve hardens 2 weeks before a tournament. "No red meat, nothing fried or greasy, and only an occasional dairy product," he says.

The mainstays: pasta, rice, tofu, and Chinese food—"chicken and vegetables, very little oil, hold the MSG." He doesn't snack much, preferring instead to eat four big meals a day.

"I eat 1½ times what a normal person eats," Chang says. "When I'm in a restaurant, people look at me strange because I'm such a small person (145 pounds) eating so much."

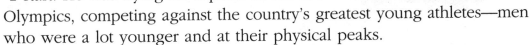

Bruce Beall, Olympic Rower

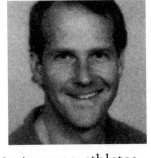

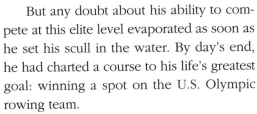

The odds were against Bruce Beall from the start. He was trying for a place in the 1984 Olympics, competing against the country's greatest young athletes—men who were a lot younger and at their physical peaks.

But any doubt about his ability to compete at this elite level evaporated as soon as he set his scull in the water. By day's end, he had charted a course to his life's greatest goal: winning a spot on the U.S. Olympic rowing team.

Although the team didn't medal, just getting a shot at the gold was enough for Beall, and an impressive accomplishment in its own right. At 32, he was the oldest oarsman on that year's team.

Now in his late forties, Beall still enjoys that competitive high, racing as often as he can in rowing and cross-country skiing events. Professionally, he has moved from an athletic position to an administrative one. After years as a rowing coach and then a fitness trainer, Beall is now executive director of the George Y. Pocock Rowing Foundation in Seattle, an organization that promotes the sport of rowing.

Not surprisingly, Beall has discovered the dangers of a time-intensive but sedentary career. When the 6-foot-5 Beall raced in the Summer Games, he weighed about 206 pounds. Today, he tips the scales at 222 pounds.

"Part of me wishes that I had more time to work out and get back in the shape I was. I know plenty of guys who feel the same way—they look back at their college or high school playing days, and they know they'll never be in that good shape again. They figure, What's the point of working out?"

But rather than giving up, Beall has taken a different tack. "Whenever I get a chance, I try to work out—you'd be surprised how little physical activity will make you feel better. It's too time-consuming to get out in a boat and row every day. But if I have enough time, I'll run or use a rowing machine for 40 minutes a day, 4 days a week."

He's also trying to watch his diet—not always with great success. "I have a real weakness for cheese. And I'll have a couple of beers once in a while, but otherwise I eat pretty well. For instance, I'm not a strict vegetarian, but I eat so little meat that I might as well be."

Beall's best advice for staying in shape? "Pick an upcoming event—a 10-K run, a cross-country ski race, whatever—and commit to it. Send in the entry fee—nothing commits guys faster than laying down their own money. If I choose an event that's a couple of months off, I've got something to focus on, to train for."

Plus, the Olympian-turned-executive is learning to always schedule his athletic commitments into his calendar, making them as important as an upcoming business meeting. "And the payoff for your exercise is great. When you compete in these organized events, you usually get some type of medal at the end." As someone who has gone for the gold, Beall ought to know.

Part 2
THE *MEN'S HEALTH* WEIGHT-LOSS FORMULA

Setting Sensible Goals

If it were strictly up to the rational part of your mind, you'd promptly file all receipts for the IRS in the same place. You'd quit playing poker with those barracudas at the corner bar. And you'd go to the gym at least 3 times a week. You know the science. Exercise will make you look better, feel better, and live longer.

Then there's diet. The part of your mind that yearns for leanness would never let you put butter on a baked potato. You'd quit eating fudge-filled, chocolate-covered granola bars. And you'd eat all your fruits and vegetables, just like your mother told you.

So much for the rational mind. Men are flesh and blood, not androids. Our logic and good intentions are forever getting mugged by a roving band of human foibles. That's why all the preaching and rules and regulations about weight loss don't work.

With so many other things to think of—your job, your family, and just having some quality time for yourself now and then—it's easy to blow off weight loss. It all seems overwhelming, not to mention dull.

That's why we created the *Men's Health* Weight-Loss Formula. It's a different approach altogether. It doesn't presume that your goal is to look like an underwear model. Nor does it presume that you have to hit a certain weight in 60 days or admit humiliating defeat. Rather, it recognizes that men have things on their minds that don't revolve around their midsections, and that the best weight-loss plan is one that's easy to follow and stick with.

The Formula is simple.

Pick a few simple, very targeted goals, then make *small* changes in your life to achieve them. Losing weight isn't rocket science. Boiled down to its essentials, it requires nothing more complicated than burning more calories with exercise than you take in with diet. This doesn't require huge changes. In fact, simple things usually work better. And it's better to have a few specific, achievable goals in mind than a whole slew of pie-in-the-sky dreams.

But first, you have to get started. For most men, that's the hardest part.

GETTING MOTIVATED, STAYING MOTIVATED

It's a phenomenon that has long worried fitness researchers. About half of the participants will typically drop out of a structured exercise program within 6 months. That drop-out rate, studies show, even applies to people who really ought to know better: cardiac patients. So when you start a training program, remember that hanging in there through the first several weeks is crucial. Your psyche is going to need major care and feeding.

Men who want to change their diets run into similar obstacles. It's tough to make changes, especially at first. It means turning a deaf ear and blind eye to the relentless propaganda campaign for high-fat eating and easy living. "This is really hard work," says Morton H. Shaevitz, Ph.D., associate clinical professor of psychiatry at the University of California, San Diego, School of Medicine and author of *Lean and Mean: The No Hassle Life-Extending Weight Loss Program for Men.*

You wouldn't try to drive cross-country without first mapping a route and figuring out how long it will take. Let's face it: If you just got in the car and started cruising blind, you'd never get there. Losing weight is like that. To accomplish goals—any goals—you have to know what they are. Moreover, the goals have to be realistic. You aren't going to lose 30 pounds in a month. Or even in 3 months.

"Some people run into inevitable failure because their weight-loss goals were unrealistic and could not have been maintained, even if achieved," says Paul R. Thomas, R.D., Ed.D., a staff scientist with the Food

THE USUAL EXCUSES

Now that you're brimming with positive thoughts, you're going to need a Dumpster for some of your old stumbling blocks—your favorite reasons for not exercising. Ready to heave-ho?

No time. This was the excuse given by two-thirds of the "less active" people surveyed by the President's Council on Physical Fitness and Sports. But the same folks found at least 3 hours a week to watch TV. Chances are, you also manage to read, go to movies, and visit the pub occasionally. You do those things because they're fun and gratifying. With the right approach, you can feel that way about exercise, too.

No energy. This is the second most common excuse. But the truth is that exercise will leave you feeling much more energized than watching *Mr. Ed* reruns.

No place to work out. Exercising does not require membership in an expensive health club. Virtually every community has public facilities for sports and fitness. Besides, you can get a great workout in and around your home with weight lifting, calisthenics, running, walking, and cycling.

and Nutrition Board of the National Academy of Sciences in Washington, D.C.

One important motivation for exercise and dieting is the knowledge that you're doing the right thing. Considerable payoffs lie ahead, and a new you is emerging. People who start taking care of themselves list among their motivations not only improved health and fitness but also better looks, improved social interaction, and psychological benefits such as confidence, self-esteem, and relief from depression, anxiety, and stress.

"Some male clients come to me very withdrawn, very timid. They will start out wearing a sweatshirt, and the next thing I know they're wearing a T-shirt," says fitness trainer Carlos DeJesus of Richmond, Virginia. "By the time they start wearing a tank top, they're there, whether they know it or not."

CLARITY IS EVERYTHING

How do you bridge the gap between what you do and what you *should* do? First, master goal-setting. Goals focus your diet and workout program and clarify what you're trying to achieve. As you attain each goal, you get that bounce of encouragement and cause for celebration.

Here's how to ensure that the goals you set not only are achievable but also take you where you want to go.

Make your goals explicit. A vague goal, such as "I want to be strong" or "I'm going to lose some weight this year" gives you nothing to shoot for. Instead, say, "I'm going to lift weights three times a week until I can bench-press 150 pounds." Or,

"I'm going to drop 5 pounds between now and Christmas."

Keep your goals within reach. You don't have to burn large amounts of fat to get the benefits. Losing as little as 10 percent of your weight will make you look better and substantially reduce health risks. "Whatever you weigh today, you can lose about 10 percent without a whole lot of difficulty," says John P. Foreyt, Ph.D., director of the Nutrition Research Clinic at Baylor College of Medicine in Houston and author of *Living without Dieting.* "A 200-pound man can drop to about 180 and then maintain that reasonably well. If you get much lower than that, it becomes harder."

Start with the basics. By making moderate changes in diet and activity—eating takeout only once a week instead of four times, for example, or walking the dog twice a day instead of just once—you'll almost automatically lose ½ to 1 pound a week. "If you have a tendency to overeat, you'll have to watch that," adds Wayne C. Miller, Ph.D., assistant professor of kinesiology at Indiana University in Bloomington and director of the university's weight-loss clinic. "Don't get dramatic. Don't go cutting calories too low and fool with your metabolism. And exercise 3, maybe 4 days a week for 30 minutes or so."

Don't get hung up on the details. There's nothing wrong with slacking now and then. Don't want to run this weekend? Don't. Stay on the couch and enjoy the game. Feel like ice cream? Have it. Enjoy. Giving in to life's little satisfactions will make it a lot easier to stick with the plan the rest of the time.

WRITING MAKES IT EASIER

It's probably inaccurate to say that most men don't know what they eat. "The bottom line," says John P. Foreyt, Ph.D., director of the Nutrition Research Clinic at Baylor College of Medicine in Houston and author of *Living without Dieting*, "is they don't care."

They should, especially if they care about their expanding waistlines. That's where a food diary comes in handy. Experts say that it's extremely helpful for anyone trying to lose weight to write down what he eats over the course of several days.

"People are more likely to succeed if they keep a food diary. That's a fact," says Dr. Foreyt. "I think it works because it sensitizes people to what they're eating. It keeps reminding them."

If you're not interested in keeping track of all the food you eat over several days, try this: Draw up a simple scorecard. Down the side of the page, set up the following categories:

- I didn't cook anything in oil or fry in grease.
- I didn't add butter or oil-based products to foods.
- All the dairy products that I consumed were low-fat.
- The meat that I had was lean red meat, fish, or poultry without the skin.

Across the top of the page, write the days of the week. Post the scorecard on your refrigerator. Each day, check off the statements that are true. Then, at the end of the week, count the checks. The more checks you have, the closer you are to living the low-fat life.

MAKING EXERCISE FUN

Changing the way you eat isn't the hardest part about losing weight; regular exercise is. Consider the average gym. The surroundings are dingy, the equipment is medieval, and the tasks are tedious. If that sounds like your workplace, let's hope you're paid well. If that sounds like your *workout,* then you won't get fired for making some changes. You're more likely to stick with a workout that's fun.

"I try to be well-rounded. I play basketball, I rollerblade with my kids, I play tennis, I go skiing occasionally. Exercise should be fun. Or at the least, it has to be tolerable," says Chris Melby, Dr.P.H., director of the Human Energy Laboratory at Colorado State University in Fort Collins. "Too many people start a program, they don't enjoy it, and they quit. I just have learned to enjoy exercise, to find the things I really like to do, and so the motivation factor is there."

Don't hesitate to shake things up. A little variety will help hold your interest in working out. If your jogging is in a rut, find a new track or a path through the woods. Or try cross-training for a while: Take up cycling, swimming, or karate.

Involve friends and family. Taking along a workout partner or a personal cheering section can be an enormous boost. People surveyed by the President's Council on Physical Fitness and Sports said that spouses were the strongest positive influence on sticking with exercise. Friends will keep you in the game, too.

"The guys I play basketball with expect each other to be there," says Dr. Melby. "We enjoy the friendship as well as the exercise—something we can do together. There's a certain amount of accountability. If you don't show up, somebody from the group is going to get on the phone and say, 'Where are you?'"

FIGHT DISCOURAGEMENT

Tyranny is no fun. If, once in a long while, you blow off a workout in favor of an ice cream cone, accept it lightheartedly. Otherwise, the sense of failure can make it harder to get yourself back on track. Focus on how much progress you've made so far, not on how far you have to go.

If you feel discouraged a few weeks into your lean lifestyle routine, don't give up—that's just a predictable part of the cycle. Your body is going through some big changes. You have to give it time.

Incidentally, forget the scales. Don't try to chart your progress by weighing in. Sure, the combination of eating better and regular exercise will shed fat, but hopefully you'll gain muscle, which weighs more. If the scales are your only measure of progress, you might end up wrongly discouraged.

How to Keep the Goals You Set

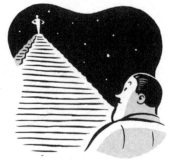

According to former U.S. Surgeon General C. Everett Koop, M.D., Sc.D., the worst enemy of weight loss in America is a household appliance. But it's not the refrigerator. "I think probably television is going to turn out to be the number one culprit," says Dr. Koop.

"Television makes couch potatoes out of people," he says. "In addition to that, I think most people who spend an inordinate amount of time in front of television eat while they watch."

It's not just eating and watching that makes us fat. Scientists agree that genetics and metabolism play at least supporting roles in what goes around our waists.

HELP YOURSELF

But biology—and television—are hardly destiny. You decide, by the foods you eat and the level of physical activity you enjoy, whether you stay lean or go to fat. "The reality is that we do have a lot of control over the outcome," says Morton H. Shaevitz, Ph.D., associate clinical professor of psychiatry at the University of California, San Diego, School of Medicine and author of *Lean and Mean: The No Hassle Life-Extending Weight Loss Program for Men.*

A study at Indiana University in Bloomington of 14 men and 21 women concluded that overweight people can shed pounds without Richard Simmons or some other weight-loss guru. The Indiana researchers concluded that people can independently change their own eating and exercise habits to reduce fat.

And this is a crucial point, says Paul Saltman, Ph.D., professor of biology at the University of California, San Diego, and coauthor of *The University of California San Diego Nutrition Book.* "It ain't the doctor's responsibility; it ain't science's responsibility; it ain't my mother's and father's," he says. "It's mine."

APPORTIONING BLAME

It's a big country. Maybe that's why our food comes in big portions, making us big.

"If you go to a good Parisian restaurant, you'll get a little 6-ounce steak. If you go to an American restaurant, they advertise one that hangs over both ends of the plate and weighs 16 ounces," says Dr. Koop. "And people tend to eat what's put before them."

Even if you already follow a healthy, low-fat diet, you still have to think about portion size. "Remember, elephants eat nothing but salad, and without dressing," says Dr. Shaevitz.

"The bottom line is that you'll put more fat on your body from 10 SnackWell's than from 5 Oreos," says Phillip M. Sinaikin, M.D., a Longwood, Florida, psychiatrist who specializes in the treatment of obesity, and the author of *Fat Madness: How to Stop the Diet Cycle and Achieve Permanent Well-Being.* "Wake up to that. Calories do count."

FAT-FIGHTING TIPS

Here are some ways experts recommend to help you lose weight and keep it off.

Give peace a chance. Switching to a low-fat diet can be like waging war. It's a tough fight, and absolute victories are rare. Wayne C. Miller, Ph.D., assistant professor of kinesiology at Indiana University in Bloomington and director of the university's weight-loss clinic, recommends a compromise position—what he calls a negotiated peace.

"We've got this internal struggle going on," Dr. Miller says. "The intellectual side is saying, 'Reduce the fat, cut out the sugar.' Then there's the emotional side saying, 'Yeah, but I like this. It tastes good.'"

LET'S GO TO THE VIDEOTAPE

The remote control has become a universal symbol for man's slothfulness. True, it is essential for the couch potato's favorite sport of channel surfing. But you're not going to burn off many calories flipping through the cable lineup, no matter how many channels are broadcast.

If you own a VCR, however, the remote could become the key to getting off the couch long enough to exercise every day.

Most men, given a choice between exercising for ½ hour and watching their favorite TV shows, will remain glued to the tube. But if you ask them why they don't work out, they say they don't have time. That's where the remote comes in.

According to Paul R. Thomas, R.D., Ed.D., a staff scientist with the Food and Nutrition Board of the National Academy of Sciences in Washington, D.C., that little switch is the secret to having it both ways: You'll have time to work out and watch your favorite shows.

"Tape the program, then watch it later and zap the commercials," Dr. Thomas advises. By fast-forwarding past the ads, you can save almost ½ hour for every 2 hours of television. "There's your ½ hour to get some activity in," he says.

Since you can't conquer your cravings outright, you need to figure out an eating plan that you can live with for the rest of your life.

"Maybe there are some things that are traditionally high in fat that you *can* give up and won't miss," he says. "Maybe there's something else you are more emotionally attached to that you just can't give up. You can have a liberal negotiated peace with that food. For example, instead of having french fries 5 days a week, have a serving 2 times a week."

Plan ahead. "On a Saturday or Sunday, we will always make something in quantity so we will have it for late evening meals when we are busy and can't get home at the regular dinner time," says Paul R. Thomas, R.D., Ed.D., a staff scientist with the Food and Nutrition Board of the National Academy of Sciences in Washington, D.C. "We can just pop it out of the refrigerator and into the microwave. We eat it along with some good bread, a steamed veggie, and a glass of fat-free milk, juice, or water."

Take your own. It's hard to eat healthy meals when you're dependent on the company cafeteria or the fast-food joint down the road. To take control of your noontime meal, make lunch a B.Y.O. affair. Packing a sandwich, some fruit, and maybe pretzels, low-fat yogurt, or snacks can save you from putting on the pounds.

Tune out. We don't think of television as being part of a high-fat diet, but it can play a key role not only in what you eat—chips and other eat-with-your-hands fare—but also in how often you eat it, says Dr. Koop.

"There are a number of strategies, ranging from watching less television and getting more activity to cutting back on the amounts of the nonessential, low-nutrition foods you eat," says Dr. Thomas.

At the very least, you may want to stock up on lower-fat alternatives so you can enjoy your tube time without packing on the weight.

Sign on for 3 months. There's no way you're going to lose weight by dieting alone. You have to get some exercise as well. It doesn't have to be rigorous as long as you do it regularly, says Dr. Miller. What is important is sticking with it.

"If people can hang in there past the third month, they've probably established some behaviors that might carry over," Dr. Miller says. "But usually, the dropouts occur around the end of the second or third month. So give yourself at least 3 months."

Eating Well, Eating Lean

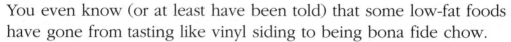

Along with exercise, eating a lean diet is the foundation of the *Men's Health* Weight-Loss Formula. You've read the diet books. You know it's time to cut back on fat. You even know (or at least have been told) that some low-fat foods have gone from tasting like vinyl siding to being bona fide chow.

So how come you have this sudden urge for a 16-ounce porterhouse?

If you've ever been on a diet that went beyond New Year's Day, you know the sinking feeling that comes as you watch your favorite foods swirling down the flavor drain. In the real world, man does not live on bread—or carrots, tofu, or celery sticks—alone. This is why most diets ultimately fail.

It doesn't have to be this way. "There are ways of eating that are healthy yet also retain their integrity," says Chris Schlesinger, chef and co-owner of the restaurants East Coast Grill, Blue Room, and Jake and Earl's Dixie BBQ, all in Cambridge, Massachusetts, and coauthor of *The Thrill of the Grill* and *Big Flavors of the Hot Sun.* "Otherwise, you end up like the Jetsons, eating nutrition as a pill."

Whether you're popping into your favorite bistro or smoking up the kitchen yourself, you can trim fat from your diet and still eat like a king. The trick, Schlesinger says, is

fine-tuning your approach to food. Always eat well—but pick your foods wisely.

"Food plays a major quality-of-life role," says Schlesinger. "I never go on a diet. If I feel like I'm eating too much, I try to eat just good things. I try to eat more fish entrées, cut down on the meat portions, and eat more good stuff. I eat six pieces of fruit a day, and I try to eat a lot of rice and beans."

You say you'd rather eat like a linebacker? Go ahead. A survey of NFL trainers showed that pro football players average six servings a day of fruits and vegetables—twice what the average American eats. The typical pregame meal includes fruits, fruit juices, pasta with low-fat sauce, pancakes, toast, scrambled eggs, and bagels. When you eat like that, your padding goes under the jersey, not under the skin.

CUSTOMIZE CRAVINGS

The only way you'll ever stick with a low-fat lifestyle is by enjoying yourself in the

SATISFYING SWAPS

There are a lot of good-tasting, satisfying foods that can help you bridge the chasm between low-fat eating and high living. On the left is the traditional, high-fat fare; on the right, some lean alternatives that are still honest-to-goodness chow.

Fatty Fare

Seafood
Breaded and fried clams (6 oz): 342 calories, 19 g fat
Breaded and fried shrimp (6 oz): 412 calories, 20 g fat
Broiled swordfish steak, in olive oil (8 oz): 600 calories, 45 g fat

American*
Chef's salad, before dressing (1½ cups): 260 calories, 15 g fat
Sirloin steak (8 oz): 523 calories, 27 g fat

Chinese*
Kung pao chicken: 490 calories, 25 g fat
Moo shu pork: 630 calories, 38 g fat
Pan-fried soft noodles: 680 calories, 36 g fat

French
Crème brûlée (4 oz): 325 calories, 25 g fat
Duck à l'orange (¼ duck): 835 calories, 69 g fat
Veal cordon bleu (4 oz): 440 calories, 27 g fat

Italian
Pasta with cream sauce and prosciutto (12 oz): 906 calories, 18 g fat

Mexican
Beef burrito with sour cream: 431 calories, 21 g fat
Chicken chimichanga: 605 calories, 35 g fat
Red beans with pork (3 oz): 320 calories, 19 g fat

Lean and Luscious

Steamed clams (20 small): 155 calories, 1 g fat
Seasoned shrimp (6 oz): 154 calories, 2 g fat
Poached salmon (8 oz): 368 calories, 14 g fat

Garden salad, before dressing (1½ cups): 50 calories, 2 g fat
New York strip steak, lean (8 oz): 478 calories, 22 g fat

Chicken and vegetable stir-fry: 245 calories, 14 g fat
Beef and green pepper stir-fry: 290 calories, 11 g fat
Shrimp chow mein: 240 calories, 5 g fat

Orange soufflé (4 oz): 155 calories, 8 g fat
Orange-glazed Cornish hen with wild rice stuffing (1 hen): 560 calories, 26 g fat
Chicken divan (6 oz): 385 calories, 18 g fat

Pasta with fresh tomato, basil, and garlic (12 oz): 520 calories, 11 g fat

Chicken burrito: 334 calories, 12 g fat
Chicken fajita: 190 calories, 8 g fat
Refried beans (½ cup): 130 calories, 2 g fat

*Typical entrée-size servings

meantime. Go ahead: Indulge yourself. What counts is fat consumption over the long haul, not what you had for dinner last night. Rather than compromise by having tough little steaks more often, "I'd rather eat one steak a month and have it be the 16-ouncer," Schlesinger says. The occasional feast won't bust your budget. Plus, it helps keep you satisfied, so you're less tempted to stray.

"Moderation is the key—not to totally eliminate fat in the diet," says Lisa Litin, R.D., a research dietitian at Harvard School of Public Health. "If you're going to have something high-fat, then you should plan ahead and control your fat intake during the other times of the day."

Besides, extreme deprivation plays strange tricks on the mind. When you deny yourself eating pleasure, you may instinctively want a reward—call it an eating binge—later on.

Lose Your Gut in a Year or Less

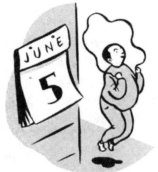

We've been talking about the importance of setting targeted, specific weight-loss goals. A great example is committing to getting back in shape in time for a high school reunion.

"I've been planning reunions for 9 years, and one of the most common things people say is that they have to lose weight," says Sunny McGinnis, president of the National Association of Reunion Managers and owner of Reunion Celebrations in Tampa, Florida. "It all boils down to people wanting to look the way they did."

There's no easy way to make the pounds disappear, to quickly regain the body you had decades earlier. What took you 20 years to put on won't come off overnight. And that's fine. The *Men's Health* Weight-Loss Formula is designed to help you lose a reasonable amount of weight in a reasonable length of time—and keep it off for the *next* reunion.

It's not impossible to drop a lot of weight in a hurry. In one study, researchers monitored 40 obese recruits who were undergoing basic training for the Singapore Armed Forces. After 20 weeks of rigorous training, the recruits who stayed with the program lost an average of 39 pounds. Average body fat plummeted from 34 percent to 24 percent.

But how many of you are willing to go into full-time basic training for the military?

GETTING ON THE FAST TRACK

"For most people, the biggest problem with losing weight for the short term is that their goal isn't to lose the weight within a year—it's to lose weight in weeks or months," says Roger G. Sargent, Ph.D., professor of public health and nutrition at the University of South Carolina School of Public Health in Columbia.

Being realistic is key. So is advance planning. If you're going to lose weight for your reunion, you'll want to begin before it's 2 months away. Even before you begin thinking about specific weight-loss strategies, here's what experts recommend.

Set a date. Yes, it would be fun to lose weight, buy a new suit, and arrive at the reunion in a blue Mercedes—all in the same 2 weeks. It's not going to happen.

"A person who weighed 150 pounds in high school and who weighs 225 now is not going to get back to 150 anytime soon," says L. Jerome Brandon, Ph.D., associate professor of kinesiology in the department of kinesiology and health at Georgia State University in Atlanta.

The point is not to be discouraged but to plan ahead. "A person may lose somewhere between 3 and 5 pounds of fat reasonably and safely in a month's time," Dr. Brandon adds. Use that as a working number. If you hope to shed 20 pounds by June, for example, get serious about losing weight sometime in January.

Make goals you can control. It's good to strive for long-range targets—in this case, that you'll lose 20 pounds by June—but don't make promises to yourself that you're not sure you can keep. When you're trying to lose weight, nothing energizes like success or brings you down faster than failure.

"My advice is to set goals that you are completely in charge of," says fitness instructor Joan Price of Unconventional Moves in Sebastopol, California. "For example, that you will exercise five times a week as long as you're able is a goal that you're in charge of. That you will lose 20 pounds by your reunion is not, since you can't control how fast you lose weight."

Be a competitor. "Nothing inspires some men more than social conditions, like com-

petition," says Bob Goldman, D.O., Ph.D., president of the National Academy of Sports Medicine and chairman of the Academy of Anti-Aging Medicine in Chicago.

So set goals for yourself. Promise yourself that you'll lose at least 2 pounds by next month. Vow that you won't look like those other overweight guys at the reunion. Or go in cahoots with another friend who's also trying to lose weight—and then do better.

"If the goal is to lose weight by a certain date, looking at it as a type of competition will work for some people," Dr. Goldman says.

Take affirmative action. One way to keep laserlike focus on your goal during a short-term fight against fat is to practice what are called affirmations. An affirmation is a positive statement you memorize and repeat, like a mantra. Doing this imprints your goal into your psyche, making you more likely to achieve your objective.

Make your affirmations short and specific, such as, "I will lose 5 pounds in the next 2 months." Write your goal on paper and post it somewhere you'll see it every day, like on the bathroom mirror. Spend a few minutes each day repeating your goal to yourself. Say it slowly, deliberately, and with conviction.

"As you repeat affirmations, try to imagine that each one is—or can be—true. Actually see yourself changing," says Dennis T. Jaffe, Ph.D., a consultant at HeartWork in San Francisco and coauthor of *Self-Renewal* and *Rekindling Commitment.*

Think about the prize. You want to look good and impress your friends. You want to fit into your blue serge suit. Maybe you just

THE MYTH OF WEIGHT-LOSS CREAMS

You may have heard about the thigh-fat-reducing creams for women. Now, there's a version for men. The idea is that rubbing the cream on your belly will cause fat to melt away. The manufacturer has trumpeted a study in which men who used the product daily lost an average of 2½ inches of waistline in 6 months.

Fat creams contain aminophylline, a caffeine derivative that manufacturers claim will cause fat cells to burn fat instead of storing it. As it turns out, however, the promise is anything but certain. "There is no scientific evidence that this is a safe or effective method for decreasing fat," says Susan Zelitch Yanovski, M.D., director of the obesity and eating disorders program at the National Institute of Diabetes and Digestive and Kidney Disease in Bethesda, Maryland.

According to the FDA, aminophylline has not been tested or approved as a fat reducer, which is why the fat creams are currently considered cosmetics, not drugs.

In other words, the one sure thing that will be lightened by a fat cream is your wallet. "The only way to trim body fat is to increase physical activity and decrease fat in your diet," Dr. Yanovski says. "You can't buy that in a store."

want to sit on a bus without crowding the person next to you. All are reasonable goals. But to keep yourself motivated throughout the year—and beyond—consider what you'll gain by losing weight.

- Physically fit men are 53 percent less likely to die premature deaths than unfit men.
- Fit men are four times less likely to die from cancer than the unfit.
- Fit people are eight times less likely to die from cardiovascular disease than those who are unfit.

Be sane. Guys who are overambitious and mount a fat-fighting operation with the same ferocity that they'd apply in a hostile corporate takeover may experience quick rewards, but they're almost guaranteed to have long-term setbacks as well.

As a rule, experts say, don't try to lose more than 5 pounds a month. Guys who try to lose more—say, 25 pounds in a month—will just become weak, or worse. "Once you lose body weight that soon, you're endangering your health," warns Dr. Brandon.

BACK TO BASICS

Once you make the commitment and set a date for losing weight, you're going to use many of the same strategies you'd use for a long-term plan, like smart eating and exercise. "But you'll do more of it," Dr. Sargent adds.

"I think that if someone wants initially to start on a program for getting in shape in a small amount of time, he should focus on doing 20 to 30 minutes of exercise every day," says Art Mollen, D.O., director of the Southwest Health Institute in Phoenix and author of *The Mollen Method.* "If you really want to get into tremendous shape, you'll need 45 minutes to an hour of good exercise every day."

Keep it fun. When you're trying to lose weight fast, don't get bogged down with a laundry list of activities that you loathe. Time is short, so stick with things you enjoy and know you'll do.

"Especially for the short term, people have to do the types of exercises that they're comfortable with," Dr. Sargent says.

"For some people, this will be biking. For others, it will be running. You have to find something that you're comfortable with in order to stick with it."

Duplicate your efforts. It takes discipline, but exercising twice a day enhances the probability that you'll burn fat fast.

"We also know that if you have limited time periods, two or three segments of exercise equal the benefit of a single bout of equal time. If I were serious about losing weight in the short term, I'd do my exer-

HIRING SOME HELP

When you're on tight deadlines, consider signing up with a personal trainer—an exercise expert who can help you get impressive results fast.

Personal trainers don't give away their time, but their rates aren't necessarily stratospheric, either. Most charge between $30 and $200 for a 50-minute session. The rate may include the use of a local gym or health club, or the trainer may work with you at home.

The advantage of working with a personal trainer is that you get personalized attention, plus you're able to work at your own pace. Before making the hire, here's what experts suggest.

Cast a wide network. You can always peruse the Yellow Pages, but a better way to find a good trainer is to ask your friends and coworkers whether they know anyone they would recommend. Or ask around at the health club.

Look for longevity. Ask prospective trainers how long they've been in business and what their experience is. You're looking for seasoned pros, not beginners trying to break into a new profession.

Ask about credentials. The oldest and most reputable programs that certify trainers are the American College of Sports Medicine, the National Academy of Sports Medicine, and the National Strength and Conditioning Association. Other good programs include the Cooper Institute for Aerobics Research, the American Council on Exercise, and the Aerobics and Fitness Association of America.

Request references. Good trainers have satisfied customers, and they won't hesitate to put you in touch. Ask to speak to three.

Take a trial run. Before signing up for a long-term program, arrange a 1-month trial period. How well you get along with this person will really determine whether you stick with the program or drop out after 2 weeks. If it's not a good match, cut your losses and move on.

cises twice a day," Dr. Sargent says. "Doubling your dose of exercise gives you a great metabolic kick. You'll put an enormous burden on your metabolism and get a great return."

Bring on the power. Serious weight loss requires serious effort—like combining aerobic exercise with strength training, points out Dr. Sargent. Aerobic exercises such as running, cycling, and walking mobilize fat throughout your body, while weight lifting builds lean muscle mass in those body parts you work hardest. More muscle tissue means faster metabolism, which enables you to burn more calories even when you're driving home.

Try the walk-jog solution. It isn't necessary to kill yourself in order to shed pounds. If you are ready to burn flab but aren't already in good shape, Dr. Sargent recommends combining walking with jogging.

Once a day, hit the road for 20 to 30 minutes. Promise yourself that you'll go the whole distance. Start out jogging until you're out of breath or your muscles start fatiguing. Walk until you've recovered, then jog some more. Do this daily, increasing the jogging time a few minutes every few days. Once you're jogging the distance, you're on the high road to slimming down.

Always be prepared. Promising yourself that you'll never miss a workout is like saying that you'll never be sick: Things happen. Keeping a packed gym bag in the trunk, however, makes it easier to work out when the urge strikes. This is particularly helpful when you're trying to lose weight fast and every workout counts.

Maximize opportunity. Exercise doesn't happen only on the track or in the gym. Every day, there are dozens of little opportunities—going shopping, walking to your car, or just going from the basement to the fourth floor—that help you burn a little more flab, says Kelly Brownell, Ph.D., professor of psychology and a weight-loss expert at Yale University.

For starters, lose the remote control and actually walk to change channels. It's not exactly a marathon, but it helps. So does getting out of the car and opening the garage door by hand, walking the shopping malls instead of ordering by mail, taking stairs instead of elevators, and walking at lunch instead of having an hour-long meal. All these small efforts add up to decent workouts, and workouts subtract pounds. When you're in a race, every step you take counts.

Eat smart. You can exercise 5 days a week, but if you're not alert to what goes into your mouth, you're not going to lose weight, says Dr. Brownell. Consider this: One quarter-pound cheeseburger, a small order of fries, and a shake has more than 1,000 calories—about the same number that you'd burn during a 10-mile run or a 3-hour game of tennis.

You don't have to be fanatical about dieting to lose weight, says Dr. Sargent. In fact, you don't need to diet at all. Just cut back on fatty foods—things like burgers, fries, and rich desserts—and eat more of the foods that you know are good for you, like potatoes, beans, fruits, vegetables, and bread.

Keep Your Gut From Coming Back

Which is harder, losing 20 pounds in 6 months or keeping it off the following year? Lots of men would say that the first is the hardest. You have the pressure of a deadline. Old habits to break. Being hungry all the time. No question, it's tough to get thin.

But the really hard part, experts say, is staying that way. Of those millions of overweight Americans who manage to lose weight, 40 to 60 percent regain it within a year. Others are luckier: They might have up to 5 years before all the pounds pile back on.

"Losing fat and keeping it off in the long term for many people is difficult, but it's by far one of the most important things you can do for your health," says Roger G. Sargent, Ph.D., professor of public health and nutrition at the University of South Carolina School of Public Health in Columbia.

HEALING MOVES

You already know that when your goal is to lose weight and keep it off, there's no substitute for eating well—consuming less fat (and less fast food) and eating more healthy things, such as fruits, vegetables, and beans. But diet alone won't take you all the way. The only way to stay fit year after year is to exercise. This is one area where there aren't any shortcuts.

Despite the health benefits of staying trim, most guys tend to overlook exercise as their number one weapon in the lifelong fight against fat. You know you should exercise. Often, you even plan to exercise. But in the hectic crush of day-to-day commitments, it's easy to just skip it.

Don't overlook the obvious. Although exercise may seem like just another obligation in an already complicated life, it's a critical part of any long-term strategy you take to lose weight, says Art Mollen, D.O., director of the Southwest Health Institute in Phoenix and author of *The Mollen Method*.

"If you want to fight fat long-term, you

must exercise long-term," Dr. Mollen says. "Do you eat every day? Of course. If you're putting energy into your system, you need to take energy out of it to maintain your weight."

Wayne C. Miller, Ph.D., assistant professor of kinesiology at Indiana University in Bloomington and director of the university's weight-loss clinic, agrees. "Anything can help you lose weight, but research shows that people who want to keep off the weight need to exercise."

MAKE HEALTH YOUR HOBBY

Don't you wish that you could approach exercise and weight loss with the same zeal you bring to your hobbies? Imagine talking about weight lifting or aerobics with the same gleam in your eye that you get when you talk about the NCAA finals or your Hawaiian vacation or a classic car that you just saw.

Unlike hobbies, which are labors of love, we tend to view exercise as being a necessary but dull part of life, like eating brussels sprouts. But there are ways to bring to exercise and fitness the same vigor you bring to your play.

Follow your heart. The best exercise for long-term weight control isn't the one that makes you sweat the most. It's the one you'll actually do, be it golf, aerobics, rappelling, or even gardening or chopping wood.

"You don't get people to change to a

FRIENDS AND FITNESS

Scuba divers, mountaineers, and even professional wrestlers depend on the buddy system. While these and other high-risk activities require partners for safety reasons, some of the same benefits of working with friends apply to you, too.

"For some people, having a buddy gives them a buzz of energy on days when they don't feel like exercising," says Jonathan Robison, Ph.D., executive codirector of the Michigan Center for Preventative Medicine and adjunct assistant professor in the department of physical activity and exercise science at Michigan State University in East Lansing.

"Any physical activity may become much more enjoyable if you can add a social component to it," Dr. Robison says.

The buddy system can be as simple as playing basketball with a group of friends from the office or as demanding as dividing up obligations for a caving expedition. Your partner doesn't even have to stand upright. Tom McMillen, former cochair of the President's Council on Physical Fitness and Sports, gets his motivation from taking his canine crew—two Labrador retrievers—for daily runs.

"If you spend your life doing everything by yourself, I question how much fulfillment you're getting," Dr. Robison says. "I always suggest that people try to do things with another person. It gives you a sense of being connected, and that's very important for good health."

healthy lifestyle by boring them. You have to make exercise fun," says fitness instructor Joan Price of Unconventional Moves in Sebastopol, California.

Get involved. Serious hobbyists become nearly fanatical when it comes to pursuing the minutiae of their interests—which is why they stick with it year after year. To turn an exercise habit into a hobby, get involved. No matter what you like, somewhere there's a newspaper, magazine, or newsletter that covers it. Check your local newsstand or magazine rack. If you can't find what you're looking for, ask your librarian for help.

Join your peers. Joining a club with like-minded fitness buffs is a great way to keep in long-term shape, says Price. Not only will you make new friends and have a regular group to hang out with but you'll also have someone pushing you to work out on the days when you'd rather slump.

Get the record straight. If you loved cars and had just inherited a '57 Chevy—a handyman special—you'd probably take pictures of the ol' clunker, then record each stage of the restoration. Treat your own chassis with the same respect.

If you take up weight lifting, for example, measure your waist, biceps, chest, and legs when you start. Take pictures of the body parts under construction. Three months later, update your records with new measurements and photos. Eventually, you'll have a paper trail documenting how your 13-inch arms were transformed into 15-inch pythons.

"We're goal-setting animals. By re-cording and monitoring our improvements, we give ourselves a pat on the back to continue," Price says.

Be a contender. For some guys, it's not victory but the thrill of competition that stokes their fires. Contact your local fitness club or check at the local sporting goods store for information on amateur competitions in your area.

Jim Schwartz, a pilot in Santa Cruz, California, first took up cycling to trim down his midsection. Then, he branched out into competition triathlons. He found that competing—and the training that precedes it—is a great strategy for staying fit and motivated.

"I think competing helps you set goals, and setting goals is important," says Schwartz, who has finished more than a half-dozen triathlons. "When you compete, it's a real emotional charge. But you don't have to be an Olympic athlete. It's more about achieving personal victory."

Diversify. When you make exercise or sports your hobby, it's like being part of a family, says Price. That means sharing similarities and differences. "For example, if you're both cyclists and your new friend likes to box, try it," says Price. "You might pick up another hobby, and at the very least, you'll be getting more exercise and broadening your horizons."

CREATIVE TRICKS FOR STAYING IN SHAPE

It's easy to talk about exercise as a way to stay in shape, but it's a lot harder to actually get around to doing it. Or is it?

Not necessarily. You don't even have to do sports, lift weights, or sweat to music. "You need to work fat off any way you can, so the more creative your solution, the better," says Steven N. Blair, director of epidemiology and clinical applications at the Cooper Institute for Aerobics Research in Dallas.

"I suspect that the traditional advice, like exercising three times a week for 30 minutes, is good for some people, but I'm not convinced that it's the best approach for everybody," says Blair.

In one study, researchers divided overweight kids into three groups. Kids in one group did a prescribed amount (and type) of exercise. Those in the second group were allowed to choose their activity, while kids in the third group did regular calisthenics and stretching. After 8 weeks, children in all groups lost about the same amount of weight. But in a 2-year follow-up, it was the ones who had chosen their activities—such as walking to and from school—who managed to keep the weight off.

"The bottom line is that you need to increase your physical activity any way you can—do something rather than nothing," Blair says.

Here are some creative approaches to staying thin, year after year.

Control the remote. If you spend every night clicking away the channels with a remote control, don't be surprised when you start resembling sofa sediment with a paunch. "The technology revolution is such that it's engineered physical activity right out of our lifestyle," Blair says. "We can do so much nowadays without even moving."

That's the trend, but it's easy to reverse. Just losing the remote control can help. Really. Rather than giving your thumb the workout, take those few extra steps across the living room and change the channels yourself. Doing this several times an hour will burn more calories than lying still, and every little bit helps.

Make use of tube time. The average 35- to 54-year-old guy watches 27 hours of television a week, or roughly 4 hours a day. If you spent even half that time doing calisthenics while you watched, you'd burn about 825 calories—more than you'd burn in an hour of cross-country skiing at a moderate pace. How about riding a stationary bike, or running on a treadmill, or pumping a stepper or a rowing machine while watching TV?

Take to the streets. You don't have to be a runner to put your legs in motion. If you live reasonably close to work, for instance, try leaving your car parked and hoofing it instead. Walking for an hour at a leisurely 3.5 miles an hour will burn about 300 calories.

Too far to walk? Try cycling. An increasing number of men are two-wheeling their way to work every day, burning about 650 calories an hour while cruising along at 13 miles an hour.

Mark the years. Rather than just plunging another candle in your birthday cake, why not take a hint from Tom Monaghan, former president and chairman of the board of Domino's Pizza in Ann Arbor,

BUILD MUSCLE FAST

With today's deadlines and commitments, the prospect of spending hours sweating in the gym—particularly as part of an ongoing, do-it-for-life plan—may be less than appealing. But there are ways to get a decent workout fast. A study by the YMCA found that people who worked out for 20 minutes three times a week with an intense weight-lifting program gained 6 pounds of muscle and lost up to 15 pounds of fat in just 7 weeks.

But you don't need a grueling workout to get stronger and leaner. A 20-minute routine of compound exercises, which involve working several muscle groups with each lift, will quickly get you where you want to be.

Do 2 sets of each exercise with weights that allow you to easily do 10 repetitions per set. Do the exercises in order, resting for 15 to 30 seconds between each exercise. Take a minute or two between sets to jog in place or do some other cardiovascular exercise. Then, start the circuit again.

Bench press. This hits most of the major chest and arm muscles, which involve some of the body's largest muscle groups. Alternate exercise: dumbbell fly.

Leg extension and leg curl. Alternating one set of each will help build the bulkiest parts of your legs—the quadriceps—and the hamstring muscles.

Seated row with tubing or seated pulley row. These exercises work nearly every upper-body muscle group, including your back, shoulders, biceps, and neck. Alternate exercise: bent-over row with barbell or dumbbells.

Leg press. This builds your quadriceps, calves, and hamstrings. It also helps tighten your butt. Alternate exercise: front lunge with or without dumbbells.

Shoulder press. This hits your deltoids, triceps, and upper-back muscles. Alternate exercise: seated military press with barbell or dumbbells.

Lat pulldown. This works those big muscles on the sides of your back—the ones that give you a V shape. Alternate exercise: pullup.

Seated dumbbell curl. Pumps up your biceps while also working your shoulders and forearms. Alternate exercise: barbell curl.

Michigan, and try your hand—and arms, shoulders, and chest—at a few pushups?

Monaghan vowed to do 1 pushup for each year of his life on every birthday. "When I promised myself to do this, I was in my early forties, and I really had to work at it," he recalls. Now, Monaghan is in his early sixties—and instead of pumping out 1 pushup for every year, he does 125 straight.

Your goal is not to beat Monaghan but simply to give yourself a yearly marker so you can see how well you're doing—and what you should strive for next year.

Make the most of vacations. It's hard to think of anything negative to say about spending a week on a sandy Mexican beach. Suffice it to say that it won't help your beer gut get any smaller. In fact, after a few days of margaritas and rich food, you can expect it to be *mucho grande* by the time you say adios.

A fun alternative to the usual lounge-about is to take an exercise vacation, a few days or weeks in which you put your muscles to work instead of to bed. Rather than tanning on the beach in Cancún, for example, you could be cycling through the countryside in Mexico or here in the United States. Take your pick. Even spinning at a moderate pace of 10 miles an hour will burn about 400 calories an hour.

If you aren't sure where to go or what you want to do, here's a start.

- Backpack through California's Yosemite National Park with Yosemite Mountaineering School, Yosemite, CA 95389.
- Try kayaking. Contact Riversport, P.O. Box 95, Confluence, PA 15424; Otter Bar Lodge, Box 210, Forks of Salmon, CA 96031; or Kayak and Canoe Institute, University of Minnesota Duluth Outdoor Program, 121 SpHC, 10 University Drive, Duluth, MN 55812.

KEEP MOVING

Any time the talk turns to losing weight and keeping it off, you're going to hear about the two cornerstones of exercise: aerobic activity and resistance training.

Aerobic exercises are those that make your body demand oxygen and burn calories. They include walking, running, rowing, aerobic dancing, and any other moderate-to-vigorous physical activity. Resistance training (weight lifting), on the other hand, is anaerobic exercise, which builds muscle mass through resistance.

Whichever workout you choose, here are a few steps to make it most efficient.

Don't lie to yourself. If you resemble Danny DeVito but want to look like Sylvester Stallone, it's time to conduct a reality check. "Understand that some goals are achievable and others are pipe dreams," Blair says. "We all come in different shapes and sizes. I've come to grips with the fact that I'll never look like a movie star. No matter how much I run, I'll always be short, stocky, and bald."

Lift for life. You probably haven't seen many 70-year-old men pumping iron at the local gym, but you may in the future. That's because experts are now realizing that weight lifting is the unsung hero of fat-fighting exercises, says Dr. Sargent.

"I feel that the only reason resistance training hasn't had the same glory attached to it as aerobics is that it hasn't had as much study," Dr. Sargent says. "You'll find that in the past 5 or 6 years the results of weight-loss studies on resistance training and aerobics have been fairly equivalent."

While advanced lifters can spend hours pumping iron, 20 to 30 minutes is enough for most guys. Begin by doing a few sets on the bench press. Then, work your way through the major muscle groups, including curls for biceps, military presses for shoulders, and leg extensions and leg curls for your lower body. Finish with some back extension and abdominal work for a complete program.

As you grow stronger and more experienced, you may want to start experimenting with different lifting styles: lifting light weights using higher repetitions, or going for more weight with fewer repetitions. According to Dr. Sargent, evidence suggests that lifting light weights more often yields greater muscle strength than using heavier weights. Regardless of the strategy you choose, lifting weights increases muscle mass, which ups your metabolism and helps you burn fat more efficiently.

Go aerobic. If experts could choose just one type of exercise to rout that Rubenesque look, they might choose aerobic exercise—roughly defined as any exercise that increases your consumption of oxygen, causing your heart rate to increase.

These days, there are more aerobic options than New York City has pizza joints: running, cycling, rowing, skiing, boxing, wrestling, basketball, walking—all of which can provide a fantastic aerobic workout.

The American College of Sports Medicine and the federal Centers for Disease Control and Prevention recommend doing 30 minutes of moderate-intensity activity, such as walking or running, every day. It doesn't have to be done all at once, however. Rather, it can be accumulated if you scatter small amounts of activity throughout the day.

"For real results, you're going to have to work at it," notes Dr. Mollen. Though you may choose to start out doing 30 minutes of exercise seven times a week, eventually you'll want to bump up your times to 45 to 60 minutes daily, he says.

Team up with team sports. Not every guy wants to be a lonely marathoner trodding for hours in self-imposed solitude. Some of us want to shoot the breeze while we're sweating away the pounds. For both the workout and the social fun, team sports are ideal.

Tom McMillen, former cochair of the President's Council on Physical Fitness and Sports and a former NBA player and U.S. congressman, still occasionally finds time to shoot hoops with friends. "I'll get together with some friends once in a while for a game or two, but it's nowhere near as often as I used to," says McMillen.

If you don't already have a network of friends active on a variety of playing fields, check the newspaper for sports leagues near you. A spot on the community softball team or bowling league might be all you need to stick to a lifelong exercise regimen.

If you strike out at finding an established community league, start a game yourself by recruiting in the office. Your coworkers might jump at the chance for some high-noon athletic antics.

Decades
of Fitness

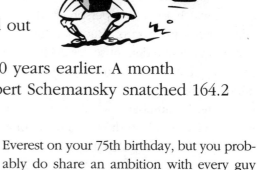

At age 45, George Foreman knocked out Michael Moorer and reclaimed the heavyweight boxing title he had lost 20 years earlier. A month before he turned 38, weight lifter Norbert Schemansky snatched 164.2 kilograms for a world record.

And as he entered his fifth decade, Ashrita Furman held the record for holding records in the *Guinness Book of Records*: 10 number one spots, all of them for athletic pursuits such as somersaulting, deep knee bends, and basketball dribbling.

So, how will biographers say that you spent *your* middle age? Give me a break, you protest, those guys are all muscular mutants! The only physical phenomenon that normal guys can look forward to is a long, slow slide toward that black abyss. Right?

Wrong.

"There's nothing special about even world-class athletes. They're human beings just like we are," says Furman, the manager of a health food store in Jamaica, New York. "At Jamaica High School, I skipped gym class all the time. I was a wimp. It's funny, because now that's where I train. My phys ed teacher can't believe that it's the same guy 20 years later."

You may not plan to swim the English Channel in your forties or scale Mount Everest on your 75th birthday, but you probably do share an ambition with every guy since Ponce de León: to stop, or at least slow, the aging process. You want to live long, well, and independently, looking and feeling good. All of this, scientists say, you *can* achieve.

THE AGING OF AQUARIANS

If you dread getting older, maybe that's because of what you see in the population around you. United States government health officials say that less than 15 percent of adults between the ages of 18 and 74 get regular vigorous exercise. The result is an epidemic of maladies related to long-term bodily neglect, such as heart disease, high blood pressure, diabetes, back problems, bone degeneration, and debilitating muscular weakness. If that sums up your concept of aging, you'll be relieved to know that a good diet and regular exercise such as strength training can help counteract all of those health problems.

You've heard of the use-it-or-lose-it

principle: Muscle that gets used stays put or enlarges; unused muscle shrinks. If you don't get off your duff, in other words, you can kiss your gluteus maximus goodbye.

A few years back, it seemed like everyone in the country was making jokes about those obnoxious television commercials in which an elderly person cried, "I've fallen and I can't get up." But with the population growing older, muscular decline is a problem that doctors and scientists are taking more and more seriously. Falls already are the number one killer of people in their eighties, according to the National Safety Council. And U.S. citizens are in for more than a touch of gray in the coming decades. Baby boomers are beginning to slide into the 55-plus category, and by the year 2030, nearly one-third of the U.S. population will be 55 or older.

"From the time that you're in your forties or early fifties, until you're in your seventies and eighties, you lose roughly 1 percent of your strength per year, or about 10 percent per decade," says Wayne W. Campbell, Ph.D., an applied physiologist at Noll Physiological Research Center at Pennsylvania State University in University Park.

GETTING OFF YOUR ROCKER

The physical advantages of regular exercise—increased muscle, better coordination, and the fat-burning power of a higher metabolism—are within the grasps of all adults, even those in their nineties.

"The studies that look at older people who are vigorously exercising show that they can maintain a more 'youthful' bodily composition with exercise programs," says Dr. Campbell. "This suggests that a very

YOU'RE NO SLOUCH

Few things will add undeserved years to your appearance like bad posture. Walking tall will not only make you look younger but it will also help ward off back pain and give you more power in sports. Further, because you breathe better upright, you'll get more oxygen and have more energy.

First, you have to learn how to walk: Tighten your belly muscles, keep your butt tucked in, pull in your chin, and don't lock your knees.

Next, strengthen your back, abdominal, and butt muscles. This exercise gives them all a workout: Lie facedown on the floor with your arms bent at the elbows and your palms and forearms on the floor, like the Sphinx. Slowly lift your head and chest up as far as you can comfortably go, keeping your palms and forearms on the floor. Then, slowly let yourself down again. When you can do this easily 10 times, try it with your arms at your sides. The next level is with hands under your chin and elbows out. Superman level is with arms extended forward, keeping an eye out for kryptonite.

large component of muscular decline is inactivity—not using your muscles enough for them to want to stick around."

In Boston, for instance, researchers studied 100 frail nursing home residents ranging in age from 72 to 98. They were put through intense hip and knee workouts—45-minute sessions three times a week for 10 weeks. The residents showed increases in muscle strength (113 percent), gait speed (11 percent), and stairclimbing power (28 percent). Four of those elderly exercisers surrendered their walkers by the end of the 10 weeks and got by with canes.

Stanford University and Veterans Affairs researchers got 25 people ages 61 to 78 to weight train for a year in Palo Alto, California. The subjects worked out for an hour three times a week, and their routines, which included 3 sets of 12 lifting exercises,

covered all the major muscle groups. The exercisers grew stronger rapidly during the first 3 months of the study and plateaued for the rest of the year. Some of the participants showed strength gains of more than 90 percent in their hip and leg muscles.

Scientists also believe that strength training can help fend off some crippling diseases. In one study, elderly exercisers lost none of their bone content over 6 months, while their counterparts who did not exercise lost 2 percent. In another study, researchers reviewed the activity levels of 6,815 Japanese-American men between the ages of 45 and 68 in the Honolulu Heart Program. They concluded that the most active guys—those in the top 20 percent, who were accustomed to lifting, shoveling, carpentry, and the like—had cut their risk of diabetes in half.

Tom Brokaw, TV News Anchor

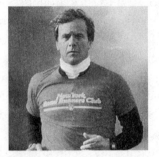

As he rounded a corner during his morning run, Tom Brokaw found himself face-to-face with a band of men brandishing weapons. In El Salvador during the war, surprising people with guns was not a great idea. "It turned out to be a Salvadoran army patrol, thank God," Brokaw recalls.

"They were heavily armed, and they were as startled to see me as I was to see them. I went back and confined my running to just around the hotel."

As anchor of the *NBC Nightly News* since 1983, Brokaw, who's in his sixties, frequently finds himself in whatever corner of the world is ready to explode. And almost always, he finds a way to keep up his daily fitness regimen, which dates back to long before the running boom of the late 1970s.

A VALUABLE LESSON

"I was a high school jock," says Brokaw, who grew up in Yankton, South Dakota. "Then I went to college, and I guess I thought that all the fitness I'd enjoyed through high school would be sustained, no matter what I did. So I kind of went on a beer-and-pizza diet and quickly ballooned up. I also started smoking."

After graduating from the University of South Dakota, Brokaw landed a television news job in Omaha. Three years later, he was married and anchoring the late-evening news at an Atlanta station when he realized that he had grown so overweight and out of shape that he could no longer take part in physical activities he had once enjoyed. He kicked smoking and took up running.

"I found out how hard it was once you get out of shape to get back into shape," says the 6-foot-tall Brokaw, who is now 185 pounds. "So I just kept working at it and working at it. And I finally got my weight down to an acceptable level. It became part of my mind-set. I've been doing it ever since."

GLOBE-TROTTING

Brokaw has worked out all over the world. While reporting from China during the Cultural Revolution in 1974, he says, "I would get up very early in the morning and run in the streets of Beijing." Chairman Mao Tsetung may have excoriated the running dogs

FAST-BREAKING FITNESS

When major news happens anywhere in the world, chances are, Tom Brokaw is on the next plane there.

Over the years, the network news anchor has come up with a number of strategies for staying healthy and fit while on the road.

Be prepared. "On every trip, I always carry workout gear," Brokaw says. "And just like getting an aisle seat on the airplane, part of the routine here for my assistants is to get me into a hotel with a gym. No matter where I am, no matter how late I arrived the night before, I try to get up early enough to go to a hotel gym and work out for 30 minutes before I go out and start the day."

Keep moving. "I've been known to run the back staircases in hotels," he says. "When I have a long international flight and there's a fair amount of airport transfer and so on, I never take moving sidewalks. I never take escalators. I always run the stairs. And I always try to do something midflight—get up and stretch and move around a little bit."

Help yourself. "On airplanes, I have a standing order for a fruit plate or a vegetarian plate of some kind. That helps. Then, when I get where I'm going, I will often go out into the local marketplace and buy food—rice crackers or something like that, and a lot of fruit—and just keep it in the hotel room."

---

of capitalism, but running proletarians were another matter. Mao had decreed that the masses should exercise, and they did—en masse.

"I had a blue running suit, just like the Chinese, and I would fall in with a group of Chinese who would be running down one of the main thoroughfares," Brokaw recalls. "Suddenly, they would realize there was this round-eye with them. And they would just veer off as one and go in the opposite direction. They didn't want to have anything to do with being around me."

Another time, in Warsaw, Brokaw was running across a public square when he encountered an older couple. The man turned to the woman and, "with a real quizzical expression on his face, said something in Polish," Brokaw says. "She looked at me, then looked back at him and said, 'Jogging.' So I guess it translates into every language."

WORKING OUT

Brokaw usually starts his day with a 7:30 A.M. run through Central Park with his yellow Labrador, Sagebrush. After 2 to 4 miles, Brokaw returns home, works out with weights, and does situps and stretches.

In the afternoon, he goes to the NBC gym for a second workout on the equipment there. His favorite is the rowing machine. "What I can do on the ergometer is get into a very strong, fast rhythm and then spend a lot of time thinking about what we're going to be doing that night," he says.

One of the reasons that Brokaw works out so faithfully is to stay in shape for what he calls "the other adventurous things I like to do." A self-described Walter Mitty, Brokaw loves mountain climbing, cross-country skiing, kayaking, and hiking.

Brokaw has an additional reason for keeping fit. "I feel better mentally as well as physically if I work out. I'm able to come in here and deal with the day."

A PASSION FOR PASTA

Brokaw watches what he eats, but confesses, "I'm not a fanatic. I succumb like everybody else does to the temptations of dessert. But I try to eat a pretty healthy diet. Pasta is a very large part of my diet."

True to his Midwestern roots, Brokaw still enjoys an occasional steak, but most of his main meals are built around pasta, chicken, or fish. When traveling to exotic locales, though, Brokaw indulges his adventurous streak. "I eat everything," he says. "I wouldn't give up that part of it. I try almost everything, and I've paid the price a couple of times, too."

Brokaw is living proof that being adventurous and fit and sitting behind a desk are not mutually exclusive. Displaying the wry wit that has made him a nightly dinner companion for millions of Americans, Brokaw adds, "I like life, and I want to be around for a while."

Part 3
SIMPLE CHANGES, LASTING RESULTS

The 24-Hour Food Plan

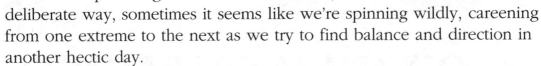

Work, play, food, rest: These are the four poles on the compass of man's life. Rather than partaking of each in a measured, deliberate way, sometimes it seems like we're spinning wildly, careening from one extreme to the next as we try to find balance and direction in another hectic day.

The report is due—cancel the workout. Can't sleep—have a snack. Kids need rides—forget the walk. It's no wonder that a lot of us wake up one day and discover that we're frustrated, tired, and overweight.

"It's all a balancing act," says Peter M. Miller, Ph.D., executive director of the Hilton Head Health Institute in South Carolina and author of *The Hilton Head Executive Stamina Program*. "Men need to learn how to adopt a set of strategies that they can use every day, making their daily activities—meals, business, exercise, leisure, and so on—work together. If they can do that, they'll go a long way toward being slimmer, healthier people with a lot more energy and a lot less stress to boot."

MORE IS LESS

Despite what your stomach would have you believe, food is not your life; it's the fuel that powers your life. But a lot of us have been topping off our tanks the wrong way—and losing energy and gaining weight in the bargain.

Although men in our society are brought up to eat three squares a day, with breakfast being the smallest meal and dinner the largest, nutrition experts say that this approach is all wrong.

"A calorie is not the same calorie at different times of the day," says Franz Halberg, M.D., professor of bioengineering, pathology, physiology, oral medicine, and laboratory medicine at the University of Minnesota in Minneapolis. Studies of lean men suggest that calories consumed at dinner are more likely to be stored than those taken in at breakfast.

Another problem with the three-a-day scheme is that it requires us to go for long periods without eating. By the time lunch or dinner rolls around, we're ravenous—and more than willing to grab the biggest, fattiest food we can find and stuff it down our gullets.

"Instead of eating three big meals a day,

a lot of men make better choices by spreading their calorie intakes over four or five meals—the three basic meals, plus one or two snacks," says Dr. Miller. With all-day grazing, you may eat more often, but you're less likely to put on weight, he adds.

Rather than alternating between feast and famine, a better strategy is to keep your metabolism running at a consistent high idle throughout the day. Here's a daylong look at how to do it.

STARTING RIGHT

When you exercise and what you eat in the morning can dictate how much energy you'll have—and how much more you'll eat—later on. "It's truly one of the most important times to eat," says Cheryl C. Marco, R.D., a dietitian and manager of outpatient nutrition at Thomas Jefferson University Hospital in Philadelphia. "Your body has been without food for several hours, and your brain is going to need some carbohydrates soon to function effectively."

To make the most of your mornings, here's what experts recommend.

Break into a walk. After 8 hours in the sack, your metabolism is running slow. So even before you eat, experts say, prime your food furnace. Get up and pull on your

STOKE SIGNALS

When you're eating, it can take up to 20 minutes for your brain to realize that your stomach is full. In the meantime, you're still shoveling it in.

To get your stomach and brain working in synch, here's what experts recommend.

Eat a multicourse meal. Having a few small courses works better than having one huge portion, says Steven Peikin, M.D., professor of medicine at the University of Medicine and Dentistry of New Jersey and author of *The Feel Full Diet*.

Eating a bowl of tomato soup 20 minutes before your main course, for example, has been shown to reduce caloric intake in the main course. By the time you reach the entrée, you're less likely to pig out, because your brain has already gotten word that you're filling up.

Don't feel that you have to eat it all. None of us is so old that we can't remember the childhood pride of being a member of the Clean Plate Club. Now that we're adults, however, it's time to let the membership lapse.

"Follow the 'taste everything, finish nothing' rule," suggests Morton H. Shaevitz, Ph.D., associate clinical professor of psychiatry at the University of California, San Diego, School of Medicine. By taking time to savor everything, he says, you'll feel fuller and take in fewer calories than if you wolf everything down.

Delay having seconds. Waiting 10 minutes before helping yourself to seconds is a tactic that gives your brain more time to catch up with your stomach. Then, see whether you really want more.

sweats. Just taking a brisk walk up the street and back for 10 to 15 minutes will get you revved.

Eat big—but eat right. "By the time you wake up, it has been hours since your last meal. Your body is literally starving for nutrients," says Marco. Since your body tends to burn food more efficiently in the morning, it's also a good time to eat well.

But traditional breakfast foods that are high in fat, such as bacon, eggs, doughnuts, and hash browns, can be your ticket back to dreamland. "Heavy, fatty foods take longer to digest. Your stomach draws more blood away from the brain. You'll have less energy and you're going to get drowsy again," says Marco.

The best foods are those that your body can quickly convert to energy—carbohydrates and proteins that keep you sharp. Good examples include dry cereal with fat-free milk, whole-grain toast with jelly (ease up on the butter or peanut butter), oatmeal, and any of your favorite fresh fruits.

Take ten at 10:00 A.M. There's no good reason to wait for lunch when your stomach is growling. Feed the beast—with a bagel and jelly, for example, or a cup of yogurt. Midmorning snacks will help keep your stomach satisfied and your brain sharp for whatever you're dealing with before lunch rolls around.

While you're taking a break, go ahead and stretch your legs by walking around a bit. This will help keep your engine running fast, so you'll continue to burn more calories even after you go back to work.

THE BATTLE OF MIDDAY

Noon to quitting time—that long stretch is when you're most likely to be bored, tired, and hungry.

"We've all been victims of that afternoon slump in energy," says Dr. Miller. "A lot of that has to do with the fact that we may have eaten a heavy meal at lunch. And sitting at a desk doesn't burn it off very quickly." Our energy levels dip, and so do our heads.

Here are a few ways to keep your metabolic momentum running high.

Lunch large. Even if you eat five or more meals a day, most food experts say that lunch should be the biggest spread. You have a long afternoon of work ahead of you, so eat accordingly. But don't gorge; big doesn't mean huge.

A good example of a power lunch may be a hearty bowl of bean or minestrone soup and half a chicken-breast sandwich with lettuce and tomato on whole-grain bread. You get enough protein and a lot of carbohydrates, but not a lot of fat. Throw in a handful of pretzels, a cup of yogurt, and an apple or some other fruit.

Stay active. After lunch, instead of going back to your desk and dozing off, fire up your system by fitting in a quick workout. If you can sneak away to the club for 15 minutes on the stairclimber, so much the better. If not, at least walk around the parking lot or down the street. "This way, lunch isn't going to sit so heavily on you. You'll feel refreshed and better able to sail through the afternoon," says Dr. Miller.

Eat again. Usually around 3:00 P.M., our

TARGETED EATING

Food does more than just fill us up. We also eat to satisfy moods and emotions. "When we're depressed, we make ourselves feel better with some big, sugary treat," says Bob Arnot, M.D., medical and health correspondent for *NBC Evening News*.

Dr. Arnot refers to this impulse as feedback eating—a primitive response to feelings and sensations. A better approach, he says, is to practice what he calls feed-forward eating. This means looking ahead at tasks you'll be doing and then eating specific foods to help you perform them more efficiently. For example:

Brain work. Eating grains and high-protein foods such as fat-free milk, yogurt, and lean meat helps keep your mind and body alert, Dr. Arnot says.

Physical activity. Eating protein provides needed material to build muscle, while slow-burning carbohydrates—such as grains, rice, and legumes—aid in muscle repair.

Rest. Cut back on mind-reviving protein and load up on carbohydrates instead.

bodies' natural rhythms kick in and we start to feel drowsy. Let your drooping eyelids serve as a signal to have another snack—something that's going to wake you up, not put you to sleep. Yogurt, pretzels, or fruit will provide quick, low-fat bursts of energy and help head off a ravenous appetite later on.

"That's important: At the end of the day you don't want to feel starved for dinner, or you'll make bad food choices," says Dr. Miller.

Hit the gym. To keep your metabolism running high, you should get at least 30 minutes of exercise 3 days a week. Do plenty of cardiovascular exercises—stair-climbing, walking, running, cycling—to keep your heart rate up. That way, you'll burn more calories. It's also a good idea to resistance train, either on a circuit trainer or using free weights. As you build more muscle, you burn more calories—ap-

proximately 50 more calories a day for every pound of muscle you gain. Keep pumping.

Feed within 15. Maximizing muscle is key to keeping fat in the fire. Experts recommend enhancing muscle repair and replacing muscle energy stores by consuming a combination of carbohydrate and protein foods within 15 to 20 minutes after your workout.

"After a workout, you're going to need to replace the muscle's energy stores to assist with muscle repair," explains Becky Zimmerman, R.D., a dietitian at the National Institute for Fitness and Sport in Indianapolis.

She recommends eating about 0.5 gram of carbohydrates for each pound of body weight. In a 150-pound man, that means 75 grams of carbohydrates, or a little more than 2 cups of pasta. You'll find protein in low-fat dairy products, in lean meats such as chicken or turkey, and in whole-grain products, beans, and rice.

Not only will eating soon after workouts help maximize muscle repair, it will also fill you up, so you'll be less likely to stuff yourself later on.

GOOD NIGHT

The traditional routine is to get home from work, kick off your shoes, loosen your tie, and enjoy a big dinner. You work hard; you deserve it, right? Maybe not. Your just desserts may be your unwanted gains.

"If there's a time to drop eating, it's probably the time when we eat the most, which is in the evening," says Marco. "There's some evidence that calories eaten in the evening are more likely to be stored as fat—they're not used as efficiently by the body as they would be at other times."

Evening is usually a time to relax, catch up on some reading, do a little channel-surfing. But when you're winding down your day, you can still keep fat away—even after you've gone to bed. Here's how.

Have a dinky dinner. Some men consume 80 percent of their daily food intake at the dinner table and at night. As a rule, dinner should account for no more than 40 to 50 percent of daily calories, says Morton H. Shaevitz, Ph.D., associate clinical professor of psychiatry at the University of California, San Diego, School of Medicine and author of *Lean and Mean: The No Hassle Life-Extending Weight Loss Program for Men.*

Regularly eating between three and five meals a day will help keep you from loading up in the evening. But even when you are hungry at night, keep your dinner light. Focus on fish or fowl. Eat no more than 4 to 6 ounces of red meat no more than twice a week, and load up on vegetables, legumes, pasta, or rice instead.

Eat before 8:00 P.M. Research suggests that the later you eat, the more likely it is that your body will store the food as flab. So whether you're eating a three-course meal or just a light snack, do it early in the evening, experts say.

Sleep with sweets. Some men crave sweet bedtime snacks, possibly because sugary foods tend to elevate blood levels of tryptophan, an amino acid that is involved in sleep.

"The mistake you could make is satisfying that sweet craving with something huge, like a piece of pie or an ice cream sundae," says Martin B. Scharf, Ph.D., director of the Sleep Disorders Center at Mercy Hospital in Cincinnati. To get the sweet without the flab, go for something low-fat: hard candies or licorice, for example, or a scoop of frozen yogurt.

Get busy. "Let's think about this. You've just eaten dinner, your biggest meal of the day. Are you really hungry just a few hours later, or are you just bored?" asks G. Alan Marlatt, Ph.D., professor of psychology and director of the Addictive Behaviors Research Center at the University of Washington, Seattle, and an expert on food cravings. He recommends doing something—anything—that takes your mind off food. "Meditating works for me. Or get dressed and go for a walk. Play a game on the computer. Do anything to distract you until the urge passes."

Lose Your Gut at Work

In the context of work, the words "trimming the fat" probably make you wonder when the ax is going to fall—and whom it's going to hit. Relax. We're not talking about layoffs here. The problem is corporal fat—and the need to do some serious downsizing.

Let's face it: When you're pulling 12-hour days, work comes first and everything else—including a decent meal—comes a distant second. Daily workouts get postponed in the crunch of conference calls and strategy meetings. Meals come to you courtesy of the doughnut tray, the vending machine, and the greasy spoon down the road. Your desk is transformed into a workaholic's table for one.

The battle of the bulge isn't fought only over office goodies and order-in lunches. No matter how far you've moved in your career, you probably haven't budged from behind your desk—with predictable results. If only there were some way to give your nose a break and press your gut to the grindstone instead.

SECRETS OF EXECUTIVE SUCCESS

Staying on top of fitness can seem like a second career, another activity in an already jam-packed day. "The main enemy to most men's fitness is the fact that their jobs are very time-consuming things that involve sitting and not moving a lot," says Peter M. Miller, Ph.D., executive director of the Hilton Head Health Institute in South Carolina and author of *The Hilton Head Executive Stamina Program.*

There's another obstacle as well: your mind-set. "A lot of men still don't see the advantage of making time during the day to get a proper meal and to exercise," says Dr. Miller. "If more men scheduled these things into their days—like any other important appointment—they'd find that they have more energy and are more physically fit, without cutting into their job performance."

Indeed, a basic fitness program will make you feel better and work sharper, and will help you lose weight and look better in the eyes of the corporate bigwigs.

BETWEEN-MEETING EATING

You skipped breakfast so you could get an early start on the day—and get first crack at the glazed goodies in the cafeteria. Your

WORKING IN YOUR WORKOUT

The trouble with most of us busy drones is that we always put exercise at the outer fringes of the day—either late in the evening after work or at an ungodly early hour of the morning. The more marginal exercise becomes, the easier it is to blow it off.

"The point is not to treat fitness like some inferior part of our day," says Peter M. Miller, Ph.D., executive director of the Hilton Head Health Institute in South Carolina. "You really need to make time during the business day for some physical activity."

Scheduling an appointment for exercise? Well, why not? In *The Hilton Head Executive Stamina Program*, Dr. Miller outlines some simple steps for incorporating a workout into your corporate routine.

Jot it down. Since exercise is now an official part of your business day, pencil it into your calendar or planner. You'll be more likely to treat it like any other appointment: too important to miss.

Keep others in the loop. Tell friends, coworkers, and family members about your exercise time. Once they understand that you're treating it like business—that is, something that can't be skipped—they'll be more supportive and less likely to interrupt.

Keep your eyes on the goal. Yes, exercise will help you lose weight and look better. More important from an office point of view, it will help you work harder and with more energy.

lunchtime strategy meeting ran long, so you put your heads together, made a policy decision, and ordered a bevy of salami torpedoes from the sub shop around the corner. At sunset, with a stack of paperwork still to file, you decided to postpone dinner—until you swung into a drive-thru on your way home and ordered the Belly Buster Bonus Meal.

"Work always gets in the way of eating a decent meal," observes Dr. Miller. "But if you wait to eat until you're starving, you make terrible food choices." What's more, you set yourself up for a ride on the energy roller coaster. "You go and go until you run out of fuel, then everything crashes down

around you: your energy, your stamina, and your mood," he says.

To keep your business day running at peak efficiency and with a minimum of fat, Dr. Miller recommends eating several small meals several times a day and packing those meals with complex carbohydrates, the kind found in fruits, vegetables, and grains. Not only will your energy level be higher but you'll also be less likely to bite into a fattening quick fix. Here are some excellent food fixes.

Brown-bag it. For a real power lunch, pack your own. "If you take your own meals to work—even once or twice a week—you're more in control of your food choices, and you can eat a bit healthier," says Patti Tveit Milligan, R.D., a dietitian in San Diego and nutrition columnist for *Selling* magazine. So pack a sack before you crash and hit the sack—for example, a nice lean-meat sandwich with lettuce and tomato, some pretzels, and a piece of fruit.

Make yourself a super hero. Whether you make your own lunch or order it from the deli, try to stock sandwiches with the leaner meats: turkey, chicken, even lean roast beef. "Stay away from the cured meats, such as salami, pepperoni, and corned beef," advises Milligan. They have hidden fat. Top your sandwich with some lettuce and tomato for filling fiber. And go easy on the mayonnaise—a single tablespoon holds 11 grams of fat. "Mustard, ketchup, even barbecue sauce is a better choice," says Milligan.

Take up snack-packing. Foraging in the break room for an afternoon snack will almost guarantee you membership in the Lard-Butt Brigade. So anticipate trouble—and beat it by bringing your own grub.

"If you keep a stash of healthy snacks in your briefcase or your desk drawer, you're going to resist the temptation of fattier foods that are available at work," says Dr. Miller. Some of the best daylong noshables are fruits and vegetables. Not only will they help keep you full, but their stores of carbohydrates quickly translate into ready brain food. And fruits are ready-wrapped, so they're easy to pack.

It's also a good idea to pack your desk with snacks that keep, such as graham crackers, animal crackers (your kids will never miss them), raisins, rice cakes, dried fruit, or pretzels. And lay in a few dried-soup packets for when you need a more substantial energy fix.

Ditch the doughnuts. Some office snacks will twist the needle off your personal fat meter. Doughnuts, for example, are veritable sponges of fat, containing 17 grams of

WHEN FAT HOLDS YOU BACK

Fat does more than slow you down on the basketball court. It can take you off the corporate fast track as well.

In one study, researchers at the Harvard School of Public Health found that people who were overweight tended to complete fewer years of school and make less money (in some cases, more than $9,000 less) than their leaner peers. In addition, men who were overweight were 11 percent less likely to marry than those with thinner physiques.

Another study found that overweight workers had up to 40 percent more problems doing simple tasks quickly, such as dialing the phone or working the computer. Workers who were heavy were 3.5 to 4.1 times more likely to develop abnormal nerve conduction in their wrists that is a characteristic symptom of carpal tunnel syndrome.

fat in some cases. When the urge for a round, doughy object with a hole in the middle strikes, opt for a toasted bagel and jelly instead.

Snack early and often. "I suggest that men have a snack at least twice during the workday—once around 10:00 in the morning, and again around 3:00 in the afternoon," says Dr. Miller. Those are the times when our appetites tend to rear their insatiable heads. "A couple of pretzels or a piece of fruit can really take the edge off so you won't be making bad food choices at a regular meal."

Do the same for evenings when you're forsaking dinner for work. "It's too easy to fall into the trap of eating a big meal late. Instead, make yourself a snack when you'd normally eat dinner," says Dr. Miller. "That should tide you over until you can get home and have something sensible."

Pour another drink. The average work environment is a dry one, and it's common for men to mistake thirst for hunger—and raid the vending machine when all they really wanted was a drink. "Everyone should be drinking about 8 glasses of water a day," says Milligan. "If you keep a bottle at your desk and just sip from it all day, you probably won't feel as hungry."

WORKING LATE AND WORKING OUT

Everyone else has punched out for the day, but you're still slaving away on that year-end report. By the time you leave work, you barely have energy to flip a quarter into the toll basket, never mind hit the gym for some much-needed exercise.

"Because most work schedules don't leave us time to work out at night, it's important for the working man to make sure that he's moving and getting exercise during the day while he's at work," says Dr. Miller.

We're not talking here about a full-blown aerobics drill in front of the water cooler. Just going through your daily activities a bit more vigorously can get blood pumping and your metabolism kicking in more efficiently. A study at Tufts University in Medford, Massachusetts, showed that men who frequently shifted in their chairs, paced around the office, or even got excited about a good idea burned up more calories over a 16-hour period than when they got $\frac{1}{2}$ hour of solid exercise.

So while that report is printing or you're waiting for a 10-page fax—or even before you hit the front door—take a couple of minutes to try these at-work exercises recommended by experts.

Park and walk. Remember how hard you worked to get that parking space by the door? Well, give it up and promote yourself to the back parking lot. That will give you a chance to stretch your legs before you embark on the 9-to-5.

"I would try to park as far away from the building as possible and then walk or jog in," suggests Dr. Miller. The quick rush of physical activity will boost your metabolism, helping you stay lean and energized. If you take public transportation, get off one stop before your office and hoof it the rest of the way.

Take the stairs. Elevators are great for

hauling a tray of cappuccino up three floors or making an impromptu sales pitch to a captive audience. But for the quick transit from your desk to a meeting with the guys upstairs, skip the elevator. "If we're talking about a distance of one or two floors, it's really kind of lazy to take an elevator," says Dr. Miller. "I always take the stairs—it's actually a lot quicker, too."

Use your downtime wisely. There's time in every workday when there's not a lot happening. Rather than use your free time to walk to the lunchroom, use it to burn a few extra calories. For example:

- Find an open office door. Stand with your feet straddling the edge. Grab the inside knob with one hand, the outside knob with the other, and slowly lean back until you encounter resistance in your arms. Then, bend your knees and let your body sink down until your arms are fully extended and your thighs are parallel to the floor. Slowly pull yourself up with your arms and push slightly with your legs. Repeat 10 to 12 times.

- To burn a few extra calories without leaving your desk, stand up straight, with your feet about 3 feet apart, and grab the edge of your desk. Keep your right foot planted and your right leg straight, point your left foot to the side, and slowly bend your left knee until your left thigh is parallel to the floor (don't let your knee extend past your foot). Hold for a count of three, then push back to starting position and repeat on your right side. Repeat 10 times.

- Nothing burns fat like a good one-legged squat. Stand facing the seat of a handy chair—the kind without wheels, please. Lean over and grip the armrests or the sides of the seat. Bend one leg and lift your foot off the floor behind you so it's suspended in midair with your shin parallel to the floor. Then, slowly bend the knee of the leg on which you're standing, and squat about 6 to 8 inches until you feel tension in the front of that thigh. Slowly raise back to the starting position. Repeat 10 times, then do the other leg.

- Do some quick situps. Situps aren't much fun, but if you do them right, they're an incredibly effective way to boost your metabolism and rev your energy. Plus, you can do situps anywhere there's room to lie down. (Just be sure to close your office door first.)

  To get the most from your efforts, don't jerk yourself up and forward, experts advise. You want to lift just your shoulders and upper back off the floor, not your whole torso. It may seem like a less demanding exercise, but it's not. It just cuts out the wasted motion and the wasted time that's typical of the traditional situp. And when you're working out at work, every second counts.

  Spend 10 seconds curling upward and another 10 seconds easing back down. The slower you go, the more muscle fibers you call into play, and the more definition you get.

Putting Snacks to Work

A hankering for a good snack can strike at any time—and often does. Between meals, before bed, in the middle of the night—sometimes your stomach just won't take no for an answer. Maybe it doesn't have to. Although experts once chastised between-meal munchers for having weak characters, they now agree that an occasional yes to snacks is in order.

The catch, of course, is that whatever your nosh of choice happens to be, it had better be at least relatively good for you. That's tough. The average guy, 9 times out of 10, will bypass the celery or figs and reach instead for a beer and a large bag of chips. "What more is there?" asks Matt Marton, a newspaper photographer in Oshkosh, Wisconsin, who's in his thirties.

CRUEL COMFORT

Marton is hardly the only man who's misguided about munching. When it comes to snacks, our appetites are wide-ranging. The Snack Food Association estimates that, for example, Americans consume about 5 billion pounds of salty snacks a year—more than 20 pounds per person.

Clearly, more is involved than just the occasional midmorning hunger pang. Experts speculate that our urge to snack is also driven by some deep-seated psychological needs. "We might be bored or feel angry or depressed. Or we might feel that we deserve a reward," explains Marcia Levin Pelchat, Ph.D., a food-cravings expert at the Monell Chemical Senses Center in Philadelphia. "Then we turn to certain foods that, in our experience, make us feel better."

To the woe of his waistline, however, a guy who craves comfort in the kitchen probably isn't setting his sights on broccoli spears. What he wants, Dr. Pelchat says, is fat: a quart of ice cream, say, or a pepperoni pizza. That's when snacking bites back.

NEW-STYLE NOSHING

But snacking, experts say, can also be good. Pause for a moment to let that sink in. What Mom never told you, and what more and more researchers are recommending, is noshing: eating several small meals—meals between meals, as it were—throughout the day. Forget the old rule of three squares a day. That went out with lava lamps.

"One of the most important stamina

rules is that your body needs its fuel in moderate doses throughout the day to keep energy nutrients optimally available," says Peter M. Miller, Ph.D., executive director of the Hilton Head Health Institute in South Carolina and author of *The Hilton Head Executive Stamina Program.* "I actually counsel people to eat four or five times a day."

At first, you may think that following this advice would make you a fat man rather than a healthy one. The idea isn't to stuff yourself, Dr. Miller adds. Nor do you want to fill up on junk food. "What I am suggesting," says Dr. Miller, "is that you reduce the amount of food you eat at any one time so that you can spread the same amount of calories more evenly over the day."

This type of snacking has a number of advantages. Because you never let your tank run completely empty, you're less tempted by whatever junk food happens to cross your line of sight.

An additional benefit is that eating more often—a better term might be *grazing*—keeps your metabolism running high. By eating smaller meals more often, you can help keep your metabolism more constant, leveling the energy peaks and valleys that dot the daily landscape. This means that even though you may be eating more than you did before, you're less likely to put on weight. "You end up burning calories very efficiently," says Dr. Miller.

It's important to note, however, that the benefits of grazing won't apply when your snacks of choice resemble photographer Marton's culinary bombs, like chips and beer.

Instead, when your stomach roars between meals, silence it with high-octane snacks such as fruits and vegetables. You should never again walk out of the house in the morning without stuffing an apple or a banana in your briefcase.

For that matter, carry a stash of carrot or celery sticks with you to handle the midafternoon slump, the time of day when you're most likely to fall prey to the siren call of the vending machine. Snacking on fruits and vegetables helps keep your pump primed with a fuel mix that's rich in complex carbohydrates.

Dr. Miller says that our diets should be about 60 percent carbohydrates, 15 percent protein, and no more than 25 percent fat daily. "Rather than having a steak and fries for lunch, for example, you would do much better ordering a fruit platter, a salad, or perhaps pasta fra diavolo."

PUTTING SNACKS ON TRACK

While it's admirable—noble, even—to dedicate yourself to a healthy, five-or-more-a-day meal plan, you're bound to feel the need for some extracurricular eating now and again: an almond-studded chocolate bar, for example, or a bacon cheeseburger.

There's nothing wrong with enjoying the occasional guilty snack. The problem for most of us is that one serving has a way of turning into two, which then become four. Naturally, this has consequences. Like when your cholesterol suddenly shoots higher than your bowling score. When your profile begins to resemble the Michelin tire man. When your afternoon slump lasts well into evening.

"Too much sugar is going to give you an energy high that won't last very long," warns Dr. Miller. Granted, if it's a mood-altering substance you're craving, you could do a lot worse than having an extra dessert now and again. But you can also do better. Here are some munchies that have the hallmarks of the great snacks: They're chewy, crispy, creamy, or crunchy. And whether you need a sweet, sour, or salty taste, one of these snacks will likely satisfy your craving—without putting on the pounds.

Give sweets to the sweet tooth. Although sugar has long been demonized as a dietary saboteur, by itself it's fairly innocuous, says Dr. Pelchat. It's when sugar is combined with calorie-laden fat, as in chocolate or buttery desserts, that it starts weighing in with trouble.

"If you have a balanced diet otherwise, it's really okay to indulge in something sweet once in a while," says Dr. Pelchat. To satisfy your sweet craving, you could try hard candies. They have zero fat and last

FEED THE FAT TOOTH

Some call it a sweet tooth. Others refer to it as an uncontrollable case of the munchies. But regardless of the name, nearly everyone has experienced an occasional craving for some delectable, not-to-be-denied kind of food.

Although men's food cravings are highly individual, they do have one thing in common: They're hardly ever healthy.

Research has shown that while men are more likely to crave salty, sour, or spicy foods than sweet ones, "what you're really craving is fat," says Marcia Levin Pelchat, Ph.D., a food-cravings expert at the Monell Chemical Senses Center in Philadelphia.

To prove the existence of the fat tooth, researchers at the University of Michigan in Ann Arbor asked obese men which foods they like the most. Here are their choices.

1. Steaks and roasts
2. Ice cream and frozen desserts
3. Chicken or turkey
4. Doughnuts, cookies, and cakes
5. Spaghetti and pasta
6. White bread, rolls, and crackers
7. Fish
8. Pizza
9. Cheese
10. Potatoes, excluding fried

STEALTH SNACKS

To hear those sandal-wearing, granola-eating health nuts tell it, anything that's not organically grown or covered with ugly lumps is probably going to rot you from the inside out. That goes double for whatever you were planning to have for your afternoon snack.

It turns out, however, that their wholesome snack choices aren't so wholesome. Take granola. It may be rugged enough to withstand a 2-month trek in Nepal, yet a single cup packs more than 30 grams of fat. By comparison, a full-size Hershey bar has 13 grams. (Tell those nut-and-twig eaters to chew on that.)

Below are the grams of fat found in one serving of some common junk foods as well as in their "healthy" counterparts.

"Not-So-Healthy" Snack	Fat (g)	"Healthy" Snack	Fat (g)
French fries (20)	17	Bran muffin (4 oz)	20
Peanut butter cup (2 large)	14	Sunflower seeds (1 oz)	14
Potato chips (10)	7	Frozen yogurt (1 cup)	8
Chocolate mint patty (1 large)	4	Cottage cheese (4 oz)	5

longer than a sugary-sweet cookie. If you want something a bit more al dente, candies such as Gummi Bears, jelly beans, and licorice will also satisfy the craving without the fat glut.

Shop for substitutes. When you do have a craving for something rich—a thick slice of German chocolate cake, for example—check out the low- or reduced-fat varieties in the grocery store. There are a lot available, and many actually taste pretty good.

Just don't eat the whole box. It's nice to think that a "reduced-fat" label somehow suspends the laws of reality, but fat or no fat, you're still consuming calories.

Don't be a cereal killer. Although the chocolate-covered sugar bombs you used to scarf down while watching Saturday morning cartoons won't fit anyone's criteria

for a healthy snack, there are a lot of good-tasting cereals that will keep you satisfied without pushing out your belt. A high-fiber wheat-flake cereal has minuscule amounts of fat. Add fat-free milk and fresh fruit or—what the hell—a sprinkling of sugar. You'll satisfy your urge for a nice, sweet, crunchy snack and get some valuable nutrients and grains all in the same bowl.

Top your popcorn. Air-popped popcorn is perhaps the least appetizing staple of the weight-watching set. But with a little creativity, it can also be a taste treat, even without the butter. Try sprinkling on a little grated cheese, or even hot spices such as pepper or chili powder. You can even toss in some cinnamon or a handful of raisins.

Get the fat-free sensation. Real snacks provide more than just a sweet taste. There's also a certain texture—the chewiness of a caramel, for example, or the creaminess of a chocolate mousse—that adds to their charm. To combine both sweetness and the right sensory experience, try fig bars. Some have no fat at all, and even those that do contain fat are healthier than their cousins over in the candy aisle.

Scoop up some sherbet. One snack food that men love intensely is ice cream. To satisfy your ice-creamy cravings, try sherbet, which can contain about one-third less fat than most ice creams. Some frozen yogurts are pretty low in fat, too. But check the labels: Some brands of frozen yogurt contain as much as 8 grams of fat per serving. (As a rule, experts say that you should avoid desserts with more than 3 to 4 grams of fat per serving.)

Say hello to Jell-O. Wonderfully squishy and eminently slurpable, flavored gelatin fits the mold when you're hankering for a sweet snack with zero fat. Or if your tastes lean to pudding, check the dairy section. Some are now made from low-fat milk. The full-fat kind, by contrast, can have four times as much fat.

Go crackers. Much as you love those salty, cheesy, savory snack chips, try switching to something with more natural flavor and a lot less fat. For example, cracked wheat crackers, rye crisps, and even flavored rice cakes have plenty of the crunch and hearty taste that guys want out of any self-respecting snack chip. The divi-dend is that they're healthy snacks with little sodium and fat.

Break bread before bed. Although no one recommends cracking a loaf of French bread every night at bedtime, there are advantages to having a healthful late-night snack. Your body starts processing carbohydrates—such as rice, potatoes, and bread—immediately, so they don't hang around all night.

Furthermore, carbohydrates help speed tryptophan (a sleep-inducing amino acid) to the brain, says Judith Wurtman, Ph.D., nutrition researcher in the department of brain and cognitive science at Massachusetts Institute of Technology in Cambridge. In other words, they'll fill you up and help you sleep. "Diets that don't contain enough carbohydrates usually turn people into insomniacs," she adds.

But earlier is better. Though a midnight carb feed won't transform you into the Hindenburg overnight, insatiable nighttime gluttony can cause its own problems. Many experts believe that food eaten at night has more of a chance of being stored as body fat than the same food eaten in the daytime. This is likely because while you sleep, there are fewer bodily functions occurring that require energy, explains James O. Hill, Ph.D., an obesity researcher at the University of Colorado's Center for Human Nutrition in Denver. The net result is that "more of the food you're eating is going into storage," he says.

How to Control the Social Scene

Oscar Wilde once said that he could resist anything except temptation. And as every waistline warrior knows, once you're out on the town, temptation abounds. Whether you're on a dinner date, at a party, or out with the guys, there's going to be food. Good food. Food to which you don't want to say no. Food you're not even aware you're eating until the bowl is empty.

Let's face it: Every invitation to go out includes a second, hidden invitation to eat fat. And as we all know from basic social etiquette, it's impolite to snub an invitation.

Maybe we should all be a little ruder.

"Socializing and eating often go hand in hand," says C. Peter Herman, Ph.D., a professor of psychology at the University of Toronto who has studied the intricacies of social eating. "The problem is, when you're with your friends, you often don't pay attention to what you eat."

Or to how much you eat. "You eat more at meals with friends than at any other time. And if you have a drink or two—which is pretty likely—that makes keeping track of your food intake harder," adds Dr. Herman.

Sometimes, it seems like there are only two options: Become a lean, fit man with no

friends, or be a stand-up, eat-anything kind of guy who looks like a manatee on legs.

But there's a third choice. With a few simple maneuvers, you can have a social life and evade fat, not only at restaurants and bars but wherever friends and food meet.

DINING OUT—NOT PIGGING OUT

Most restaurants do their best to provide the perfect space for a casual meal, a business lunch, or maybe a candlelit dinner for two. But these same cafés and bistros also overdo it: They almost always give you way too much food, and that food almost always has way too much fat in it.

This doesn't mean that you have to restrict yourself to water and a salad, however. Eating should be a pleasure, after all.

BAR CHART

If you have a beer gut, don't blame it all on the beer. On any given night out, even the designated driver will toss back at least a few shots of fat—from nachos and peanuts to those salty little fish-shaped crackers.

Just how bad is pub grub? See for yourself.

Two Beers with . . .	Calories	Fat (g)
1 cup peanuts	1,146	72
7 Buffalo wings	1,028	44
8 nachos supreme	861	31
4 fried cheese sticks	512	12
30 corn chips	447	9
10 potato chips	397	7
1 pickled egg	382	5
1 cup popcorn	333	2
1 beef jerky stick	330	1

So here's an eight-course plan for cutting fat from your menu without sacrificing your social life.

Begin with the soup. When you're starving, the soup can seem more like an obstacle between you and the main course than something to be savored in its own right. Think again. That steaming bowl of consommé can get between you and another—and presumably fattier—appetizer.

"Soups do a good job of filling you up," says Steven Peikin, M.D., professor of medicine at the University of Medicine and Dentistry of New Jersey and author of *The Feel Full Diet*. A study at Johns Hopkins University in Baltimore found that a tomato-soup appetizer reduced overall calorie consumption during a meal by 25 percent.

While just about any clear soup or broth is low in fat, you may want to steer clear of the creamier variety. "They're pretty high in fat," Dr. Peikin warns.

Graze on some greens. Like soup, a green salad will take the edge off your appetite, meaning that you'll be less likely to need a whole chicken and a side of ribs to feel satisfied. "Besides the vitamins and minerals, the fiber in the leafy greens and vegetables will be quite satisfying," says Dr. Peikin.

Be careful what you toss on the tossed salad, though. "You can ruin the healthiest salad with just a few sprinkles of some fatty toppings," cautions Dr. Peikin. These include sliced hard-boiled eggs, bacon bits, and even seeds or nuts, any one of which can double the fat content of a salad.

Dress with discretion. Nothing is tackier than overdressing. That goes for something as elaborate as a dinner party or as simple as the salad in front of you. Most chefs agree that putting anything more than 2 tablespoons of dressing on your salad is like dumping ketchup on a filet mignon: It masks the true flavor of the food and shows that you're probably not ready to be taken out in public yet.

Of course, your good breeding isn't going to help if the waiter has a heavy hand. To make sure that your salad doesn't arrive at the table already drenched, ask for the dressing to be brought on the side. That way, you can control exactly how much goes on.

PREPARING FOR THE MAIN EVENT

Be it at the ballpark, the bowling alley, or the beach, fun-spot food offerings will likely be fattening. As a golden rule, it's best to take your own munchies. Besides saving money by avoiding extortionary concession stands, you'll also spare yourself unwanted calories.

At the movies. Movie popcorn smells great and tastes great. It's also made at some theaters with coconut oil, which is 86 percent saturated fat. Put another way, one medium-size bucket may contain 50 grams of fat—and that's before you add the butter.

In the bleachers. There's not much you can eat at the ballpark or stadium that isn't going to knock your diet over the center-field fence. Nachos, roasted peanuts, chili-cheese wieners—they're loaded with fat. They're also irresistible. So go ahead and have a hot dog with your light beer. Then make it a point to stick with pretzels for the rest of the game.

At the bowling alley. Most bowling establishments stopped evolving in the early 1960s, which means that the menu is pretty much limited to fatty snack-bar and vending-machine fare. About the best you can hope for is to find some pretzels in the machine or a turkey sandwich at the snack bar.

On the trail. Hiking is one of the healthiest social activities you and your intrepid cronies could pick. You can make it one step healthier by booting the beef jerky and trail mix out of your pack—both have fat aplenty. For a trimmer trailside treat, try dried fruit, suggests Patti Tveit Milligan, R.D., a dietitian in San Diego and nutrition columnist for *Selling* magazine.

At the ski lodge. When you're trying to warm up after a morning of hotdogging on the black diamond slopes, it's tempting to snowplow into a big basket of fries or some steaming mozzarella sticks. For a better hot lunch, get a bracing cup of coffee, tea, cocoa, or apple cider, and a plate of pasta. If all else fails, treat yourself to a hamburger—that's right, a hamburger, without cheese. Yes, it has fat in it, but far less than those other fried goodies.

At the beach. Experts say that when we think we're hungry, we're often really thirsty. And despite all those waves, nothing dries you out like a day at the beach. So between volleyball games, while you're soaking up the rays and drinking in the view, take a minute to quench your thirst from that big jug of water you brought along. Or try a combination of half water and half juice, suggests Milligan.

Incidentally, don't put all your faith in the vinegar-and-oil dressing: It has about as much fat per 2-tablespoon serving—approximately 16 grams—as the blue cheese. It's best to order low-fat dressing, but don't feel guilty for getting the full-fat kind. If you don't overdo it, you're not going to move up a waist size, regardless of the dressing you choose.

Read between the lines. That wonderful menu prose makes it easy to forget that "lightly kissed with our own savory sauce" usually means "slathered with butter." When something is described as batter-dipped, fried, sautéed, or creamed, that's a giveaway that there are gobs of fat in it. "The same goes for food that's described as having lots of gravy," adds Barbara Whedon, R.D., a dietitian and nutrition counselor at Thomas Jefferson University Hospital in Philadelphia. "If you can't tell how much fat is in the sauce or gravy, you can always ask for it on the side."

Entrées that usually contain the least fat are those that have been grilled, broiled, baked, roasted, or steamed. Don't hesitate to ask how a dish has been prepared. If restaurants want to print their menus in a foreign language, they should be willing to provide the translation.

Cast a wide net. It's hard to resist a hankering for a thick, juicy steak, but sometimes a fish steak will hit the spot just as well. "A nice piece of grilled salmon or tuna can be very satisfying," Whedon says. "It can be just as filling as the same portion of beef—and it's healthier for you."

Eat more vegetables. Even if you don't normally chew the parsley that comes stuck to your plate, the vegetables accompanying the meal are more than a colorful distraction. "A lot of meals come with a baked potato or another vegetable as a choice of side dish," says Dr. Peikin. A starchy spud or another high-fiber vegetable will be plenty filling. Keep in mind, however, that many restaurants serve their veggies dripping with butter or some other fatty sauce. "Ask them to serve it on the side or leave it off entirely," Dr. Peikin says.

Don't desert dessert. "If you've been making good choices throughout the meal, it's okay to have some kind of dessert. And if you're out with someone, it's certainly very social to share the dessert with a date or a friend," Whedon says.

"Quite a few restaurants offer some kind of low-fat dessert, even if it's as simple as sherbet or sorbet," she adds.

Invite a like-minded friend. Experts have long recognized that people who eat their meals with others consume more chow than those who dine alone. Indeed, research has shown that buddies with gargantuan appetites have a way of encouraging—consciously or not—their tablemates to keep up.

This doesn't mean that the only way to lose weight is to spend the rest of your life eating alone. Experts have noted that those who are diet conscious are just as likely to imitate friends who eat with restraint as to imitate those who stuff it in with both fists. So go ahead and set the table for two. Just be sure to invite someone who eats at your pace.

TRIMMING TACTICS AT THE TAVERN

Be it bowling night, a postgame party, or a down-and-dirty pub crawl, it seems like many male social activities involve at least some booze and a bowl of snacks.

Where there is alcohol, there are calories—7 per gram, to be precise. In many beers, that can add up to more than 150 calories, as much as in a handful of tortilla chips. And that's before you help yourself to any of the wonderful greasy, salty foods that go down so well with a couple of brews.

This isn't to say that you have to become a teetotaler or wire your jaw closed every time someone passes the peanuts. But you can make smarter choices to ensure that when you belly up to the bar, your belly isn't resting on the bar.

Don't cruise on empty. When you're meeting friends after work, it's tempting to skip supper and make up for it with a round of Buffalo wings and some potato skins. "Don't set yourself up to gorge on those fatty bar snacks," says Whedon. Instead, try to eat something low-fat before you start carousing. If your local taproom doesn't serve meals, suggest meeting somewhere else for dinner first.

Skip the nuts. When you drink, your body naturally loses salt, which is why you readily reach for salted peanuts. The problem is, the average guy can down a couple of handfuls—which contain more than 70 grams of fat—before he's blown the foam off his first beer. Do yourself a favor and ask the barkeep if he has any other pub grub, such as pretzels and popcorn, which contain a lot less fat.

Beware the calories on tap. The average imported brew has about 170 calories per glass, while domestics weigh in at about 140 calories. "Some of the domestic light beers have even less—and they don't all taste as bad as guys think," says James Horan, longtime bar manager of Boston's Statler-Hilton Hotel.

Be particularly wary of specialty brews: Some pack a serious punch. You can't spot them by their color, either. Brown, yellow, red—color doesn't make any difference in terms of either calorie count or alcohol content, says John Hansell, editor and publisher of *Malt Advocate,* a magazine for beer and whiskey aficionados.

Here's how to tell what you're getting into: Hold the brew up to the light and see how much light passes through. In general, the less translucent it is, the thicker it probably is. If it's thick, that means more barley went into creating it, thus more sugars and, inevitably, more calories.

You can also tell by tasting it. If it has a malty flavor, chances are that it's a highly caloric beer. You don't have to give up your favorite brew. Just keep in mind that beers this rich are made to be savored in small quantities and not guzzled.

Mix drinks. Instead of guzzling your usual high-calorie brew or cocktail, try something lighter for a change, Horan suggests. "Some of the mixed drinks aren't so bad, especially ones with carbonated water in them." He recommends a wine spritzer. "Of course, not every guy wants to drink a spritzer with his buddies," he admits.

Traveling without Setbacks

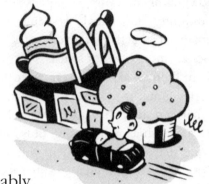

Unlike Willie Nelson, many of us probably can wait to get on the road again. They say that getting there is half the fun, but time spent traveling when you're trying to stay fit is really half the battle. It's tough to get your workout fix when you're cruising Route 66.

Arrival and departure schedules turn meals into grab-anything affairs—and let's face it, airports, bus terminals, and train stations aren't exactly famous for their salad bars. As for those roadside fast-food joints, take the letter *s* out of *fast,* and you have a pretty good idea of what you're getting.

The bottom line is that any kind of travel can turn lofty aspirations for a good diet and exercise into so much lost luggage.

HOW TO TRAVEL LIGHT

Experts acknowledge that keeping trim while traveling can be as frustrating as trying to refold a road map, but it's not impossible.

"Being away from home is not a license to gain weight," says Morton H. Shaevitz, Ph.D., associate clinical professor of psychiatry at the University of California, San Diego, School of Medicine and author of *Lean and Mean: The No Hassle Life-Ex-*
tending Weight Loss Program for Men. "It may be a bit more difficult to keep up a fitness routine, but you've got to convince yourself that whatever you do at home for your health and well-being you can do when you're not at home, too."

Whether you're stuck in some endless airport layover, trapped in a hotel with no gym, road-tripping down the interstate, or even in the midst of a well-earned vacation, with a few simple methods you can wring a fitness plan out of any trip.

PLANE TALK

Being on the go may seem fun and glamorous to the desk-bound, but anyone who travels for a living will tell you it's about as exciting as a car crash—and only a little less damaging to your health in the long run.

"I travel several weeks out of the year, and it just throws off my eating and exercising habits," says Steve Brackett, a sales manager in Des Plaines, Illinois, who's in his midthirties. "I try to watch what I eat and stick to a workout, but it's tough."

Granted, the occasional overnighter—along with the requisite airline peanuts, fattening room-service fare, and missed evenings at the health club—won't pack a lot of excess baggage into your cargo hold. But for men who travel for a living, the pitfalls can be profound.

"You're in a rush to get somewhere, so you don't have time to eat a decent meal. Or you might have a layover, where you'll be either bored or famished. Or you're arriving at odd hours, when there might not be a lot of good food choices open to you," says Patti Tveit Milligan, R.D., a dietitian in San Diego and nutrition columnist for *Selling* magazine, a publication devoted to men who travel for a living.

You may not be able to control flight schedules or check-in times, Milligan says, but you can still control what goes in your mouth.

Pack a snack. You skip breakfast to make the first leg of your flight. Then, you get stuck in a red plastic seat in an airport lounge far from anywhere, and your hurry-up morning has left you famished.

It's a bad situation, but easy to avoid. "Buy lots of little snack-size foods to pack in your briefcase or carry-on," suggests Milligan. She recommends miniature boxes of raisins or dry cereal. Fruit cups are also good, as are fig bars, crackers, or juice boxes.

"They keep for a long time, so once you pack them you don't have to worry about them. But they'll be on hand when you need to take the edge off your appetite," Milligan says. Fresh fruit is also a good traveling food, she adds.

Try terminal treats. Airports aren't exactly bastions of healthy eating, but when there's nothing else to nosh on, you can at least limit the damage. "The hot dog, burger, and nacho kiosks are really bad choices—all of that food is very high in fat," says Milligan. "You're better off getting just a snack until you can have a decent meal."

She recommends assuaging the beast within with a more-or-less healthful snack: a bagel, say, or a soft pretzel with mustard. "A lot of the cafeterias have a bowl of fruit at the end of the line—that's a good choice. And if you go into some of the newsstands, you might even find a bag of dried fruit snacks."

Look for midair distractions. Once you're on board, avoiding midair collisions with food can be a tricky maneuver. "Airlines use food and alcohol to distract you from the fact that you're in a narrow metal tube, 35,000 feet up in the air," says Dr. Shaevitz. Look for less fattening distractions, he suggests. Pack a fast-paced novel or magazine. Watch the in-flight movie. Even catching a nap is better than wolfing peanuts (and asking your neighbor if you can have his, too).

If you don't see it, ask. When the meal cart rolls by, you may not have to settle for that Salisbury steak with the vegetables swimming in butter and the fudge brownie for dessert. Plenty of airlines offer special low-fat meals for passengers who call ahead. Even if you didn't call, ask anyway. The airlines typically keep a few special meals on hand and give them out to the first people who ask.

Be a two-fisted drinker. The air in planes is extremely dry. "When we get thirsty, we often mistake thirst for hunger," Milligan says. So try to drink plenty of water during the flight.

WORKING OUT AT THE INN

Just because you've checked into a hotel for a few days, that doesn't mean you have to check out on healthy eating and exercise.

"Most hotels recognize that their guests are trying to be health conscious," says Dr. Shaevitz. Many major hotel chains offer amenities such as exercise rooms or a pool, and low-fat fare on the room service menu. To stay in shape in your home away from home, try these tips.

Lodge yourself in the exercise room. If you're going to pay top dollar to stay at a hotel that has a pool and exercise room, you may as well get your money's worth. Even if you've had a long day, just 15 minutes on a stairclimber can help you unwind. And a few laps in the pool can be the perfect relaxer before you hit the sack.

Pack your trunks. "I almost always stay at a hotel with a gym, but I never remember to bring clothes to work out in," says Brackett. Keep workout clothes, wrapped in plastic, in your suitcase. That way, you're always ready to go—and the running shorts can double as swim trunks in a pinch. Keeping the clothes wrapped in plastic helps ensure that you don't attend a sales conference in a suit smelling of tennis shoes.

Use your imagination. If your credit card is so worn out that you have to settle for a hotel with no exercise facilities, improvise. Do situps and pushups on the floor of your room. Go for a run—or even a brisk walk—around the hotel complex. Pretend that you're back in high school and do sprints on the stairs.

We're not talking only about convenience: Climbing stairs burns about 13.5 calories per minute, while pumping a stationary cycle in some smelly, mirrored room in the basement burns about 8 calories.

Skip your exercise. For a great on-the-road workout, take along a jump rope. "It's excellent exercise equipment for traveling. It fits easily in your suitcase or carry-on. You could jump rope for 10 to 15 minutes and get a good workout," says Art Mollen, D.O., director of the Southwest Health Institute in Phoenix and author of *The Mollen Method.* How good? In 10 minutes, you'll skip about 800 times, burning about 130 calories in the process.

Just be considerate of the guy in the room beneath you and restrict your rope-skipping to civilized hours.

Don't eat in your room. In the privacy of your hotel room, eating sensibly can be as tricky as figuring out the remote control. You're bored, no one is watching—hey, why not raid the honor bar or order a five-course meal from room service?

"Instead, go down to the hotel restaurant or walk to one nearby," suggests Milligan. For one thing, when you're in public instead of squirreled away in your room, you tend to eat less. Plus, just heading downstairs ensures that you'll get at least a little exercise.

EATING IN STRANGE PLACES

When you're visiting some foreign paradise, you want to do as the locals do and eat their food. But deciphering a menu in the native tongue is tough enough without trying to figure out how fattening the dish you just ordered is. Here's a quick gastronomic review of world cuisine, helpful for the next time you dine in another country—or in the ethnic neighborhood near your hotel.

Cuisine	Good for You	Bad for You
Chinese	Wonton soup, steamed vegetables or rice, fish	Deep-fried egg rolls, barbecued pork ribs, fried rice
French	Consommé, vegetable salads, crusty bread (easy on the butter), anything grilled, broiled, or roasted	Croissants, any creamy sauce
Greek	Pita bread, rice, fish, chicken, tzatziki (yogurt and cucumbers)	Feta cheese, phyllo dough, nuts, olives, anchovies
Indian	Chapati (baked bread)	Poori (fried bread), samosas (fried pastries)
Italian	Pasta, tomato sauce with garlic, sherbet	Antipasto, parmigiana, Alfredo or other creamy sauces
Japanese	Natto soup, chicken teriyaki, sushi, anything yakimono (broiled) or nabemono (boiled)	Tempura, miso soup, anything agemono (deep-fried)
Mexican	Soft corn tortillas, grilled fish, chicken fajitas, salsa	Crispy tacos, chorizo, refried beans, tortilla chips, guacamole, sour cream

If you're getting in on the red-eye and all the eateries are closed, go ahead and eat in your room. "But order just a snack," says Dr. Shaevitz. Your best bets are lighter foods that won't keep you awake, such as fruit trays, salads (dressing on the side, of course), cereal, or even a bagel and jelly.

HEALTHY HOLIDAYS

When guys go on vacation, they tend to take off from every kind of work—including the work it takes to stay in shape. After all, it's not every week that you get to lounge in some sun-dappled paradise, letting the cabana boys see to your every gustatory whim. It's vacation, for crying out loud. You're entitled to indulge a little.

There's a good point here. And if your vacation is the kind that includes plenty of physical activities, such as skiing, hiking, or scuba diving, you can probably take a vacation from your usual workout routine.

"But if your trip is basically sedentary with lots of eating opportunities, such as a cruise or a visit to a resort, exercise should be mandatory," advises Dr. Shaevitz. You can still bask in the glories of surf and sun and squeak in time for fitness before the next round of margaritas.

Go ahead, live a little. One of the biggest joys of traveling is eating. Just don't do it in a big way three or four times a day.

"I suggest that travelers have a couple of micromeals and one bigger meal where they indulge a bit more," says Dr. Shaevitz. If you have cereal for breakfast and a salad for lunch, then have a four-course meal for dinner. This way, you can watch your food intake and still be a bit decadent.

Do as the natives do. Traveling isn't much fun if you can't sample some of the local cuisine. But that doesn't mean that you have to eat the fattiest of foreign foods. If you're in an exotic locale, sample the indigenous fruits, vegetables, and other local low-cal fare.

"When I went to Paris with my family, lunch often consisted of picking up three or four pieces of fruit at a local outdoor stand, a large bottle of sparkling water, a loaf of crusty French bread, and just a few slices of cheese, which we'd share amongst the four of us," says Dr. Shaevitz. Avail yourself of the culture. As often as not, you'll find some pretty healthy choices.

When in Rome, roam. At least once a day on your vacation, get off your beach towel and do some sight-seeing. Stretch your muscles; expand your horizons. You'll have plenty of time later to lounge by the pool with a bottomless cocktail.

STAYING ON THE ROAD TO FITNESS

You might think that a speeding ticket would be the worst thing you could pick up on a road trip, but ounce for ounce, drive-thru food is probably worse. For travelers who rely on ground transportation, riding the roads and rails is almost always an order-to-go proposition fraught with dietary perils.

"If you're driving or taking a bus or train somewhere, there's not much you can do except sit and eat. And when you do stop for meals, it's almost always at some roadside restaurant that offers fast—and not very healthy—food," says Milligan. Here are some ways to keep those excess pounds from hitching a lift with you.

Pack munchies for the miles. Instead of relying on the vending machines and bags of junk food in gas stations and rest stops, pack your own munchies for the road. "Fresh fruits and raw vegetables are the best choices, but you can also pack low-fat crackers or dried fruit, or low-fat granola or sports bars," suggests Milligan.

Stretch your legs. After a few hours on the road, your butt is bound to fall asleep, and the rest of you may soon follow. A brisk walk around the rest area or truck stop will not only keep you awake, it will also help burn some of those calories you picked up at the last fast-food emporium.

Leave the station. Unlike airports, where you're usually stuck in the outlands, bus terminals and train stations are usually in the heart of town—and you don't have to mess with security checks to get in and out. So leave the vending machines behind and seek out a local restaurant or corner grocery. That way, you can eat well and also get in a little sight-seeing.

Beating the Holiday Trap

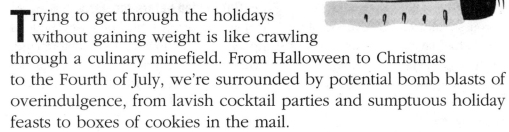

Trying to get through the holidays without gaining weight is like crawling through a culinary minefield. From Halloween to Christmas to the Fourth of July, we're surrounded by potential bomb blasts of overindulgence, from lavish cocktail parties and sumptuous holiday feasts to boxes of cookies in the mail.

We try to rein in our cravings, but all it takes is one misstep, an excessive meal or two—and we could blow up.

CAUGHT IN THE HOLIDAY VORTEX

Keeping a steady weight can be tough at any time of year, but the holidays, experts agree, pose particular risks. Research has shown that we put on weight when we put on our party hats. In a study of Christmas revelers, for example, Swedish researchers found that people who were otherwise in good trim typically put on almost a pound over the Yuletide season. Some gained as much as $2\frac{2}{3}$ pounds.

"It's not just the sheer amount of rich food and treats that starts piling up around the holidays, it's the fact that you're also socializing with friends and relatives and paying less attention to what you're eating," says Barbara Whedon, R.D., dietitian and nutrition counselor at Thomas Jefferson University Hospital in Philadelphia. "It all starts to add up."

Nor are you likely to get much relief from overly hospitable hosts who plead with you to eat, please eat, just a little smidge, just another bite, just a taste, just one more helping.

"Even if you're not especially hungry at a big dinner, there's always some social pressure to eat—this is your host's best recipe, and you wouldn't want to offend her," Whedon says. "It can be a complicated situation, and a lot of people give up and overeat."

FIT FOR FEASTS

There's no reason that you should become a holiday hermit, a sad soul consigned to watching the festive gorging from the culinary sidelines.

No one should have to entirely forgo the traditional holiday spread we get to enjoy only once or twice a year. Be it a

Thanksgiving turkey with all the trimmings or a sizzling Independence Day barbecue, you have every right to eat your fill. But it's possible, Whedon says, to eat well without blowing your good intentions in the process. "Don't obsess about it—you won't enjoy the holiday if you're frantic about eating too much," she adds.

What you should do, however, is plot your moves before laying a napkin in your lap. That way, you can enjoy the holidays—and the good food that goes with them—without carrying around the weighty consequences later.

Don't starve ahead. It's natural, when a major spread is pending, to think about skipping a few meals to leave room for the big event. Problem is, this makes about as much sense as giving up sex for 3 weeks to enjoy 1 good night. Your appetite may be stronger, but your enjoyment of the experience won't be much improved.

"By dinner, you'll be starving, so you won't be making good decisions about what you eat," Whedon adds.

Get loaded before the party. Instead of eating light before a big holiday event, load up with some low-fat food beforehand. "This curbs your appetite, so you can make better choices," says Whedon.

Some good choices for preemptive snacks include soup and bread, pasta and vegetables, or even a few pieces of fruit. Carbohydrates quickly convert to body fuel. Since your body can store only a limited amount of this fuel, your appetite is going

REINVENTING YOUR HOLIDAY ROUTINE

Eating, drinking, napping, channel-surfing—if these pastimes sum up your holiday routine, it's no wonder you're having a hard time keeping the weight off. But with a little creative retooling, you can curb fat and have fun at the same time. For example:

Last Year . . .
Watched the game on TV with the guys
Watched *A Christmas Carol*
Cleaned out the buffet table
Ate turkey smothered in gravy
Got up from the table and took a nap in the recliner

This Year . . .
Organize a game in the backyard
Go out and sing Christmas carols
Help clean up the buffet table
Eat turkey smothered in cranberry sauce
Get up from the table, go for a 15-minute walk, and then take a nap in the recliner

to lose some of its insistence. In comparison, your body can store about 50 times more fat before your stomach says, "Full."

The idea isn't to make yourself so full that you won't be able to cram in another mouthful later. But by taking in at least some calories before the big event, you'll take the edge off your appetite and help keep yourself from going overboard.

Exert cocktail control. Studies have shown that alcohol makes people hungrier. At the same time, it lowers their inhibitions, so they're more likely to gorge. "The more you drink, the less you care about what you're eating—especially if you're drinking on an empty stomach," says Steven Peikin, M.D., professor of medicine at the University of Medicine and Dentistry of New Jersey and author of *The Feel Full Diet*. To keep alcohol from crashing your party, he recommends drinking only water or some other low-cal, nonalcoholic beverage until after the dinner bell rings. Or at least stick with a low-cal alcoholic beverage such as a wine spritzer.

Reward yourself later. There's nothing wrong with having a beer or a glass of wine with your dinner, Whedon adds. "By waiting for the meal, you're not drinking on an empty stomach, so you're controlling your appetite better," she says. So revel in the holiday spirit. Drink a toast to your host—and to your own good health.

Wet your appetite. "Drinking generous amounts of water is, overwhelmingly, the number one way to reduce appetite," says George Blackburn, M.D., Ph.D., associate professor of surgery at Harvard Medical School. "Many people think that they're having a food craving when in fact they're thirsty," he says.

As a rule, experts say, you should drink at least eight glasses of water a day. And when you're planning a big feed, pouring in a few extra ounces will help keep your appetite under control.

Eat the chow, skim the fat. While not all holiday calories can be easily trimmed away, there are ways to limit the damage. If you're eating turkey, for example, a serving of white meat has less than half the fat of a comparable serving of dark meat. If you're having a roast, trim away the visible fat, including the crispy bits—they're nothing more than burned fat.

Go easy on the salt. Guys who are concerned about their blood pressure already know enough to watch their salt intakes—but the possible evils of sodium aren't restricted to those with high blood pressure. Salt may make you want to eat more, perhaps by boosting levels of hormones that stimulate appetite. So if you want to spice up your food, try vinegar, lemon, dried herbs, or other low-sodium alternatives instead.

Give up the skin. Much as you might love the crackly skin on the holiday bird, it can really cook your goose. One serving of white-meat turkey without skin, for example, contains a little more than 3 grams of fat; one serving with the skin has more than 8 grams. Whedon recommends discreetly peeling the skin off the bird and setting it to the side of your plate.

Be careful with add-ons. Don't cover

WINNING THE DRINKING GAME

When it comes to putting on weight, alcohol is a dangerous accessory. It inhibits your inhibitions. It makes you careless about what you eat. And it also packs more than a few calories of its own.

It can be tough to say no when it's the boss who's buying the rounds or when your buddies are quaffing and want you to quaff along. But according to James Horan, longtime bar manager of Boston's Statler-Hilton Hotel, there are ways to resist the pressure without making a scene.

Make it last. "Get a big beer and sip it all night," Horan advises. "The guy you're with won't feel like he's drinking alone—he'll think you're keeping up."

Cede the victory. Don't even try to match a guy drink for drink. Admit right off the bat that you're no match for his prowess. "It should satisfy his honor," Horan says.

Befriend the barkeep. If you want to keep your drinking under control, don't hesitate to approach the bartender beforehand. Tell him that when you order a gin and tonic, for example, what you really want is sparkling water. Or ask him to reduce the alcohol in your mixed drinks. "Then slip him 5 bucks," says Horan. "He'll be your friend after that."

your plate with a whopping serving of stuffing and a wash of gravy. Both gravy and stuffing are often made with organ meats, which are extremely high in artery-clogging fat and cholesterol.

Go for the greens. The cornucopia of vegetables at the holiday table will satisfy just about any taste. At the same time, vegetables fill you up, so you eat less fat. "They're a good choice as long as they're not dripping with a cheese or butter sauce," adds Dr. Peikin.

In fact, don't look on greens as being only a supporting player. By giving them star billing, you'll naturally eat less of the fattening foods you're trying to avoid.

Always keep something on your plate. During the holidays especially, an empty plate is to the host what a red flag is to a

bull. "No one believes that you're full if your plate is empty. But if your plate still has a bit of food on it, that sends the signal that you've had all you can possibly eat," says Whedon.

While you're at it, make sure that the little something left behind is your least favorite dish. Otherwise, you're more likely to forget yourself and eat it, thus devouring your antifat shield.

Enjoy your just desserts. It's no easy task to forgo a delicious slice of apple pie or a heaping helping of baked Alaska. So don't even try. Enjoy yourself. "You don't want to overdo it, but you don't want to deny yourself completely, either," Whedon says.

What you *can* do is avoid those desserts that you can pig out on at any time of the year. For this special day, focus on holiday treats. "If you can't resist having more than one dessert, limit yourself to just one or two bites of each treat. Or share it with someone—it's better than eating the whole thing by yourself," says Whedon.

Skip the sofa. Your war against weight doesn't end at the dining-room table. Once the feast is over, the temptation to sink into the nearest chair can be almost overwhelming. By staying on your feet and getting a little exercise—a fast walk, for example—you'll fight off the stupefying urge to sleep, and you'll burn a few of the calories you just consumed. "It won't make up for all of the food you just ate, but it will help your body burn more calories," Whedon says.

Go easy on yourself. Don't despair if your appetite occasionally gets the best of you. It's a holiday, you're surrounded by great food, and all your friends and relatives are eating like kings. You'd have to be Superman to always keep your appetite under control. So cut yourself some slack if you slip a little in the discipline department.

"You can compensate for the calorie load by choosing lower-fat foods for the next day or so and by being more physically active," Whedon advises.

On the other hand, don't let a momentary lapse lead you further down the road of culinary temptation.

GOING LIGHT AT A HEARTY PARTY

Although meals make up the biggest fat threat around the holidays, parties and other social events can be pound-packing experiences, too.

"Parties are just as damaging to someone trying to watch his weight as big dinners are," Whedon says. "All that finger food looks small, but it's very big in fat."

What follows is a safer way to work the room—without lingering too long at the bar or over the hors d'oeuvres.

Begin with the buffet. Although this is usually where a party's heartiest—and heaviest—fare resides, you should be able to scavenge at least a few good-tasting items that don't contain fat in the double digits.

"Some good choices are things like shrimp cocktail, fruit salad, and any vegetable that's light on the dip," Whedon says. And don't forget the pretzels, which are also low in fat. "If there's a cold-cut platter, stick with turkey, ham, or lean roast beef," she adds. By contrast, other meats, such as bologna, salami, and pepperoni, and most cheeses are extremely high in fat.

Eat fruit, not fruitcake. Foods high in fiber are good choices when you're cruising the buffet line, for a couple of reasons. You have to thoroughly chew fibrous foods such as apples, pears, oranges, and carrots, which means you'll eat them more slowly. The longer it takes you to eat, the fuller you can feel. Plus, the fiber in those foods takes up more room in your stomach, leaving less room for fattier choices.

Turn up the heat. Adding a dash of spicy food to your meals increases metabolism, allowing you to burn some of those holiday foods a little faster. At the same time, spicy food decreases appetite. So when you're at that holiday cookout, ladle on a little extra barbecue sauce or add jalapeño peppers to your burger. And seek out buffet sauces such as hot mustard, cocktail sauce, salsa, or horseradish.

Watch your hands. It feels awkward while mingling not to have a drink or snack in hand. "It's kind of a social security blanket," says Dr. Peikin. "The problem is, you're going to consume whatever you're holding." He recommends cruising the room with a glass of water or a nonalcoholic beverage in hand. Or if you're walking and noshing, make sure the chow is low-cal.

Keep moving. When you don't know many people at a party, it's tempting to hover where there's food—at least that's one place you feel at home! It's better to move on, Whedon says. "It's amazing how much less you eat when the food is not right in front of you."

Dressing Lean

Those last 10 pounds are taking longer to burn off than you'd hoped. Or maybe you have already lost 10 pounds and are looking forward to looking a little better. In either case, wearing proper duds can help make the most— or, since we're talking about size, the least—of your physical attributes.

It has been said that clothes make the man. But as any tailor can tell you, the wrong clothes make the man look fatter. Chances are that your closet is filled with mistakes—clothes that looked good in the store but not on you. Take that Hawaiian shirt. You thought it would hide your gut, but instead it made you look bigger than a roast pig at a luau. Or those snug jeans: They held everything in—until you bent over. Then they revealed a major crack in your fashion foundation.

On the other hangers are those special clothes that make you look 20 pounds lighter: a loose sweater, those gray pleated pants, a jacket cut just so. If you could just put your finger on exactly what makes them work, you would always look like a million bucks—without having to spend that much.

SIZING UP THE PROBLEM

In our society, women have a definite edge over men, fashionwise. "Early on, women are taught to recognize which clothing styles look good on them, which ones make them look fat, and why. Men aren't," says Keith Scott, general manager for Giorgio Armani in New York City.

It's never too late for men to learn the sartorial sleights-of-hand that can make even less-than-perfect physiques look terrific. Here's what you need to know.

When in doubt, go big. Men sometimes buy too-tight clothes in the hope that they'll hold the flab in. They don't. Stuffing yourself into smaller sizes will only make the fat more prominent. When shopping, look for clothes that feel comfortable or even roomy (but not baggy). If the item that you're trying on feels snug, go to the next size up. In most cases, bigger will make you look thinner.

Keep your clothing quiet. "On jackets and shirts, large designs like paisleys, boxy patterns, and wide horizontal stripes cause the eye to move from left to right," Scott notes. In other words, when someone looks at you in that checked shirt, they're going to

QUICK CUTS

There are a number of strategies that clothiers use for "thinning" body parts, from double chins to big feet. Here's a quick primer.

Problem Area	Don't Wear	Do Wear
Double chin	Tight collars, which squeeze extra flesh upward	Pointed collars, which make your chin look longer and thinner
Big waist	Narrow, tight jackets or pants that emphasize bulk	Pleated pants and jackets with shoulders broader than your hips, which create a slimmer profile
Large behind	Heavy, textured fabrics such as corduroy, which accentuate your bulk, or no-vent jackets that ride up and expose the seat	Thinner, flatter-looking gabardine or worsted wool pants, or a vented jacket
Fat feet	Light-colored shoes with thick soles, which make size 12s look like 24s	Dark shoes with thin soles, such as black or dark-brown oxfords

focus on your girth, not your length. So stick with solids or small, subtle patterns.

Go vertical. While horizontal stripes make you look broader, vertical stripes coax the eyes to travel up and down. This will help you look tall and lean even if you're not. "In this case, a nice pinstripe shirt can really have a slimming effect," says Scott.

Tie one on. A tie can be a large man's best friend, giving a thin, vertical line to any outfit, Scott says. Keep your neckwear subdued and simple, he adds. "The trend has been toward solid, neutral colors, with maybe a faint pattern."

Live in layers. Paradoxically, some men look thinner when they pile on more clothes—a trick known as strategic layering.

"Basically, instead of one layer—say, a shirt and pants—you drape on something extra: a big sweater, for example, or a flannel button-down that you wear over a T-shirt," Scott says. The layering "distributes" your weight over your body instead of making it look concentrated in the middle.

Don't tuck and cover. Wearing oversize shirts tucked in results in excess material inside your pants. This gives you a big bulge—and not the flattering kind, either. "Wear it untucked with a T-shirt underneath," advises Scott.

Wear high collars. Wide collars are right for the retro look, but when you're trying to look slim, go high, advises Marvin S. Piland, men's clothing consultant for Saks Fifth Avenue in New York City. Like stripes, high collars cause the eye to travel upward, away from a thick neck or barrel chest.

Put your clothes on a diet. "As a matter of common sense, the heavier fabrics look heavier, the lighter fabrics are lighter," says Scott. So if you want to create the illusion of thinness, "cotton, twill, linens, even flannel can be much lighter-looking choices," says Scott.

Please with pleats. Pleated pants tend to make men look thinner by concealing the belly bulge, Scott says. "Plain-front pants are all right if you're thin, but they can be a real problem on bigger men," he adds.

When wearing pleated pants, however, the pleats should lie flat. If they spread out or if the pockets flare open while you're buttoning the pants, go for the next size up.

Beware of bold buckles. We all need to hold our pants up, but the last thing a big guy needs is a big belt with a matching buckle. For one thing, a big buckle acts like a bull's-eye, drawing everyone's gaze to your belly. Also, wearing a wide belt makes you look wider.

Use a thin belt—one not much wider than your thumb, Scott advises. It will keep your pants on without drawing attention to the equator.

Put yourself on suspension. If you're a big guy, a belt can cinch up flab and make it more prominent. As an alternative, strap on some suspenders. They'll hold up your pants just as well and give you a smoother line. Limit your choice to subdued, solid colors, though. Rainbow suspenders won't lend you any character and will focus attention on the area you're trying to hide.

Tommy Moe, Olympic Ski Champ

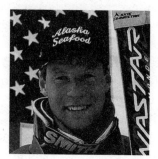

Ask the pundits: Not one of them expected great things—or *anything*—from the U.S. Alpine Ski Team heading into the 1994 Winter Olympics in Lillehammer, Norway. *Sports Illustrated*, in its Winter Olympic preview issue, dismissed the team as "woeful," dubbing it a "lead-footed snowplow brigade."

Tommy Moe, who had placed a disappointing 20th in the men's downhill at the 1992 Olympics, was determined to prove the critics wrong. "It bugged me a little, because I really didn't think we deserved it," the Alaskan, who is in his mid-twenties, recalls. And prove them wrong he did.

At Lillehammer, in 5°F weather, in front of about 30,000 stunned spectators, Moe rocketed down the icy track on a flawless run that earned him the gold medal in men's downhill. In doing so, he led a charge that earned the U.S. ski team five medals in the first 10 days of the Olympics—including another medal for Moe, who took the silver in the Super G competition.

Two weeks after slamming the ski team, *Sports Illustrated* ate its words, featuring Tommy on the cover. And a proud American public was calling for Moe.

BUILDING MOE-MENTUM

Moe owes his success to an absolute knowledge of his abilities. His coaches have marveled at the speeds he can handle—upward of 90 miles an hour—and his razor-sharp precision executing turns at that velocity. But Moe is the first to admit he wouldn't have the control or the ability without an eclectic fitness regimen that keeps his mind and body honed as sharp as a ski's edge.

"When I'm training for the winter, I try to follow a 6-day program. Monday, Wednesday, and Friday are my weight-training days. On Tuesday, Thursday, and Saturday, though, I mix it up with some other sports to get a good aerobic workout," he says. For Moe, that could mean anything from hiking to kayaking.

Although he advocates doing as much of a total-body workout as possible, Moe devotes most of his weight training to his legs, abdominals, and lower back. "They're the foundation. People think it's just the legs, but you use your back and torso a lot—it's where your center of balance is." So Moe strengthens that center with plenty of crunches, sidebends, and leg lifts.

Then, he subjects his legs to a battery of grueling exercises: leg curls, squats, tuck jumps, and box jumps—where Moe literally jumps on and off a foot-high box as many times as he can in a minute. "The jump exercises are great for the leg strength you need when you have to change position quickly on a run," he says.

When he's not competing, Moe has little trouble staying in skiing shape. "I just try to do a lot of activities that require the same skills I use in skiing—balance and reaction time, especially." Moe's favorites include kayaking and mountain biking. "The kayak fine-tunes your balance because you always have to be careful not to tip over. And in either sport, you always have to be looking ahead, reading the terrain, because stuff is flashing by really quickly," he says. But Moe's most important off-season workout is the minimum 3 hours a week he spends on inline skates. "It's about the closest thing to skiing—it really helps me keep in form."

FUEL TO BURN

Moe's 5-foot-10, 200-pound body is ideal for skiing, and he helps keep it that way with a surprisingly average diet that most of us would be glad to follow.

"Basically, I eat whatever I want. For breakfast, I'll have cereal, bread, bagels, pancakes, even eggs. I eat lots of fruit. For dinner, I love pasta or steak," he says. "When I'm in Alaska, I'll eat tons of salmon and halibut. And I gotta say, I like drinking a beer after a hard day of skiing—it tastes pretty damn good."

But don't be misled by his omnivorous attitude. "As a skier, I need a lot of calories. It helps keep an extra layer of insulation on me so the cold won't interfere with my performance," he says. And although Moe eats what he wants, he still watches out for the saturated fats that could clog up his high-performance heart. "I'm not big on butter. I don't eat a lot of bacon or mayonnaise. And yeah, I'll have a steak, but I make sure it's a good lean cut, and I cut the excess fat off," he says. Even with his "extra layer of insulation," Moe's body fat is just 8 percent.

Although Moe may allow himself a few dietary excesses, when it comes to his overall fitness regimen, he doesn't cut himself any slack. "If you want to get anywhere, you always have to push yourself as hard as you can," he says. "Whether you're doing a rep or a set, or taking a hill on skis or a mountain bike, you have to push it, you have to challenge yourself. Try to do a little bit more than you think you can. Don't give up. Keep pushing, keep digging."

Joe Lewis, Former World Karate Champion

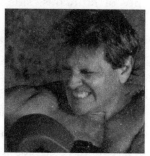

Joe Lewis is the Muhammad Ali of karate: simply the greatest. He learned karate while serving in the Marines, earned a 10th-degree black belt, and trained with Bruce Lee. In his fighting career, he garnered more titles than a small library and was voted "The Greatest Karate Fighter of All Time."

But Lewis doesn't preach a dogma of discipline when it comes to exercise. Now in his fifties, he's as much a philosopher as he is a fighter. And his words of wisdom pack as much power as his jabs and kicks.

"I don't go over all the health reasons for working out. You hear that junk every day from medical experts and so-called experts," Lewis says in his light North Carolina accent. "For me, exercise is trying to balance out the phenomena of hard work and having fun; follow me?

"Too often, guys go to the gym and it becomes a duty. Anything that's a duty, you tend to become irresponsible with, and that's no way to motivate yourself," he says. "People used to think I was rude because I didn't talk to anybody in the gym. I came in, worked out, and left. That was okay for me, but for most other people, working out should be fun."

FROM FARM BOY TO WORLD CHAMP

Lewis grew up with four brothers. His father was a full-time college professor who still worked the family farm every day. Lewis's father preferred an old-fashioned way of life: He plowed the soil by hand instead of using a tractor, and when he got sick (which he rarely did), he relied on home remedies and avoided doctors.

"If he were about to come down with a cold, he'd buy a bag of oranges and sit down and eat nearly every one of them," Lewis says.

At 14, Lewis began weight lifting with the same dedication and zeal that he would later apply to karate. "I always thought that a muscular body was a beautiful body. It has an aesthetic appeal. It has power," Lewis says. "Even as a boy, that look appealed to me. I'd run to the store just to pick up the muscle magazines."

VARIED WORKOUTS

Joe Lewis mixes up his training regimen to keep things fun. Plus, he never forces a workout. "I let my body have a say-so in my daily schedule, so my workouts vary. I just listen to my body," he says. Lewis lifts weights once a week and practices martial arts several times a week. Here's a typical week's workout.

Weight-Lifting Routine

Upright rows	2 sets, 10 reps
Lat pulldowns	2 sets, 15 reps
Incline bench presses	2 sets, 10 reps
Bench presses	2 sets, 10 reps
Dumbbell flys	2 sets, 30 reps
Leg extensions	2 sets, 15 reps
Leg curls	2 sets, 15 reps
Situps with a twist	2 sets, 20–30 reps
Leg raises	2 sets, 30–50 reps
Stretching	15–20 min

Martial Arts Routine

Stretching	15 min
Heavy bag	4 or 5 rounds of 3 min each (punching)
	4 or 5 rounds of 3 min each (kicking)
Double-end bag (7" size)	3 or 4 rounds of 3 min each
Shadowboxing	15–20 min
Defense shadowboxing	1 or 2 rounds of 3 min each
Stretching (total body)	15–20 min

By 19, Lewis beefed up to 225 pounds. He also joined the service. After a few weeks of seasickness en route to Okinawa, he dropped 10 pounds and took up martial arts, training under three native instructors.

"Around that time, I got turned off to weight lifting a little bit because I started getting stretch marks on my thighs and chest," he says. "They kept getting bigger and bigger, and I didn't like that. I thought they were disgusting. It's not necessary to blow your body up like a balloon."

Lewis eventually received his black belt in Shorinryu karate, a Japanese martial art. He gained an enviable reputation for his prowess by teaching fellow servicemen hand-to-hand combat in Vietnam. In 1966, at age 24, he became the amateur world karate champion in the point-fighting system. By 1971, he migrated to kickboxing and became the U.S. heavyweight champ. (Kickboxers fight continuously with full-contact blows, much like boxing; point-fighters fight with controlled blows to score points by hitting specific body parts.)

Before long, Lewis was making action movies, cohosting a talk show on martial arts, and appearing in the popular media. His career culminated in 1983, when he was voted "Greatest Karate Fighter of All Time" in a *Karate Illustrated* magazine survey. Nine years earlier, he had had a similar honor bestowed on him by the French publication, *Karate*.

FIGHTING THE GOOD FIGHT

Lewis doesn't fight competitively anymore. But he still appears at karate functions around the country. He also makes training videotapes. He has produced more than 20 of them on everything from fighting technique to weight lifting for martial artists. Like him, they're folksy and no-frills but packed with the wisdom that he has acquired through the decades.

Lewis's biggest project these days is giving self-defense seminars, especially to senior citizens. He has won two North Carolina Governor's Awards for his educational efforts in crime prevention.

When he's not on the road, Lewis works out several days a week by mixing weight lifting and martial arts. "I mix it up a lot. You have to. That's part of making it fun," he says.

As for diet, Lewis sticks to what he likes best, tempered with common sense. "I'm turned off by the traditional American breakfast of eggs and bacon. I've conditioned myself to like foods that are good for me. I try to eat a salad with my meats, and I eat red meat only once a week or so. I also eat my food plain—no garnish, butter, or salt."

Lewis's only quirk is that he eats his dessert first and salad last. "It started when I was a kid," he says.

But whether he's eating lunch or throwing a punch, Lewis's message of empowerment shines through everything he does. "My motivation comes through a personal feeling of responsibility, a feeling of personal empowerment. Weight lifting and martial arts can give you this confidence, too," he says. "But the most important thing to remember is that it's better to do some workout some of the time than to do nothing all the time. If you can balance the hard work by having fun, you're going to stick with it."

Tom McMillen, Former Congressman and Basketball Star

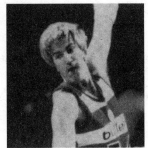

When he was cochair of the President's Council on Physical Fitness and Sports in Washington, D.C., Tom McMillen encouraged Americans to exercise and lead active lives. It was his official mission as well as a personal one. And the former NBA star and three-term Maryland congressman firmly believes in practicing what he preaches.

Instead of running for elective office—or running the hardwood in arenas nationwide—McMillen, now in his forties, can be seen almost every day running with his two Labrador retrievers.

"I run with them, or they run me," McMillen says. "They sometimes go off the beaten path and try to pull me here and there. That's a minor problem. I can usually adapt to that."

McMillen first became involved with the President's Council on Physical Fitness and Sports in 1970 when as a standout high school athlete he was named to the organization by President Nixon. He went on to play basketball at the University of Maryland and was a member of the 1972 Olympic basketball team.

A first-round draft pick by the old Buffalo Braves in 1974, McMillen enjoyed an 11-year stint in the NBA before retiring in 1986. That year, voters in Maryland sent him to the U.S. House of Representatives for what was to be the first of three terms. Later, in 1993, President Clinton named him to cochair the fitness council along with Olympic star Florence Griffith Joyner.

Keeping a busy schedule and maintaining a healthy diet is tough, but McMillen has made it a priority. A typical day starts with "a very light breakfast—a banana, toast, maybe some cereal, orange juice, coffee," he says.

For lunch, he usually has a vegetable patty, turkey sandwich, or salad. "At dinner, I eat tomato-based pasta, fish, or chicken," McMillen says. "Occasionally, once a month, I'll eat meat."

As a professional athlete, McMillen was

always in great shape—running and lifting weights to help survive the grueling NBA schedule. What he learned on the road he continues to use. "I look for hotels that have health clubs," he says. "I look for hotels where there's an ease of exercise, where you can run nearby."

It was during his NBA days that McMillen started running the stairs at hotels when he was stuck in some frozen city during the dead of winter. "That's the way I would get a workout, because it was too cold to go outside," McMillen says. "Steps were a great way to do that."

In addition to aerobic workouts, McMillen hits the weight room about every other day. One thing he doesn't do much of is play basketball. "My regimen today isn't so much competitive sport–based as it is in-dividualistic," McMillen says. "I've evolved away from that, going out and playing a round of basketball. I just try to do some-thing every day. That's the key, to just go out and exercise every day."

Part 4
FITNESS: WHAT TO EXPECT, WHAT TO IGNORE

What to Expect from Your Body

For poker players, "luck of the draw" has a ring of finality to it. You can discard once and hope that your hand will improve—then you're stuck. In real life, you're dealt a body with certain genetic characteristics. But unlike in poker, you get to upgrade your hand as much as you please, and no one calls it cheating.

In other words, you don't have to settle for hand-me-down genes.

"We inherit a certain amount of our body type from our parents, and that genetic constitution has a big impact on our body weight, our height, and our percentage of body fat," says Chris Melby, Dr.P.H., director of the Human Energy Laboratory at Colorado State University in Fort Collins. "But in addition to that, we have the behavioral factors that interact with our genetic constitution: what we eat, how much we eat, and how much we exercise or don't exercise."

The idea is not to get obsessed with looking like one of those rippling hunks in the magazines. It would be much more productive to check out your own body's characteristics and develop a reasonable, tailor-made training program.

"I get irritated with Madison Avenue and the fashion magazines that suggest that people all need to look very lean when in fact they may not be genetically set up to be that way," says Dr. Melby. "They're told that they don't have much value unless they are. And that's really a travesty."

THE BASIC SHAPES

Fitness professionals recognize three basic body types: endomorphs (round), mesomorphs (muscular), and ectomorphs (lean).

In one study, Dutch researchers put 21 sedentary men through a weight-training program of 14 exercises twice a week for 12 weeks. Ten of the men were slender, and 11 were solidly built. The two groups showed comparable strength gains and fat loss during the training. But while the solidly built group showed considerable muscle buildup, the slender group showed none—even though their strength had increased equally. The scientists theorized that the two groups were genetically different, either in their potential to build muscle or in the speed at which their bodies adapted to training.

A massive ongoing research project at Arizona State University in Tempe, involving five colleges and 650 subjects, indicates that 5 to 10 percent of people who work out are destined to show only modest gains. Most of the research subjects show moderate improvement in training programs, and another 5 to 10 percent are those fortunate souls who respond like genies released from bottles. Part of the reason for these differences is that performance factors such as maximum oxygen uptake, lung capacity, muscle fiber, and body type are influenced by genetics.

A man's body shape, by the way, is not a foolproof indication of his health or fitness level. "A person's outward appearance doesn't necessarily match his 'inward appearance,' his body composition," notes Wayne W. Campbell, Ph.D., an applied physiologist at Noll Physiological Research Center at Pennsylvania State University in University Park.

"You could be an extremely fit-looking person and still have a low amount of muscle and a high amount of fat if you carry

DIFFERENT BODIES, DIFFERENT STRENGTHS

Babe Ruth knew what his talents were, and they didn't include marathon running. Here's a list of activities that are best suited to specific body types. Maybe you're a champion in search of the right sport.

Endomorph	Mesomorph	Ectomorph
Walking	Sprinting	Cycling
Cycling	Cycling	Basketball
Swimming	Football	Nordic skiing
Alpine skiing	Ice hockey	High jump
Baseball	Basketball	Pole vault
Ice hockey	Track events	Tennis
Rowing	Windsurfing	Volleyball
Football	Racquetball	Weight training
Basketball	All types of skiing	Long-distance running
	Weight training	
	Baseball	

it well. On the other hand, you can be very not-fit-looking or pudgy, yet really be solid and mostly muscle," Dr. Campbell says.

CUSTOM BODYWORK

All three body types—endomorphs, mesomorphs, and ectomorphs—can be improved with diet and exercise. Here are training strategies for each.

Endomorphs

These are the Babe Ruths of the world, large-framed and relatively high in body fat. They may or may not be well-muscled. Endomorphs are naturals at powering through moderately intense, long-haul activities such as cycling, Alpine skiing, rowing, and football.

Disadvantages: Their metabolisms often are slow, meaning that they have to watch what they eat. They're also more vulnerable to heart disease and injury to their knees and ankles.

Training tip: Follow a low-fat diet, about 70 percent carbohydrates, 10 percent protein, and 20 percent fat. Burn calories with moderate aerobic exercise. Also, tone and build muscle with weight training.

Mesomorphs

The Carl Lewis types are medium-framed and naturally well-muscled. They respond best to strength training and don't have to work overly hard to stay in shape.

Disadvantages: They're vulnerable to weight gain if they don't eat carefully. Their considerable musculature makes them a tad weighty for long-distance running and swimming.

Training tip: Go for a low-fat diet that's higher in protein: 60 percent carbohydrates, 15 percent protein, and 25 percent fat. Split your workouts evenly between aerobics and strength training.

Ectomorphs

Think of Kareem Abdul-Jabbar—light-framed, low in both fat and muscle. Ectomorphs are energetic, nimble, and naturals at endurance. It doesn't take much of a workout for them to keep trim, and they're less prone to heart disease.

Disadvantages: They have to work harder to build muscle. Also, envious endomorphs and mesomorphs hope these sleek guys choke on their Twinkies.

Training tip: Emphasize carbohydrates and moderate amounts of protein to keep those muscles primed and working. Aim for a diet that contains 65 percent carbohydrates, 15 percent protein, and 20 percent fat. Work out with weights to build muscle, and make sure you get light aerobic activity to keep your heart honest.

How Movement Melts Fat

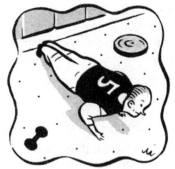

By the time most of us have reached middle age, we find that paunch has replaced our punch. That a beer belly now conceals our stomach muscles. That our chests, hidden behind baggy "athletic-cut" shirts, have become shadows of their former selves.

The ticket to fitness, experts say, is exercise. It's the one proven way to get trim and stay that way without resorting to liquid meals or the latest in fad diets.

WHY EXERCISE WORKS

We often say that exercise melts fat, as if fat were cool butter and exercise a warm frying pan. But that analogy isn't quite accurate. What really happens is even better.

"When you exercise, fat is metabolized in the muscles as energy," explains L. Jerome Brandon, Ph.D., associate professor of kinesiology in the department of kinesiology and health at Georgia State University in Atlanta. "There's no such thing as melting fat. You're burning fat as energy."

Yet fat doesn't go willingly into the fire. Like us, it fights for a sedentary life—which is why the pounds we accumulate are so hard to get rid of. To burn just 1 pound of fat, for example, "you're going to need to burn 3,500 calories," Dr. Brandon says.

You'd have to walk 30 miles in order to burn that much energy. "That's a lot of calories," says Dr. Brandon.

Although sustained exercise is a highly efficient way to drop pounds, more moderate approaches also work. Consider, for example, that hypothetical 30-mile walk. You could do it all at once. Or you could spread it out, walking a mile a day for 30 days. This will ultimately burn the same pound of blubber as a more concentrated approach—assuming, of course, that you're not porking out on spareribs in the meantime.

Done consistently, exercise will help keep fat off for the long haul, says Wayne C. Miller, Ph.D., assistant professor of kinesiology at Indiana University in Bloomington

MENTALLY FIT

Exercise is only as good as you make it. Focusing on two power workouts a week is a lot better than doing four sloppy ones. The test below will tell you whether you have staying power or whether you tend to wimp out. It will provide an estimate of your self-motivation, based on the self-motivation inventory developed by Rod K. Dishman, Ph.D., professor of exercise science at the University of Georgia in Athens.

1. I get discouraged easily.

Very unlike me	5	Somewhat like me	2
Somewhat unlike me	4	Very much like me	1
Neither like me nor unlike me	3		

2. I work no harder than I have to.

Very unlike me	5	Somewhat like me	2
Somewhat unlike me	4	Very much like me	1
Neither like me nor unlike me	3		

3. I seldom if ever let myself down.

Very unlike me	1	Somewhat like me	4
Somewhat unlike me	2	Very much like me	5
Neither like me nor unlike me	3		

4. I'm not the goal-setting type.

Very unlike me	5	Somewhat like me	2
Somewhat unlike me	4	Very much like me	1
Neither like me nor unlike me	3		

5. I'm good at keeping promises, especially to myself.

Very unlike me	1	Somewhat like me	4
Somewhat unlike me	2	Very much like me	5
Neither like me nor unlike me	3		

6. I don't impose much structure on my activities.

Very unlike me	5	Somewhat like me	2
Somewhat unlike me	4	Very much like me	1
Neither like me nor unlike me	3		

7. I have a very hard-driving, aggressive personality.

Very unlike me	1	Somewhat like me	4
Somewhat unlike me	2	Very much like me	5
Neither like me nor unlike me	3		

Scoring

Add you answers to get the total. The lower your score, the more likely you are to quickly lose motivation and drop out of an exercise program. If your score is 24 or lower, you'd better get a motivation fix—fast.

and director of the university's weight-loss clinic.

"I think the critical role for exercise is in weight maintenance," Dr. Miller says. "Almost anything can help you lose weight, even a quack diet. People who continue exercising are the ones who maintain their weight loss."

HIGH-INTENSITY WORKOUTS

By far, the best exercise for burning fat, experts say, is aerobic exercise. *Aerobic* means with oxygen, and aerobic activities are those that raise your heart and breathing rates for an extended time.

"All exercise is good, but you need to elevate your pulse to 50 to 75 percent above its resting rate to burn fat effectively. Aerobic exercise does this," says Art Mollen, D.O., director of the Southwest Health Institute in Phoenix and author of *The Mollen Method*.

In addition to burning more fat, strenuous aerobic exercise keeps weight off by boosting metabolism—upping your rpm, as it were. When your motor idles faster, you burn more fuel, even when you're not driving.

To begin losing weight with exercise, here's what experts recommend.

Do it till you're breathing hard. As we've seen, aerobics is a total-body fat burner that supercharges your metabolism and ignites calories faster than normal for up to 2 hours after exercising.

Some of the best aerobic activities are running, swimming, and cycling. These and other aerobic workouts are most effective when done for a minimum of 30 minutes, three times a week.

Make a long-term investment. Unless your goal is to lose weight once and then never eat again—a strategy that weight-loss experts don't recommend—fighting fat is an enduring commitment.

In order to succeed, you have to view exercise realistically and plan your regimen accordingly. If you hate the loneliness of running, for example, don't jog. Join an aerobic dance class instead, or take up squash or tennis with a friend.

Score with realistic goals. Losing weight takes time, and keeping it off takes a lifetime. Trying to do it all at once will only make you frustrated and fat. Instead, define a big goal, then achieve it by reaching smaller ones.

If in the big picture you want to lose 50 pounds, shoot first for more modest goals, like losing a pound or two a week. Every day, take it a little bit further and don't backslide. You'll lose weight a lot more efficiently—and ultimately, faster—than by jumping on a crash plan that's sure to fail.

Hang in for 3. You wouldn't expect to get that big promotion overnight, would you? So why expect more when it comes to losing weight? "I find that the break-off point for exercise for most people is about 3 months," Dr. Miller says. "If you can hang in there past the third month, you've probably established some behavior that might carry on, so give yourself at least 3 months."

Targeted Weight Loss: Why It Fails

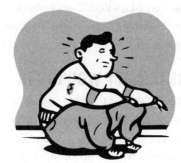

Situps drive a lot of men crazy. They're hard to do in the beginning and they don't get a whole lot easier later on. And the results aren't always evident. Men who embark on situp routines to trim their midsections are invariably disappointed. The reason is simple: This type of approach is called spot-reducing, and it doesn't work.

"In reality, there's no such thing as spot-reducing," says Art Mollen, D.O., director of the Southwest Health Institute in Phoenix and author of *The Mollen Method*. "You can do 300 situps a day, and they won't give you a washboard stomach. You'll probably have a stronger stomach, but it won't necessarily look it."

HITTING THE TROUBLE SPOTS

Spot reduction sounds good in theory: You work extra hard on specific body parts to cut fat in those areas. For example, a guy might try squats to reduce his caboose or labor over leg lifts to lighten heavy thighs. While it's possible to build muscle at these and other target sites, fat burning just isn't that precise.

In one study, for example, researchers measured the forearms of 20 tennis players who were on the courts at least 6 hours a week. They found that while the players' racket arms had better-developed muscles than the "inactive" arms, they didn't contain significantly smaller amounts of fat.

"Fat is a metabolic fuel that the body uses to produce energy," explains L. Jerome Brandon, Ph.D., associate professor of kinesiology in the department of kinesiology and health at Georgia State University in Atlanta. But the fuel tank, as it were, isn't located in one place. Instead, it consists of millions of individual fat cells spread throughout your body. So even when you're killing yourself with crunches, your body is drawing fuel from those myriad cells in more or less equal amounts. That's why spot-reducing doesn't work.

Yet most guys do want to banish belly fat—or at least firm up the bellies they already have. Abdominal exercises may not be a great way to lose weight, but when they're combined with an overall fat-fighting regimen, they will get your middle under control. Your abdominal muscles will be stronger and you'll stand straighter, says Wayne C. Miller, Ph.D., assistant professor of kinesiology at Indiana University in Bloomington and director of the university's weight-loss clinic. "In that vein, you'll

HOW MUCH EXERCISE?

If you're like most men, you've occasionally cast a covetous eye on some forbiddingly rich, triple-decker dessert and asked yourself, How far would I have to run to work off that one piece of cake?

Wonder no more. Thanks to Bob Abelson, Ph.D., of Redondo Beach, California, a health and fitness instructor certified by the American College of Sports Medicine, you can now see for yourself exactly how much exercise you'll need to burn off the calories in 16 common foods and drinks.

The chart is based on a 150-pound person. Actual calories burned may vary depending on your weight.

Food	Exercise (min)			
	Running (7.5 mph)	Aerobic Dance	Walking (3 mph)	Cycling (9 mph)
Breakfast				
Bacon (2 strips)	6	13	22	13
Egg muffin sandwich	22	44	77	46
Oatmeal (⅔ cup)	7	13	23	14
Lunch				
Cheeseburger (¼ lb)	39	78	136	82
Cheese pizza (5-oz slice)	11	22	38	46
Hot dog on roll	22	44	77	23
Dinner				
Beefsteak (3 oz)	25	50	87	73
Beef burrito	35	71	123	52
Macaroni and cheese (1 cup)	33	65	113	68
Snacks				
Chocolate cake (2-oz slice)	19	38	66	39
Doughnut (filled, 2.5 oz)	21	41	71	43
Potato chips (1 oz)	11	23	39	24
Pretzels (1 oz)	8	17	29	17
Beverages				
Beer (12 oz)	11	23	39	24
Martini (dry, 2.5 oz)	11	21	37	22
Soda (12 oz)	11	22	38	23

look fitter, like you've lost maybe 5 to 10 pounds," he says.

Here are a couple of moves to firm up your midsection.

Work out at crunch time. Stomach crunches and situps, where you lie on your back, knees bent, and curl your upper torso until your shoulders leave the floor, are great for toughening your midriff and building a strong muscle base. "If you work on the abdominal muscles enough, you can reduce some of the hanging and sagging," Dr. Brandon says. "Your stomach doesn't have to hang out. You can firm it up."

Try doing 3 sets of 10 to 15 crunches per set. To give your muscles time to recover, be sure to allow a day of rest between workouts.

Again, crunches won't strip away fat. But when you finally do get serious about overall fitness training and dieting, you'll have a rippling set of abs just waiting to be revealed.

Get the bends. Doing sidebends is another great way to firm up your abs. Start by holding a lightweight dumbbell, say 20 pounds, in each hand. Then, slowly bend sideways at the waist, first to the left, then to the right. Do 3 sets of 10. As your muscles strengthen, gradually increase the weight and the repetitions. To maximize toning (as opposed to adding muscle bulk), it's best to stick with light-to-medium weights and to go for the maximum repetitions within the suggested 10.

The Role of Sweat

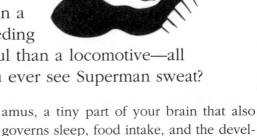

Superman could leap tall buildings in a single bound, fly faster than a speeding bullet, and flex muscles more powerful than a locomotive—all with no sweat. We're serious. Did you ever see Superman sweat?

Unlike the Man of Steel (or at least the actors who've portrayed him), you don't have someone standing by with a terry towel to blot you dry between scenes. Whether you're participating in a fast-track aerobics class or walking up five flights of stairs, you've probably been getting a little damp around the collar—as well as under your arms, on your chest, and between your shoulder blades.

But don't let sweat dampen your mood. Although perspiration may necessitate having a few extra shirts on hand, it's your body's built-in radiator. Sweating keeps you cool when things get hot.

"Plus, the nice thing about sweat is that you know you've worked out hard," adds Michael N. Sawka, Ph.D., chief of the thermal physiology and medicine division of the U.S. Army Research Institute of Environmental Medicine in Natick, Massachusetts.

THE MECHANICS OF MOISTURE

Sweat is more than just a little surplus moisture. It's controlled by the hypothal-amus, a tiny part of your brain that also governs sleep, food intake, and the development of secondary sex characteristics such as chest hair.

Although some parts of your anatomy get wetter than others, just about every square centimeter of skin—a centimeter is an area about the width of a paper clip—contains an average of 100 sweat glands. Guys with more sweat glands will get wetter than those with fewer. Clearly, nature intended you to sweat.

The sweat itself comes from two types of glands. The apocrine sweat glands, which are the largest, are concentrated in your armpits and groin. The second type of sweat glands are the eccrine glands. These cover your entire body except for your lips, your nipples, and portions of your genitals. Numbering about 3 million, they produce up to a quart of sweat a day. This fluid is thinner than apocrine sweat and is mainly water, with small amounts of salt, potassium, urea, and lactate. Its major role is to assist in ther-

SWEATY SITUATIONS

Men are most likely to sweat when it comes to affairs of the heart. The makers of Dial deodorant say that according to their "Big Sweat" telephone poll of 1,000 American adults, emotional factors are the ones most likely to turn our pits into leaky pipes. Here are the top five sweat producers and the percentage of guys who were affected.

1. Public speaking	45%
2. Getting divorced	45%
3. Getting married	44%
4. Interviewing for a job	44%
5. Going on a first date	34%

moregulation—to prevent your body from overheating.

KEEPING COOL

When you're active, capillaries close to your skin dilate. As bloodflow increases, your skin temperature rises. Though your body can dissipate some of this heat through convection and radiation, there's still a tendency to overheat. Sweat picks up the slack, particularly when you are exercising and need to blow off heat in a hurry.

When you sweat, the fluid evaporates from your skin's surface, carrying away excess body heat. But sometimes, even heavy sweating won't keep you cool. "As you exercise, about 80 percent of your energy goes into heat," Dr. Sawka explains. In extremely hot situations—for example, running a marathon on a muggy day in July—your body may not be able to dissipate the heat effectively. If you don't give yourself a cool-off period, this can lead to

heat exhaustion or even heatstroke, which can kill you.

FLUID FACTS

Despite what the $750 million antiperspirant and deodorant lobby tells you, sweat is good. But if you find yourself exuding large amounts of moist machismo, there are a few things you should know.

Don't be fooled by fluids. A lot of men, equating sweat with melted fat, thrill to the sight of perspiration dripping from their tired brows.

But you may as well grab a towel. "When you sweat, you lose water weight," explains L. Jerome Brandon, Ph.D., associate professor of kinesiology in the department of kinesiology and health at Georgia State University in Atlanta. In other words, although you may lose as much as 5 pounds during a workout, you'll gain it all back as soon as you take a few drinks of water.

Don't suit up to sweat out. Although

wearing a plastic exercise suit will make you sweat more, it will have no effect on your long-term weight. "People who exercise in these sweat suits are foolish," says Dr. Sawka. "The suits put you at risk for heat exhaustion or heatstroke—they're the worst thing you can wear."

Keep the tank filled. To prevent your body from overheating, it's critical to replace the fluids you lose during exercise. If you've sweated out 2 pounds in water weight after a workout, for example, you should replace it with its fluid equivalent—about 32 ounces of water, Dr. Sawka advises. Weighing yourself before and after exercising will tell you how much fluid you need to take in.

Don't bother with commercial sports drinks, he adds. Unless you're into some serious training, like long-distance running, high-impact aerobics, or hours of cross-country skiing, plain cold water is all you need.

Watch for warning signs. During times of heavy exertion, it's critical to watch out for heat exhaustion or heatstroke—potentially dangerous conditions that can cause symptoms ranging from headache and dizziness to a weak, rapid heartbeat.

While heat exhaustion can be relieved by resting, cooling off, and drinking fluids, heatstroke is a medical emergency. The two conditions can be similar, but with heatstroke, you get extremely hot, plus you stop sweating. If this happens, get out of the heat and call the pros immediately. While awaiting treatment, lower your temperature with alcohol rubs or ice packs or by immersing yourself in cold water.

Don't do as the Romans did. Roman rulers thought that salt was vital for health, so they paid their soldiers partially in salt. (It's from this ancient practice that we get the word *salary* and the phrase "worth his salt.") Today, the dangers of getting too much salt—the risk of developing high blood pressure, for example—are well-known. This goes for increasing salt intake during exercise as well. "There's enough salt in the American diet as is," Dr. Sawka says. "People do not need to supplement."

Story Musgrave, M.D., Former Astronaut

Story Musgrave has cycled around the globe at 5 miles a second. His idea of power walking is striding several thousand miles above Earth while carrying more than 400 pounds of space suit on his back. A physician, an exercise physiologist and, for 30 years, an astronaut, Dr. Musgrave flew five missions and logged more than 850 hours in space.

This starship trooper helped design the Skylab space station and flew on four space shuttles, including the ill-fated *Challenger,* which he rode during its maiden voyage. More recently, Dr. Musgrave thrilled Earth-bound viewers with his orbital acrobatics during the televised repair of the Hubble Space Telescope. On that jaunt, Dr. Musgrave went extravehicular—outside the ship—three times, successfully recalibrating the telescope so that it could scan deep space.

"Let me tell you, weightless though you are in space, that 480-pound suit still has plenty of inertia. You've got to be in some kind of shape to deal with it," he says.

Although he's no longer an astronaut, Dr. Musgrave, who's in his sixties, still tries to keep his weight to 152 pounds. His strategy is a combination of low-fat eating and a variety of aerobic exercise.

"When I work out, I try to mix it up a lot," says Dr. Musgrave. "I do 25 minutes on the stair machine, 20 minutes on the rowing machine, 30 minutes of high-grade fast walking on the treadmill. Then, I throw in circuit training." Outside, Dr. Musgrave runs 3 to 4 miles a day. "To get more of a workout, I run on grass at the golf course near my home. And I run on my toes. It's less efficient in terms of speed, but it's a great toner."

Dr. Musgrave's regimen emphasizes cardiovascular benefits, and with good reason. "Good cardiovascular fitness was the one thing that allowed me to keep going up in space and to work long hours at mission control, decade after decade. It really helped me keep up endurance. And as an astronaut, in the shuttle or at mission control, you don't need to have a lot of muscle, but you've got to have the stamina. When I was on the ground, communicating with a crew in orbit, I pulled 16-hour days and longer. I needed to be in good shape in order to stay sharp and alert."

In those high-stress situations, Dr. Musgrave admits, he gave in to some down-to-earth weaknesses. "Long about midnight, I'd break down and just eat whatever junk food I could find. Anything with sugar—doughnuts and cinnamon rolls especially. I figured that if I behaved the rest of the time, I was allowed to have some junk when I really wanted it."

But in general, Dr. Musgrave says, he still adheres to simple dietary rules. "I watch my fat intake. I watch the salt. I try to eat plenty of grains—the carbohydrates in them really keep you going for the long haul."

David Bradley, Author

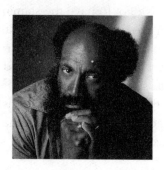

David Bradley's life is jammed. The acclaimed author sometimes works on more than one book at a time while he freelances for newspapers and magazines, lectures at various colleges and writers' organizations around the country, and even works on a movie deal.

He splits his time between two homes: one in Philadelphia, another in La Jolla, California. He spends many nights in hotels and is often on the road or in the air.

But he manages to find time to run—for at least an hour on most days. And he lifts weights a couple of days a week. For Bradley, skipping workouts because he's too busy is not an option. Now in his mid-forties, Bradley has been running for more than 25 years.

"The only serious time I have been down is when I was injured," says the author of *South Street* and *The Chaneysville Incident*, which won the 1982 PEN/Faulkner Award. In 1980, Bradley blew out a knee after competing in numerous marathons. The injury did take away some of his competitiveness. But it didn't stop him from running.

"The idea that I might not ever run again is just not there. Even when I have been sick and not able to run for a couple

of weeks, there's always the question of how soon I can get back to it. I think that's just something that comes with a lot of years of doing it and realizing that it's part of my life," says Bradley.

THE BIG DECISION

Hard as it is to imagine, Bradley's life is actually less hectic than it once was. In the mid-1970s he worked as an editor at J. B. Lippincott in New York City, spending about 70 hours a week at the office. He was under tremendous stress, but he managed to go to a track over by the East River and run 3 days a week. Sometimes, if he was lucky, he could fit it in after work. But he couldn't run too late in the evening. "In New York, you don't want to be going over there at 7:00 or 8:00 at night," Bradley says.

Time flew by, and so did the miles. Looking back, he can't figure out exactly how he fit it all in. But eventually, the frenzied pace caught up with him. His running had become stressful. He felt pressured to run faster so that he could get other things done.

Faced with a choice between running and work, Bradley decided to quit his job.

"I had been editing a book on running (*The Joy of Running*). The author (Thaddeus Kostrubala) was writing about running marathons. I decided that I wanted to do that. Something had to go. So the job gave," says Bradley.

CREATIVE RUNNING

Though his new life of freelance writing and lecturing allows Bradley to pretty much set his own schedule, it doesn't give him tons of free time. Just traveling to various speaking engagements involves sitting in airports, on airplanes, and in cars—all time that could be spent running. And writing novels isn't exactly a speedy process.

So it's a good thing that Bradley can work while he runs.

"What I do for a living, of course, has a lot to do with thinking. You can think anywhere. You don't have to be doing anything with your hands while you are thinking. In fact, I think it is more beneficial to be away from the word processor while you are trying to work through various problems. As those things come up in your mind, you work through them without having to commit to the paper or the word processor," says Bradley.

Often, Bradley sits at his keyboard and types. Then, silence. Maybe it's a character who needs to say something but has con-tracted verbal amnesia. Or a plot that has run out of options. Or maybe it's a speech that needs a third main point. The silence all means the same thing: It's time to run.

It takes about 20 to 30 minutes before the answers start coming, before the characters start talking, the plots start turning around, and the outlines start changing.

"In your mind, you have an outline somewhere. You get committed to that. You are sitting there trying desperately to work it out," Bradley says. "Then, you get away from it. You go out and run for 15 to 20 minutes, and suddenly it hits you that you don't have to do it that way at all. Things that you have not thought of, things that are hard to think of while you are in the middle of something, come to you."

Bradley is not sure why the running technique works. Maybe it's because it makes him so relaxed. Or maybe it's the endorphin rush. Or maybe it's the fact that when he's on the run, no idea is a bad idea.

"It's just the inability to act on something. In society, we tend to act on our ideas immediately. We're under a lot of pressure to do that. And running is a context where you can't act immediately. You are 5 miles out. Before you can do anything, you have to come 5 miles back. It just forces you to go through things or to rehearse things," Bradley says.

The same thing can't be said for weight lifting. Bradley doesn't think up characters, plots, or outlines while he pumps iron. But working out with weights has helped him save time on the job. "The weights are good for meetings. If I know that it is going to be a tense or difficult situation, I will work out ahead of time. That way, I blow off a lot of the tension that I anticipate," he says.

After lifting weights, Bradley can walk into a meeting feeling calm, prepared to present his side in a nonthreatening manner. And all concerned can discuss options and come to a consensus rather than increasing the tension to such a level that everyone begins hurling invective.

"People ask me if I work out because I want to live forever. I tell them that I work out because I want *them* to live forever," Bradley says.

MAKING TIME

Even though both aspects of his exercise routine help him do his job, Bradley still struggles to fit them in. When on the road, he sometimes splits weight lifting into multiple workouts. For instance, during a spare 15 minutes, he'll do pushups. During another break, he'll do crunches.

Over the years, Bradley has gotten pretty creative at turning a hotel room into a miniature gym. He uses chairs to do decline pushups. And he uses chairs and other furniture as his weights.

"It's kind of hard to come up with something that is the equivalent of a 220-pound bench press. But it can be done. I do military presses with chairs. I hold the chair over my head. If a maid happens to come in at that moment, things can get a little weird," Bradley says with a laugh.

But Bradley can't break up his running routine. If he doesn't have enough time to run, he walks instead.

"It doesn't do me any good to run for less than an hour. It just doesn't. It isn't worth it," Bradley says. "I'm trained to run a distance of 10 to 12 miles. Three miles just gets me going. It's not really a lot of fun for me to run under pressure. I like to do it away from pressure. So when I'm really pressured and I don't have the time to do it right, I'll put running off. But there's a limit. Sooner or later, I'll say, 'Sorry guys, I gotta go.'"

Part 5

HOW TO BURN CALORIES EVERY DAY

Walking

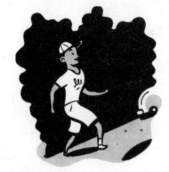

One reason that more men don't exercise regularly is the perception that it's a sweaty, muscle-burning business.

It can be, but it doesn't have to be. Research shows that *any* type of movement can burn substantial numbers of calories.

Your idea of exercise is going for a long walk? Keep doing it. It's a very effective way to lose weight.

Steven M. Newman is a case in point. A former newspaperman from Ripley, Ohio, he set out in 1983 on a journey that spanned 20 countries and 5 continents. Newman, now in his forties, walked around the world alone, setting a Guinness record and logging more than 22,000 foot-punishing miles.

But roaming did more than just secure the itinerant's name in history. Newman has discovered what many experts have been preaching: Walking is an easy, inexpensive, and enjoyable way to trim your midsection.

A SMALL STEP FOR MAN, A BIG STEP FOR FITNESS

"We used to believe that you had to walk briskly before you would gain any health benefits," says John Duncan, Ph.D., professor of clinical research at Texas Woman's University in Denton. "But we now know that metabolic changes occur at very moderate exercise intensities and that

those metabolic changes confer health benefits."

Bob Abelson, Ph.D., a health and fitness instructor in Redondo Beach, California, who's certified by the American College of Sports Medicine, can vouch for that. A geophysicist who started out at a staggering 400 pounds, Abelson devoted his life to walking after it helped him lose more than 200 pounds, most of which he has kept off since 1983. Like Newman, he's a true believer. "You'll have better endurance, sleep better at night, and you'll probably perform better in bed and have better overall personal health," he says.

ON THE RIGHT PATH

Once you decide that it's time to put on your walking shoes, you'll want to make the most of your first—and future—steps. Here's what experts recommend.

Pick proper tools. Shoes can be your best friends or your worst enemies. An ill-fitting pair of shoes can spell blister city, while good sneakers or walking shoes can make you feel like you're striding on air. All-purpose athletic shoes will do in a pinch, but you'd be better off considering a good walking shoe, says Dr. Duncan. They have firmer heels that are beveled to help keep your feet stable. They also have good arches for support and sturdy lacing to keep your feet from sliding forward and back.

Ban the rays. Unless you're doing all your walking at night, you're going to want sun protection. Wearing a cap and shades and sunscreen will help keep your skin from looking like a football when you're 70. If you avoid the sun altogether by walking at night, wear reflective clothing and carry a flashlight, suggests Dr. Abelson.

Time your trek. Walking is fun, sure, but you'll want to know that it's working. To stay motivated, experts say, try keeping track of your progress. Many beginners start out walking a mile or two at a time and then work up from there. When one day you discover that you've gone 5 miles without struggle, congratulate yourself—and set your sights on the next goal. An easier strategy is just to wear a watch. For example, start walking for 20 minutes at a time. When that gets easy, gradually increase your workouts by 15-minute increments. Whenever the distance (or time) you're walking gets easy, bump to the next level, says Dr. Duncan.

And remember, the total number of miles walked is more important for fat burning than the distance walked during any one stretch, Dr. Abelson adds. Don't let the goal to walk farther each time overshadow the goal to walk regularly.

Set a schedule. If you always walk on the same days and at the same times—say, Monday, Wednesday, and Friday from 6:00 P.M. to 6:45 P.M. and Saturday from 8:00 A.M. to 9:00 A.M.—you'll be less likely to think of it as an expendable activity, says Dr. Duncan. Otherwise, you may find yourself canceling walks due to more pressing concerns—like watching *Star Trek* reruns.

TRACK FACTS

Here are some facts and findings to ponder the next time you're on the road.

- There must be something about walking that gets the brain stirred up. Great thinkers who loved to walk included Hippocrates, Aristotle, Bertrand Russell, Harry Truman, Charles Dickens, and Walt Whitman.
- If you can't walk fast, walking longer has the same effect. If you weigh 150 pounds, for example, and cover 1 mile at 4 miles per hour, you'll burn about 110 calories. You can burn the same amount by walking 1.1 miles at 3 miles per hour.
- If you walked 45 minutes a day, four times a week for 1 year, you'd burn about 18 pounds. And that doesn't include weight you'd also lose through sensible eating.

Take your time. Although some guys do everything at a competitive pace, when it comes to walking, slow and steady is what burns pounds.

In one study, researchers asked three groups of people to walk 3 miles a day, 5 days a week. Those in one group walked at a heart-pumping 12-minute-per-mile pace. Those in the second group walked a 15-minute mile, while those in the third group ambled along at 20 minutes per mile.

"We were as surprised as anyone to find that it was the slowest group that lost the most body fat," says Dr. Duncan. "And they lost the most despite the fact that the 12-minute-per-mile walkers burned 53 percent more calories."

Save it for lunch. Studies have shown that brief bouts of exercise can help give your appetite a time-out. So rather than filling up on bratwurst during your lunch break, first take a 15-minute walk. When you come back, you'll feel more energized but probably less hungry than when you started, says Dr. Duncan.

Get an earful. A lot of walkers say that wearing a Walkman makes the time pass pleasantly. You can groove to your favorite tunes or catch up on the latest books on tape. Or just enjoy the silence. "Walking is a great time to work out a lot of your mental chores," Newman says. If you do play tunes, just be sure to keep the volume low, so you can hear traffic or passing cyclists coming from behind.

Take a hike. Who says that walking has to be on flat ground? If you want a bigger challenge, turn your walking into hiking by heading for the nearest hills. "I guarantee that you'll lose pounds real fast," Newman says.

Expand your horizons. "Take the time to stop while you're walking to talk to other people," Newman says. "If you take an interest in the people around, you won't be like the runners and joggers who pass right on by."

To get the maximum cardiovascular benefit, Dr. Duncan suggests that you walk with people at a slow enough pace to carry on a conversation. This way, you don't have to stop to socialize.

At Home and in the Yard

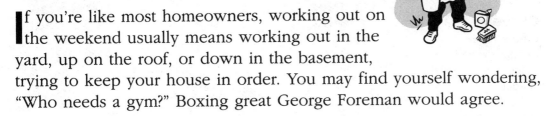

If you're like most homeowners, working out on the weekend usually means working out in the yard, up on the roof, or down in the basement, trying to keep your house in order. You may find yourself wondering, "Who needs a gym?" Boxing great George Foreman would agree.

In 1994, when Foreman regained his heavyweight title after 20 years, the middle-age boxer made yard work an integral part of his comeback workout. To help hone his legendary punching power, Foreman spent hours at his Texas ranch working with a pick and shovel.

"I'd measure out 5 feet square and I'd dig. I'd keep digging until I got that hole maybe 4 feet, then I'd cover it up and go on to another. Then, I'd get a wheelbarrow and push rocks back and forth," Foreman says.

After that, Foreman went to the woodshed, where he'd chop logs with a hatchet. "When people would say I was out there working on the ranch, I was really training," he says.

Who's going to argue with the champ? Doing chores makes for a strenuous workout—hauling firewood into the mudroom, raking a square mile of leaves, yanking the lawn mower to life. Who needs weights?

FIT FOR LIFE

Actually, not even George Foreman relies exclusively on yard work for power in the ring—it's just an addition to a more formal workout. And that formal workout is what gives him the strength to spend all those hours digging and refilling ditches.

"This is one of the reasons why men should be on a regular fitness program—not just to look good and be in shape for their favorite sports but also to be in shape when it comes time to do some real physical work," says John Amberge, a certified strength and conditioning specialist and director of corporate programs for the Sports Training Institute in New York City.

Here are a few exercises designed to help you avoid some of the most common domestic pitfalls.

Twist for side strength. Amberge says that reverse trunk twists are great for your oblique abdominals—those muscles you use for push-and-pull activities such as raking leaves or wrestling with the lawn mower.

SCORING YOUR CHORES

Don't worry about missing formal workouts because you spent the whole week doing odd jobs around the house. You may well have burned more calories doing chores than engaging in your favorite weekend activity. Check out the chart below and see for yourself.

All numbers below are based on calories burned per hour for a 180-pound male.

Chore	Calories Burned	Activity	Calories Burned
Carpentry	270	Sex	240
Chopping wood	414	Golf	411
Digging (with shovel)	701	Cross-country skiing	666
Gardening (digging, hoeing)	576	Tennis (singles)	522
Mowing lawn	486	Brisk walking (3.5 mph)	432
Painting	378	Bicycling (15 mph)	600
Trimming hedges	378	Inline skating	550
Washing car	270	Volleyball	396

To do them, lie on your back on the floor, with your arms straight out to the sides and your palms down. Bend your knees, placing your feet flat on the floor. Now, with legs and feet together, slowly lower your knees to the left until your left thigh touches the floor. Hold for a moment, then raise your legs back to the starting position and switch sides. Do 15 to 20.

Row to mow. Mowing is another great outdoor exercise that burns plenty of calories—assuming that you're using a push mower, of course. But to take advantage of the benefits, you'll need to do more than twists. Spend some time training your upper-back muscles, too, using one-arm dumbbell rows, says Chip Harrison, strength and conditioning coach at Pennsylvania State Uni-versity in University Park. You'll know that you're working those muscles when you can pull-start your mower in one yank. This exercise also helps when it comes time to rev up the chain saw in the fall.

Stand with a dumbbell in one hand, and bend at the waist. Place the knee and the hand opposite the one with the dumbbell on a bench or chair for support, keeping your back parallel to the floor. Your other knee should be straight but not locked. The arm with the dumbbell should hang freely. Raise the dumbbell until it touches the side of your chest. Hold for one count, then lower. Do 8 to 12 repetitions, then repeat with the other arm.

Work on your pick-up muscles. For the muscles in your middle back and shoulders—so handy when you're rearranging your crates of stuff in the garage—try upright rows with a barbell or dumbbells, says Amberge.

Stand upright, holding a barbell in both hands with your palms down in a narrow grip. Your arms should be fully extended in front of you, the barbell at your upper thighs. Allow your shoulders to relax slightly, but keep your back straight. Pull the barbell straight up and tuck it under your chin. Your elbows should be pointing up and out. Hold briefly, then lower the weight.

Flex your hips. When you're hauling junk around, your abdominal and hip flexor muscles carry their share of the load as well. You can exercise them with flat-bench leg lifts.

Sit on the end of a flat exercise bench and grab the sides for support. Put your back flat against the seat of the bench, but raise your neck and shoulders slightly. Extend your legs parallel to the floor, slightly bend your knees, and raise your legs until they form a right angle to your body. Hold for a moment, then slowly lower them until they're at a 45-degree angle, halfway to the bench. Do 2 sets of 10 to 12 lifts.

Dig your work. George Foreman can tell you: If you want strength, digging can give it to you, in spades. But ounce for ounce, digging is also one of the most exhausting—and potentially injuring—chores you can do. "Besides the strain that shoveling can have on the heart, it can also injure the back if you don't do it correctly," says Scott Donkin, D.C., a chiropractor in Lincoln, Nebraska, and author of *Sitting on the Job.*

When you take spade in hand, put your dominant hand as far up on the handle as possible. Your other hand should be about 18 inches down from the top of the handle. Push with your legs and arms, not your back or shoulders. Once you have your load of dirt, hold your head up and be sure to pivot your feet when you turn to deposit it—don't twist your back or your knees.

Golf

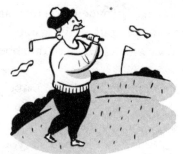

It has a reputation for being a lazy man's sport, but golf is great exercise. You'll walk about 2 miles playing the average 9-hole course. An 18-holer will take you 4 miles. Walking 1 mile at a normal pace, assuming you weigh 170 pounds, will burn roughly 365 calories.

Moreover, the game can be a heck of a lot of fun. "Golf is an excellent activity to promote health," says John Duncan, Ph.D., professor of clinical research at Texas Woman's University in Denton. "Call it a pleasurable pursuit where you get exercise by accident."

One study found that golfers who played three times a week showed dramatic improvements in their cholesterol levels. The game is also good for business health. In a survey of top executives, 80 percent considered golf an excellent way to make contacts. Gaining clout while losing weight and improving cardiovascular health—what could be better?

EXERCISE ON THE LINKS

The National Golf Foundation estimates that as many as 1 in 10 Americans plays golf, and upward of 2 million take their first swings every year. To get the best workout when you're on the greens, here are some tips you may want to try.

Can the cart. Some clubs put a lot of pressure on players to use the carts. "Golf-cart rentals make money for golf courses," explains Edward Palank, M.D., spokesman for the Professional Golf Association (PGA). Don't give in. Your goal is to get some fresh air and exercise. "Insist on your right to walk," he says.

Pass on the caddy. To maximize the physical burn—and save a couple of bucks in the bargain—always carry your own clubs. "The benefit to carrying your own clubs is that you'll expend more energy and burn more calories," says Dr. Palank.

Be a night owl. If getting in to play during peak weekend hours is a challenge, try going at night. Many courses are well-lit and open until late. Also, many unlit public courses offer discounted twilight rates: all the golf you can get in from 4:00 P.M. to sunset for a fraction of the full-course rate. So break out of work early and do a fast-paced nine holes.

HONING YOUR GAME

Perhaps more than any other sport, golf requires talent—not to dazzle colleagues, necessarily, but simply to progress to the next hole. It's hard to keep your weight-loss plan under par when you're wrapping an iron around the nearest tree. Here's what experts advise to take the kinks out of the links.

Start with a stretch. You might think that a round of golf is about as stressful as raising a Tom Collins, but lack of flexibility is a leading cause of back injury on the PGA Tour, says Lewis A. Yocum, M.D., assistant medical director of the PGA Tour and PGA Senior Tour.

To prevent injuries, get in the habit of loosening up and stretching before you hit the first tee, says Ralph Simpson, physical therapist with the PGA Tour. He recommends stretching your upper body for several minutes, including your arms, shoulders, chest, neck, and back. Finish up by stretching your calves and hamstrings and the rest of your lower body. Improving flexibility may not improve your swing, but it'll keep you from throwing something out of whack on the 18th hole.

Perk up with putt-putt. Statistics show that 47 percent of your score in an average golf game comes from putts and half-swings. This means that you should spend at least half of your time practicing these shots instead of just whacking away at the driving range. Many public courses have putting greens and chipping areas, so you can practice your short game for a modest fee. An hour of quiet practice is good for your soul and your game.

Choose a lower number. When choosing which club to hit with, be realistic and choose one size lower than what you think you'll need. (The lower the number of the club, the farther it hits.)

"Nine times out of 10, people wind up hitting the ball short," says Brad Faxon, the eighth-ranked money winner on the 1992 PGA tour. Choosing a club that hits slightly longer than you think you'll need will help keep your swing smooth.

Work on your posture. Many golfers bend over too far or stand too straight when swinging. The posture that most pros teach is a comfortable, athletic one with knees slightly bent, feet comfortably apart, and arms hanging freely from the shoulders. Your weight should be on the balls of your feet. Your backswing should be a slow coiling motion, followed by a forward release of energy carried through the ball with full follow-through.

Dancing

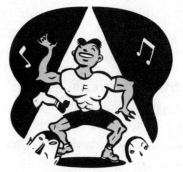

Fred Astaire, you'll never be—and John Travolta, you never want to be (at least not in his white-suited *Saturday Night Fever* incarnation).

Yet between those two poles of the male dancing pantheon is an enviable position: that of the good dancer.

And truth to tell, you wouldn't mind being there—a light-on-his-feet kind of guy, well-known for his ability to cut a rug.

Instead, it's more likely that you'll cut out in the middle of an evening of dancing, suffering as much from exhaustion as from embarrassment. Meanwhile, your dance partner spins on like a whirling dervish, oblivious to your near cardiac arrest, your aching feet, and your bruised ego.

A TOUGH EXERCISE WITH MUSIC

Professional dancers have incredible physiques, and even occasional dancing can build just about every muscle in your body and help you lose weight.

"There's a lot of movement. You're using muscles that are different from the ones you normally use," says Dan Downing, a power lifter and accomplished ballroom dancer in Allentown, Pennsylvania. "I've been doing both for years and I love them. It's a strange combination, but they go well together." Lifting may tighten muscles, Downing says, but dancing helps keep those muscles supple and limber.

"Dancing is very demanding. It can be as energetic an exercise as sprinting," adds Dennis Rogers of Westfield, New Jersey, treasurer for the National Dance Council of America and a dance instructor for more than 40 years. While dancing itself is a great cardiovascular exercise, it doesn't hurt to do other aerobic exercises as well. If anything, they'll make you a better dancer. "You see a lot of dancers at the competitive level who will do aerobics and other exercises. They're training for dancing," says Rogers.

To improve your dance technique and your health, begin with these simple steps.

Sign up for classes. Men are often reluctant to join aerobic dance classes, but how about plain old dancing? In nearly every city, you'll find dozens of classes in ballroom and country line dancing. "Dance lessons are a great form of exercise—and it's something you can do with your partner, too," says Rogers.

Focus on your partner. One reason that men tend to be tense on the dance floor is because they're self-conscious. Put it out of your mind. For one thing, people aren't

PUT ON YOUR DANCING SHOES

If you're not wearing the right shoes, dancing can be pretty bad for your feet, to say nothing of your dancing form. And you can't wear just any old thing when you dance. "Some shoes feel good until you try dancing in them," says Dennis Rogers of Westfield, New Jersey, a dance instructor for more than 40 years. "People talk about wearing their dancing shoes—it's a good idea to have a pair."

Don't go out and ask your shoe salesman for a pair of dancing shoes, though—just pick a pair that has plenty of cushioning. "A hard-soled, stiff shoe is going to hurt and it limits your agility," says Rogers. For casual dancing, you'll be better off with a thick-soled walking shoe.

But what if it's a black-tie affair, and you have to wear the nicest-looking, least comfortable shoes you own? Or you're going out line dancing and those cowboy boots are painful just to look at?

In that case, pad them yourself with insoles, which you can find in any drugstore and most supermarkets. "Just a little padding adds a lot of comfort, and it will show when you dance," says Rogers.

watching as much as you think. They're more interested in improving their form than in worrying about yours. And you probably don't look anywhere near as clumsy as you think you do. So forget about everyone else and just pay attention to your partner, Rogers says.

"I can tell you as a dance instructor that the more you focus on yourself and your partner, the better a dancer you'll be. And the better you are, the less you'll care if other people are watching you," he says.

Stay loose. Whatever the dancing venue, wear loose clothing. If you're doing line dancing, wear relaxed-fit jeans. If you're at your brother's wedding, loosen your tie or cummerbund. "The more constricting the clothes, the less maneuverability you'll have. You'll get hot and wear out faster," says John Amberge, a certified strength and con-

ditioning specialist and director of corporate programs for the Sports Training Institute in New York City.

Drink a lot of water. Whether you're under the blaring lights, caught in the press of gyrating bodies, or gracefully gliding across the ballroom with your partner, it's only a matter of time before your body will start screaming for fluids. "If you don't drink water often, you'll eventually wear yourself out," says Rogers. "That's why at professional dance competitions they have water stations set up all around the dance floor." Take a break every 10 to 15 minutes and drink some water. Keep alcoholic beverages to a minimum; alcohol will make you more dehydrated.

Take up aerobics. If you want to be a hot shot at the dance club, go to the health club first. "Stairclimbers, rowing machines, treadmills, stationary bicycles, and cross-country ski machines are all excellent aerobic tools that improve your cardiovascular health," Amberge says. They tone your legs and other crucial dancing muscles.

Stretch. Professional dancers often stretch before competition, Rogers says. You probably should too—even if it's just a night of country swing dancing. If you haven't been dancing in a while and your legs and hips are feeling a little bit tight, spend about 15 minutes doing some basic total-body stretches, then concentrate on your lower body.

Not only will you dance better that night, you also won't feel so sore the next day. And when your partner suggests going out again the next night, you won't have to give her a song and dance about why you can't make it.

Jumping Jacks

Before the stairclimbing machine, before the NordicTrack, before the full-body aerobics workout, there was that cornerstone of calisthenics: the jumping jack. From gym class to football practice to boot camp, it has been a part of most guys' lives. It's a great exercise. It gets your pulse racing and, more important, gets you warmed up for other types of exercise.

Jumping jacks are primarily a cardiovascular calisthenic that benefits the heart and lungs far more than specific muscle groups.

"Jumping jacks get the system up and running, a warmup for a more strenuous workout," says Steven McCaw, Ph.D., associate professor of biomechanics at Illinois State University in Normal. "They are deceptively hard on the body." Swinging your arms and legs through a quick range of leaping motions can cause a lot of stress to joints, especially your shoulders and hips.

"If you use wrist or ankle weights, when you swing your arms or legs, the weights at the ends of your limbs generate a great deal of momentum and will become really heavy, which could cause an injury," cautions Chip Harrison, strength and conditioning coach at Pennsylvania State University in University Park. "You should just rely on the vigor of the exercise to warm you up. Jumping jacks are the kind of activity you want to do before you launch into heavy flexibility work or before you go out running."

A few sets of jumping jacks can be as pulse-raising as a quick stint in an aerobics class.

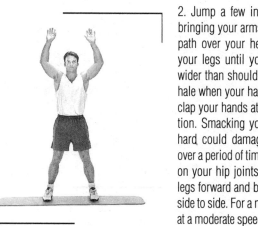

1. Start with your arms at your sides, your feet together, and your back straight. To work your calves a little more, stand up on your toes. Inhale before you jump.

2. Jump a few inches off the floor, bringing your arms in a wide circular path over your head and spreading your legs until your feet are a little wider than shoulder-width apart. Exhale when your hands are up. Lightly clap your hands at the top of the motion. Smacking your hands together hard could damage your shoulders over a period of time. To make it easier on your hip joints, try splitting your legs forward and backward instead of side to side. For a mild warmup, do 20 at a moderate speed.

Pullups

Just this once, think of yourself as one big dumbbell. Pullups are a simple exercise that strengthens your shoulders with minimal equipment. All you need is a sturdy chinning bar that lets you hang about 6 inches off the ground. Oh, and you need your body to supply the weight.

Chinning bars are standard equipment at gyms and playgrounds, or you can pick one up at a sporting goods store and mount it at home in a door frame or in the basement.

"Pullups will increase the strength in the shoulder muscles, the upper arms, and the upper-back muscles," says Bob Viau, a Baltimore physical therapist and trainer. "Your body weight determines how much you will progress." If you want more of a workout from your pullups, you can always add weight to your body. Wrap a chain around your waist and hang a weight from it. Or try ankle weights.

If you're new to pullups, try doing just two or three at first and see how you feel the next day. If your muscles are sore, take an extra day's rest before resuming. If you're having trouble completing a pullup, keep trying until you go all the way up and down. That full range of motion makes the exercise more effective, Viau says.

As with any other type of weight lifting, pullups should be done in a steady motion. "A lot of people feel that getting that last rep in and jerking themselves up is a benefit," Viau says. "It's not: You could sustain an injury."

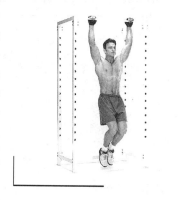

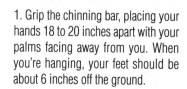

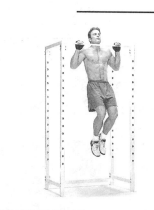

1. Grip the chinning bar, placing your hands 18 to 20 inches apart with your palms facing away from you. When you're hanging, your feet should be about 6 inches off the ground.

2. With a slow, steady motion, pull yourself up until your chin is higher than the bar. Then, lower yourself to the starting position. Exhale on your way up, and inhale on your way down. Don't let your body swing. Try to keep your back slightly arched backward.

Jumping Rope

If you want to burn fat, boost your cardiovascular capacity, tone muscle, and improve agility and rhythm, you could sink a thousand bucks into a fancy home gym. Or you could buy a jump rope.

A 165-pound man jumping rope can burn 14.2 calories in a minute, or 852 calories an hour. That's more calories burned than by jogging or cycling.

Ken M. Solis, M.D., author of the book *Ropics: The Next Jump Forward in Fitness*, offers these pointers.

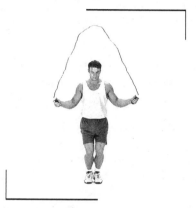

- Give yourself enough rope. When you stand in the middle, the ends of the handles should just reach your armpits.
- Land on the balls of your feet, not on your toes or heels. Then, roll back toward your heels and push off again. Jump only an inch or less off the ground. Wood, vinyl tile, or low-pile carpeting make the best jumping surfaces.
- Your wrists and forearms should do the turning,

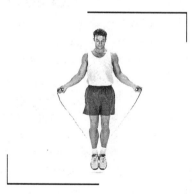

not your shoulders. Your arms should stay at your sides, with your elbows tucked in.

- Wear well-padded cross-trainer or aerobic shoes. Running shoes generally won't do.

Here's how to do basic rope jumping.

1. Start with a handle in each hand and the rope behind you, your feet together. Use your wrists to swing the rope up and over your head. Keep your hands at waist level and your elbows tucked in.

2. As the rope nears your feet, jump up an inch to let the rope pass underneath. Land on the balls of your feet. Aim for about 130 skips per minute—just over 2 skips a second.

Tom Peters, Management Expert and Author

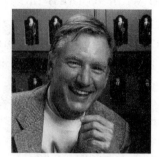

Another exhausting 5-day management seminar behind him, Tom Peters eased his 5-foot-11, 220-pound frame into a hotel chair and began reading comment cards from the participants—standard procedure after each event. Among them was a two-sentence note from the chief financial officer of a huge health-care organization.

"Tom is a walking heart attack," it said. "Will give him a free stress test anytime he wants one."

The message cut through the management expert like a pink slip on Friday at 5:00 P.M. Peters knew that he was overweight and that his face turned beet red when he got worked up during a seminar. Heck, he'd even spit sometimes while talking to high-powered executives. And worst of all, he never could quite find time to exercise.

The next morning, Peters got up and took a nice, long walk—and liked it. Two days later, he bought and read *Aerobic Walking* by Casey Meyers. "Life is weird. Why after X number of years of being a very irregular exerciser that particular line hit me, I have no idea. But with the exception

of taking a 30-day hiatus a couple of times, I haven't stopped walking since," he says.

TRADING FITNESS FOR SUCCESS

It's not as if Peters had been standing still. His first book, *In Search of Excellence*, has sold more than 5 million copies, and he also authored the bestsellers *A Passion for Excellence*, *Thriving on Chaos*, and *Liberation Management*. One of the nation's foremost authorities on business management, Peters wrote a syndicated newspaper column, penned forewords for more than 30 books, wrote articles for publications from *Business Week* and *The Economist* to the *Wall Street Journal* and *Harvard Business Review*, and founded the Tom Peters Group, three training and communications companies headquartered in Palo Alto, California.

But as we all know, busy doesn't mean fit. And when it came to physical activity, an occasional racquetball game was all the exercise this management expert could swing. And even then, it wasn't managed very well. "Nothing about it was planned—it was a function of when a buddy had some free time," he says.

Peters's extensive travel schedule didn't help. With 150 to 160 management seminars a year—and stops in such far-flung locales as Düsseldorf, Paris, and Bangkok—keeping in shape was that much more difficult. Peters doesn't like jogging ("God bless the people who do," he says); hotel gyms aren't for him either. The bottom line is that, aside from the considerable energy he expended during the seminar, he wouldn't do much of anything.

And, although he rarely found himself overeating at mealtime, minibars seemed to get the best of him—particularly on Monday nights. "Lord help me during Monday Night Football," says Peters. "It's hard to stay away from the cashews. If memory serves, cashews are about 1,000 calories a bite, and you get your first 1,000-calorie hit when you just take the top off the bottle."

ON THE RIGHT PATH

But speed walking—or dork walking, as one of Peters's friends likes to call it—was a perfect marriage of his busy schedule and his disdain for more formal exercise.

An early riser, Peters often decides when to walk based on the "terror quotient" of the city he's visiting. "I don't like walking in some cities when it's pitch-dark and the middle of December," he says. "So I usually wait until dawn, or sometime between. It's a great way to start the day when I'm going to be in an intense seminar. I discovered that if I didn't do it at the crack of dawn, the statistical odds of me doing it went way down."

When he's at home—be it in Palo Alto or at his 1,300-acre working farm in Tinmouth, Vermont—Peters prefers an afternoon jaunt. "It probably doesn't happen more than 20 percent of the time, but I'll work until 1:00 P.M. and then take an hour walk to decompress," he says.

Just how long Peters walks also varies. Staying in cities like Cincinnati or Chicago only seems to allow 25-minute treks; a walk at home could last 90 minutes. "If it's a rotten, snowy day in Chicago and the wind is roaring off the lake and the temperature is -7°F, I'll go out for 10 minutes, and 10 minutes is just fine. It's the act of doing it and the consistency that's important," he says. "There's a feeling of arrogant, egocentric self-satisfaction about having beaten your way through a blizzard. The crappier the weather, the more I like it."

And the walk itself? Definitely "not a thing of beauty," he says. "I think that I have reasonably good arm form and body posture, but speed walking doesn't look too good unless it's being performed somewhere like the Olympics."

Unlike in the Olympics, you'll never see Peters in a pack of other speed walkers. "If I ran into my best friend on Earth in the lobby of the hotel and he said, 'Do you want to walk together?' I'd certainly walk around town with him, but I wouldn't speed walk with him. That's my private thing that has nothing to do with any of my 6 billion fellow human beings."

WALKING FOR INSPIRATION AND PERSPIRATION

In addition to all the physiological benefits of speed walking—Peters says that he's read that it works more muscles, burns more calories, and is easier on the joints than jogging—it has also become a source of inspiration for him.

"When I wrote my column, I would guess that roughly 40 percent of them were written on my walks—especially when I was totally out of ideas," he says. "Forty-eight hours before the damn thing was due, I would say that it's this walk or else. You walk until you get an idea. That didn't always work, but it worked reasonably well."

On topics relating to business and management, Peters is unabashedly outspoken. A biography provided by Peters describes him as a "gadfly, curmudgeon, champion of bold failures, prince of disorder, maestro of zest, professional loudmouth, corporate cheerleader, lover of markets, capitalist pig." But he rarely chooses to share his enthusiasm for walking with others.

"I remember disliking being beaten up by the you-have-to-exercise people," Peters says. "If someone asks me about it, I'll tell them. But my shtick is business and business management."

Still, Peters credits walking with energizing his life and making him happier as well as healthier. "Walking really makes a physiological, chemical difference," he says. "If you crawled around the block, it would still be incredibly valuable. There's nothing more fun. It's rung just about every bell that you can find in my church spire."

Not only that, but he's 25 pounds lighter and has passed the last three stress tests without a hitch.

"A few years ago, I tried to find that guy to thank him, and I never did. But I did take him up on his offer," says Peters. "Just not on the freebie."

Bob Arnot, M.D., NBC News Medical Correspondent

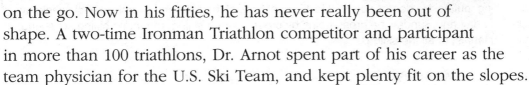

As a medical and health correspondent for NBC News, Dr. Bob Arnot is constantly on the go. Now in his fifties, he has never really been out of shape. A two-time Ironman Triathlon competitor and participant in more than 100 triathlons, Dr. Arnot spent part of his career as the team physician for the U.S. Ski Team, and kept plenty fit on the slopes.

But like a lot of men, Dr. Arnot reached a point where he figured that the onset of middle age and the demands of a fast-paced career were conspiring against him—and he'd have to say farewell to his former fit self.

A news assignment in Africa in 1994 changed all that. The assignment exposed him to the twin perils of cholera and dysentery. "When I came back from that extended trip, I was feeling even older than my age." That's when he said, "Physician, heal thyself!"

And he did heal. Dr. Arnot began interviewing medical and exercise experts from all disciplines, trying to devise the best possible health-and-fitness regimen for himself. He ended up writing his findings in the book *Dr. Bob Arnot's Guide to Turning Back the Clock*. In the process, Dr. Arnot

also transformed his 6-foot-4 frame into a trim, 200-pound paragon of fitness, with 7 percent body fat and 14 pounds of new muscle.

Today, when he competes in his favorite sports, Dr. Arnot leaves guys half his age in his dust. "I did it by taking charge of my health, my fitness, by not listening to those old paradigms," he says. Instead, he began eating better and came to appreciate the need for a powerful workout routine. "My friends and I were lifelong aerobic animals. We always disdained bodybuilding—and that was a big mistake. I tell people now, if there's a fountain of youth, it's the heavy metal in your local gym," he says.

FUELING HIS WORKOUTS

Dr. Arnot's workout begins early, with his commute to work in New York City. "I live in East Harlem, about 4 miles from the office. I'll either ride my bike there or use in-line skates. I do it every day, even in the winter. I keep a rack of clothes in my office and I change there."

Every day, Monday through Friday, Dr. Arnot hits the gym. He starts with an hour on the Alpine Trainer, a beast of a machine that looks like a stairclimber on steroids. "The steps are three times as long as your average climber. It also has plenty of bars on it where I can lay my papers and medical journals and work while I'm working out," he says.

Then, he spends about 40 minutes cycling and at least 40 minutes lifting

HEAVY ON THE METAL

For a man who was once indifferent to weight training, Dr. Bob Arnot follows a surprisingly punishing routine. He does 4 sets of 8 to 12 repetitions of the following exercises each weekday. On Saturday and Sunday, he cross-trains by cross-country skiing, mountain biking, kayaking, playing tennis, or alpine skiing.

Monday
Pullups
Incline rows
Horizontal rows
Upright rows

Tuesday
Military presses
Deltoid machine
Vertical rows
Shrugs
Abdominal machine
Lower-ab crunches
Rotary twists

Wednesday
Bench presses
Incline presses
Flys
Cable rows
Triceps presses
Leg presses
Lunges

Thursday
Biceps curls
Preacher curls
Cable curls
Abdominal machine
Lower-ab crunches
Rotary twists

Friday
Triceps dips
Triceps pulldowns
Triceps inverted preacher curls
Leg presses
Lunges

weights. "I favor a weight-training regimen where you work a different group of muscles each day of the week. On Monday, for instance, you focus on just back exercises. Tuesday, maybe it's shoulders and abs. That way, you have a good variety to your workout and you'll never be too sore."

Dr. Arnot doesn't let an assignment get in the way of a workout, either. "When I'm on the road, I'll take my bike and my skates and tour the cities I'm in. I also try to stay in hotels that have exercise rooms or a fitness club nearby."

Exercise, however, is only half the answer, Dr. Arnot believes. "Being powerfully fit is as much about eating the right foods as it is about pumping weights," he says. "The more men learn to fuel for their workouts, the more powerful they'll be."

Dr. Arnot favors a diet heavy on slow-burning carbohydrates—foods such as high-fiber cereals, fruits, and whole grains—and proteins, including yogurt, fat-free milk, and lean meat. "Proteins build muscle. Slow-burning carbs keep your blood sugar steady, so you won't crash during a workout," he says. And after a stint in the gym, Dr. Arnot immediately tops off the tank with a protein-filled sports beverage. "This is a controversial area, but it's had tremendous results for me."

Most men would probably have serious qualms about Dr. Arnot's self-imposed restrictions—his diet is extremely low in fat, with no red meat or alcohol. "But my nutrition allows me to do what I want, when I want—and with the energy of a 19-year-old," he says.

FOREVER YOUNG

For the older guy who wants to get in shape, Dr. Arnot says it's never too late. But the earlier you start training, the longer you'll enjoy the benefits.

"Don't let yourself be programmed into believing that you can't beat the kids at their own game. If you're willing, you can have the heart, lungs, and body of a man 20 years younger than the date on your birth certificate." A big part of that, he says, is attitude. Dr. Arnot is living proof, actively competing in sports that most older men wouldn't even think of trying. "It's all part of being in better shape physically and mentally—don't be afraid to try new things," he says.

Don't be afraid to use your head, either. "A lot of young guys don't pace themselves, don't take the time to learn the proper technique of a sport or exercise—and don't have the buying power to afford the best training and equipment money can buy." Older athletes have three advantages, says Dr. Arnot: wisdom, experience, and a bigger wallet. "Use them," he says.

Doug Foreman, Entrepreneur and TV Personality

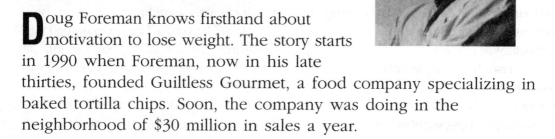

Doug Foreman knows firsthand about motivation to lose weight. The story starts in 1990 when Foreman, now in his late thirties, founded Guiltless Gourmet, a food company specializing in baked tortilla chips. Soon, the company was doing in the neighborhood of $30 million in sales a year.

In the process of developing a health-related business, Foreman, of Austin, Texas, concluded that Americans were hungry for information about diet and exercise. In the entrepreneurial spirit, he decided to fill that need.

He sold Guiltless Gourmet and started the television program now called *Good Living with Doug Foreman,* 90-second TV news inserts that cover a range of self-improvement topics, from eating low-fat food to bettering relationships. In the early days, one potential client had reservations about how Foreman looked on camera. "He said, 'Well, gee, Doug is talking about how to live right—diet, exercise, and health. But it looks like he may need to lose 25 pounds.'

"It was real motivating to me to hear people say that they liked what I was doing,

but I needed to lose a little bit of weight to come across on TV. The industry says TV adds 10 pounds to you just when you get in front of the camera."

To shed pounds, Foreman started working out aerobically—bicycling and climbing stairs—1 hour in the morning and again in the evening.

In a few months, he had dropped the offending 25 pounds—and got the client. Today, the 5-foot-11 TV host weighs 195 pounds and is generally satisfied with his physique. "I would still like to have that rippled stomach," he adds. "And who knows? Maybe by summer I will. When you're not out in the sun, when you're not out there exposed, you tend to let things go a little bit."

For the most part, he practices what he

preaches. For breakfast, he has orange juice, coffee, and a bagel. "Breakfast is pretty steady, the monotonous routine. At lunch, I have either a turkey sandwich—no cheese or mustard—or a breast of chicken with steamed vegetables. In the evening, I try to stick with some type of pasta, or possibly chicken."

As an entrepreneur, Foreman thinks a lot about what motivates people. That inspired his idea for the M & M Diet.

"People would initially think that it's candy, but M & M would stand for Money Motivates," says Foreman. "I'd take 25 people and ask them to lose an average of 2 pounds a week over a 2- to 3-month period. I'd tell them that at the end of that period, I would give them $1,000 if they would lose the weight."

Foreman acknowledges that even M & M-ers—if he ever really put up the dough for such a diet—would still have to learn to eat responsibly if they wanted to keep the weight off long-term. "Yeah, that goes along with any diet," he says. "But it would at least get them started, and I think that's a big part of the whole thing—getting started."

Part 6

THE AEROBIC PLAN

The Fastest Way to Burn Fat

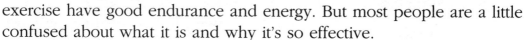

Even men who are serious about fitness have a hard time defining aerobic exercise. Everyone knows that it's good for the heart and lungs, and that people who run, bike, or get other forms of aerobic exercise have good endurance and energy. But most people are a little confused about what it is and why it's so effective.

This haziness has a way of derailing many aerobic fitness programs. Exercise without focus is like driving without a map: fine if you want to meander, not so good if you want to get somewhere fast. You need to understand aerobic exercise if you're going to reap all the benefits it has to offer. Don't think of it as dull physiology. See it as inspiration. Because once you understand the basics of aerobic exercise and the wonders it can bring to your waist, you'll wonder why you didn't dive into it sooner.

THE POWER OF BREATH

While the terms *aerobics* and *aerobic exercise* are often used interchangeably, they really aren't the same thing. Aerobics generally refers to aerobic dance—leotards, loud music, mirror-covered walls, and so forth. Aerobic exercise means any activity that gets your heart pumping and keeps it

pumping. Running is great aerobic exercise. So is biking, shadowboxing, rope jumping, or even, for that matter, aerobic dance.

Aerobic is derived from two Greek words meaning "air" and "life." Aerobic exercise is effort that requires an enhanced flow of oxygen to supply energy. You breathe in. The oxygen spills from your lungs into your bloodstream. Your heart pumps it to your muscles. There, the oxygen is used to break down carbohydrates, fat, and protein into the energy that your muscles need to move. You run, leap, pivot. And breathe some more.

So what exercise isn't aerobic? Examples include lifting a barbell, throwing a ball, jumping, even doing a short sprint. These exercises don't rely on your heart and lungs; they are mostly about short bursts of muscle strength. The muscles being exercised rely on the oxygen and glucose that are immediately available to them to meet the challenge. For an exercise to be aerobic, it must put continuous demands on muscles, enough to force your heart and lungs to deliver a heightened stream of oxygen for your muscles to keep churning.

By strict definition, nearly any exercise performed faster than sitting in a chair is aerobic; your heart and lungs will ratchet up a notch for even small efforts. But to produce a real benefit for your body, there needs to be some real effort involved. Effective aerobic exercise, the stuff that taxes your heart and lungs and burns calories, generally occurs when you exercise at roughly 40 to 80 percent of your maximum effort.

You need to raise your heart rate to a level that burns sufficient calories and taxes your cardiovascular system, but not so high that you can't suck in enough oxygen to fuel your working muscles. As a rule of thumb, you're exercising at a good pace when you're able to talk at the same time. If you're overdoing it, there won't be enough oxygen to fuel your muscles and limbs, and your lungs will feel as if they are being grilled on a spit. At this point, you either throttle back or pitch forward on your face.

Marvelous things happen inside your body when you start a regular aerobic exercise program. Your lungs become stronger and more efficient, enabling you to take in and dispense more oxygen. Your heart becomes stronger and more efficient, too, pumping more blood and oxygen with each beat. More capillaries are formed to ferry the oxygen to your muscles. Enzymes in your muscle fibers become more active, and your muscles are better able to use oxygen to burn fuel. Perhaps most enticing, the metabolic machinery in your muscles slowly improves its ability to burn fat. In other words, you improve two ways: inside and out.

LEAN FOR THE LONG HAUL

The great thing about aerobic exercise is that it produces stunning transformations in your heart and lungs in as little as a few days or weeks.

"The human body is a remarkably adaptive machine," says John Duncan, Ph.D., professor of clinical research at Texas Woman's University in Denton. "Just a few weeks of training can produce cardiovascular, muscular, and nervous system adaptations that make the body markedly more efficient."

Fine. But as men interested in fitness, we are concerned with deeper issues. Pushing our limits. Gleaning lessons in fortitude, perseverance, and self-destiny. Making sure that our physiques don't resemble beanbag chairs.

It's okay to be superficial. If you don't care about your looks, you're either Dennis Rodman or deceased. But if you're looking to burn calories and lose weight, there's nothing better than aerobic exercise. Equally important, aerobic exercise will keep that weight off—unlike slick diet schemes that advertise by trotting forward clients who have lost 30 pounds, but decline to show you those same folks 3

THE AEROBIC EDGE

Researchers keep finding ways in which regular aerobic exercise makes men healthier, happier, and calmer. For example:

- Scientists have discovered that aerobic exercise increases the immune system's ability to recognize invading bacteria and viruses. It doesn't matter what form of exercise you do. "The things that matter are the intensity and duration," says David Nieman, Ph.D., professor in the department of health and exercise science at Appalachian State University in Boone, North Carolina.

  Dr. Nieman looked at 150 people who had walked regularly for 12 weeks. Those who had exercised moderately, Dr. Nieman found, had half the number of colds and sore throats as the least active subjects. It's possible to overdo it, however. After 90 minutes of high-intensity activity, the body releases stress hormones that push the odds of illness in the other direction.

- When life is getting crazy, low-intensity aerobics can keep you off the window ledge. Researchers have found that people who cycle for just 20 minutes report feeling less anxiety. "You can reap the calming benefits of exercise without running yourself ragged," says Jack Raglin, Ph.D., associate professor of kinesiology at Indiana University in Bloomington.

- If you want to reduce your susceptibility to pain, try doing aerobic exercise for 30 minutes. Research has shown that pain thresholds are significantly higher after exercise, says Kelli F. Koltyn, Ph.D., assistant professor of kinesiology at the University of Wisconsin in Madison.

months later because they went right back to their corpulent selves. Aerobic exercise, combined with a smart diet, is the most effective way to ensure that lost weight stays that way.

The fat you lose with aerobic exercise has an impact beyond how you look. Excess fat has been linked to heart disease, diabetes, high blood pressure, and certain cancers. What's more, experts believe that the vilest fat, the stuff most responsible for this carnage, is the intra-abdominal fat, or visceral fat, resting out

of sight beneath your abdominal muscles.

"A lot of people are concerned with what they look like, and external body fat certainly plays a role there. But from a health-risk standpoint, it's intra-abdominal fat that you really should be concerned about," says Gary Hunter, Ph.D., professor of exercise physiology at the University of Alabama in Birmingham. "Not only does exercise make you leaner but it also makes you extra leaner in the place where you don't want fat."

Unfortunately, shedding fat via exercise

is a slow process. When you start an aerobic exercise program, your heart, lungs, and muscles may acclimate quickly. But your metabolic machinery—your body's ability to remove fat from the cells where it's stored, carry it to muscles, and then burn it up—adapts far more slowly.

Yes, aerobic exercise greatly improves your body's ability to burn fat and shed pounds, but it can take months before the fat-burning machinery is up and running full bore. There are no shortcuts. Unfortunately, most men either (a) don't realize this, (b) don't have the patience to wait weeks and maybe months for noticeable results, or (c) have seen one too many "Lose 5 Inches a Day from Your Waist!" headlines in supermarket checkout lines. This may explain why many well-intentioned exercisers eventually reduce their exercise to stuffing themselves into their pants.

Don't get discouraged. It takes time to build momentum, but once your system is in tune, you will quickly notice the difference. "Fat loss is a matter of dislodging the fat, transporting the fat, and using the fat—and all three of those take time to physiologically develop," says Ralph LaForge, managing director of the Duke Lipid Preceptorship Program at the Duke University Medical Center in Durham, North Carolina.

ADDING YEARS

While you wait for the pounds to peel away, you can take solace in knowing that aerobic exercise will deliver plenty of other benefits. Dozens of studies have looked at the link between exercise and aging and all have reached the same conclusion: Regular aerobic exercise can extend your years.

Stanford University's landmark study of nearly 17,000 Harvard alumni showed that men who burned 2,000 calories a week by walking 3 miles a day had a 28 percent lower death rate than fellow alums who exercised less or didn't do anything at all. More specifically, the researchers found that men who exercised regularly could expect to add about 2 years to their lives.

Their lives will be better ones, too. Aerobic exercise relieves depression, anxiety, and stress. It can improve your sex life and foster creativity—a potentially fortuitous one-two punch. It can help ease the sting of minor illnesses. Research has shown that the immune systems of regular exercisers can quash colds and flus more quickly. Aerobic exercise also reduces the risk of major health problems such as heart disease, high blood pressure, colon cancer, and diabetes. No other form of exercise confers as many benefits.

"Basically, aerobic exercise affords you the opportunity to turn back the hands of time," says Dr. Duncan.

EASY GAINS

Right about now you're probably thinking, "Right. All I have to do is give up my job, family, and all other interests in exchange for a fanatical exercise regimen and the personal life of moss."

True, it wasn't long ago that exercise physiologists poked their heads out of their laboratories to issue exercise prescriptions so time-consuming that no reasonable guy with a real life could possibly do them. But studies show that moderate activity provides the same health benefits as vigorous stuff. For basic health, the Centers for Disease Control and Prevention and the American College of Sports Medicine recommend that you get 30 minutes of moderate-intensity physical activity—easy walks, casual bike rides—a day. If you can't grab that exercise in a single 30-minute chunk, shorter bouts totaling 30 minutes will work just as well.

For losing weight, the American College of Sports Medicine recommends burning 1,000 to 2,000 calories a week—about 200 calories a day over and above what you normally burn.

"We used to tell people that they had to go out there and work and sweat to get any kind of benefit from exercise, but we've since found out that that isn't true," says Dr. Duncan.

Biking

Men typically shove their beloved bikes aside about the time they learn to drive, at which point they begin questing for new toys, like Range Rovers.

Time to revisit your youth. Not only is the two-wheeler the most popular mode of transportation worldwide, it's a mighty machine in the fight against fat.

Consider that an average Tour de France cyclist burns 5,900 calories in a day, compared with the 4,654 calories a pro baseball player burns in a whole season or the 3,136 calories a distance runner burns on a training day.

A study at Tufts University in Medford, Massachusetts, for example, monitored a group of cyclists using stationary bikes. After 12 weeks, the riders lost 19 pounds of fat and gained 3 pounds of lean muscle—all without dieting.

CHOOSE YOUR WHEELS

If your main interest in biking is actually getting somewhere, you'll probably find yourself using a traditional road bike or one of the new hybrids. But as far as your gut is concerned, it makes no difference whether you're riding on smooth pavement or tackling the back roads—or, for that matter, spinning away in your living room while watching B movies. As long as it has two wheels and you're doing the pedaling, you're going to burn a lot of calories very quickly.

For many men, however, traditional riding, either in the gym or on the streets, is as dull as toast. This may explain why nearly 10 million Americans now own mountain bikes.

Even if you're more interested in losing weight than in experiencing off-road thrills, there are good reasons to consider buying a mountain bike. In traditional cycling, your legs do all the work; your upper body just sort of sits there. But when you're riding your mountain bike over rugged trails, your upper body comes into play constantly—jerking the bike over logs, for example, or pulling away from free falls that suddenly materialize inches from your front wheel. And of course, the more muscles you use, the more calories you burn.

BUYING SMART

Whether you decide to take to the road or to the trails, you want to make sure that you get the right gear. Here are a few suggestions for getting started.

Buy basic. If you're like most guys, you

probably are already convinced that the only way to ride is on the latest aerodynamic, carbon-fiber, multitech wonder. But when you're biking to burn fat, all that really matters is riding, no matter what kind of machine you eventually buy.

If you want to use your bike to get fit, first you have to make sure that you fit your bike. A visit to your local bicycle shop, particularly one that features the Fit-Kit or the Serotta SizeCycle, is a good place to start.

Dress the part. Although sweats are fine when you're riding a bike with a sealed drivechain in the comfort of your living room, in the real world, baggy pants have a tendency to get stuck in the chain. Opt for cycling shorts instead. Shorts won't get sucked into moving parts, and they move when you do, which helps prevent chafing,

A PROGRAM FOR PEDALING

You don't have to brave the elements or traffic to get the benefits of biking. A stationary bike is a superb way to shed fat fast while building lean muscle.

Here's a 20-minute routine that offers all the challenges of real-life riding.

Saddle up. Sit comfortably on the saddle and bend forward. Rest your hands on top of the handlebar and relax your shoulders. This position is the cornerstone for steady, calorie-burning cycling. Adjust the resistance so that you can pedal smoothly at 90 revolutions per minute. Breathe steadily.

Jump for explosive speed. Jumps give you an intense cardiovascular workout and develop balance, coordination, and leg strength. Lean forward and rise up out of the saddle an inch or two while maintaining speed. Use your leg muscles to elevate yourself. Then sit down and pedal slower. In another 3 seconds, rise up again and repeat. Don't stop pedaling between jumps; the transition should be smooth. Do 5 to 10 jumps, building up to 30, 60, and eventually 100.

Stand for power. This builds strength in your arms, shoulders, abdominals, and calves, and it gives your legs a good stretch. Simulate a hill indoors by switching to maximum resistance. Place both hands shoulder-width apart on the handlebar, stand upright, and lean from side to side, using your body weight to push down the pedals. As you step down on one side, pull up on the handlebar on that side of the bike to exercise your arms. Do this for 1 to 2 minutes and return to the crouch.

Sit back for endurance. Build leg strength and endurance by putting your large hip and butt muscles to work. This simulates pedaling into a headwind or up a long grade. Start by increasing the resistance slightly, then move back on the saddle so that your rear is hanging off a bit. This forces you to push the pedals forward instead of down. Lean forward and keep your head low, and rest your hands shoulder-width apart on the handlebar. Pedal like this for 3 to 5 minutes, then return to the crouch.

chapping, and pinching. You needn't buy skintight spandex shorts, either. If the thought of wearing those in public terrifies you, looser touring shorts are available that provide similar padding and support (not to mention more pockets).

Ride light. Any interaction between a car and a bicycle—no matter who initiated contact—can have only one outcome. (Hint: You won't be the winner.) Make it a point to always be maximally visible, experts advise. This means wearing bright, reflective clothing and making sure that your bike is well-equipped with reflectors.

Of course, riding with a headlight at dusk or after dark is just common sense. In some areas, it's also the law.

Don't neglect the headgear. Unless you're trying to make the critical list at the county hospital, always wear a helmet to protect your brain box.

While you're thinking about protection, don cycling gloves as well. They'll protect your hands if you take a spill. Plus, they absorb sweat, dampen vibration, and give you a better grip on the handlebar.

Kick off the sneaks. When you're getting ready to ride, forget your favorite sneaks. "Soft, flexible running shoes are the worst things to ride in," says Len Pettyjohn, former director of the Coors Light professional cycling team. Make the investment in some stiff-soled biking shoes, he advises. These are designed to grip the pedal, giving you more power and helping to prevent your feet from flying off and into the front wheels or pavement.

RIDING SMART

The sun is shining, the car is parked, and you're ready to go. To make the most of your ride—and your new bike—here are a few tips from experts.

Get clipped. To get the most mileage from the same amount of oomph, experts recommend using clipless pedals. What they do is enable the upstroke on one pedal to deliver power while you're pressing down on the other. The added force can increase your cruising speed by 1 to 2 miles per hour.

Gear down. Beginning riders have a tendency to ride in high gears, which quickly tires both legs and lungs. Smart riders stay in lower, easy-to-push gears and keep the pedals revolving quickly. Strive to always keep your pedal speed, or cadence, at 80 revolutions per minute or higher. (Serious bikers often sustain more than 100 revolutions per minute.) Once your pedal speed is established, use your gears to maintain that rate as grades or terrains change. If you do it right, your pedals will turn at roughly the same rate, a little slower going uphill, a little faster on the descents.

Theoretically, it's possible to count revolutions, shift, and ride. But an easier solution is to invest in a cyclometer that also measures cadence.

Stay relaxed. "Many people ride with a really tense upper body and a death grip on the bars," says Fred Matheny, fitness and training editor of *Bicycling* magazine and author of *Weight Training for Cyclists.* "They use up a lot of energy that way." Your bike doesn't get a lot of help from your staying upright, and it's not going anywhere without you. So relax and loosen your grip.

Look up. Because of fatigue, many bikers ride with their heads down. While that gives you a splendid view of your front hub, it does create one minor problem: You're liable to run into a parked car or a wall because you can't see where you're going. So remember to always keep your head up.

Back down. Your shoulders should be relaxed, and your back should be flat—or as close to it as your body's natural shape allows. This actually helps you breathe more efficiently by opening up your chest cavity. If your back on the bike resembles Marty Feldman's Igor in *Young Frankenstein*, it could be a sign that your bicycle's top tube–stem combination is too short.

Bend your elbows. The old stiff-arm may come in handy for football running backs trying to break a tackle, but it can cause fatigue and increase your chances of crashing on a bike. If your arms are stiff, any bumps in the road will send shock waves straight through your body. Stiff arms also severely limit your ability to steer. Concentrate on keeping your elbows slightly bent. This will allow your arms to absorb road shocks and put you in position to maneuver quickly when needed.

Flutter your fingers. For cruising speed, your hands should be on top of the brake levers. This position offers the best of all worlds: It's reasonably aerodynamic, it provides stability, and it allows easy access to the levers. To accelerate, move your hands forward on the drops—the lower arms of the handlebar. For moderate uphill climbs, try moving your hands to the upper bends. And remember to ease up on the death grip. With your palms on the handlebar, occasionally flutter your fingers to stay relaxed.

Sit and slide. Once the saddle is positioned correctly, you should primarily be seated in the center for long rides. If you need a sudden burst of speed, you'll slide forward onto the tip of the saddle. If you're climbing a long, steady hill, you'll slide to the back, which cuts down on pedaling cadence but generates more power, Matheny says.

Position your feet correctly. The ball of your foot should be directly over the pedal axle. If it's too far behind the axle, you can wind up with an Achilles tendon strain.

Plan ahead. As the costs of gas, insurance, and new cars have shot into the stratosphere, more and more guys have begun biking to work. While this type of "service" (as opposed to recreational) riding doesn't require a great investment of time or money, it does create some special demands.

Clothes, for instance. Your spandex suit may work on the trail or at the club on weekends, but it's not going to impress your boss. What you need to do is drive to work in the car one day and drop off a week's worth of socks, shirts, pants, and so on. Assuming that your office also has a shower, you'll also want to take along soap, deodorant, and other toiletries.

Running

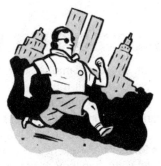

Humans have been running—for survival, transportation, or just the sheer fun of it—ever since they came down from the trees. Even today, while nature's two-footed transit system isn't the fastest or most efficient way of getting around, running is one of the best ways to get in shape fast.

"It burns fat, keeps your heart healthy, and can be done without a lot of preparation or trouble," says Art Mollen, D.O., director of the Southwest Health Institute in Phoenix and author of *Run for Your Life* and *The Mollen Method.*

You've probably known hard-core runners so enthusiastic about their sport that you weren't sure whether to join them or call the police. But you don't have to be a maniac (or marathoner—same thing) to burn pounds. You just need to do it.

"Simply running a minimum of 10 minutes every day is a very good workout," says Dr. Mollen. "It can increase cardiovascular endurance, muscle strength, and muscle tone as well as enhance the overall efficiency of your metabolism, particularly for someone just starting out."

CHEAP AND EFFECTIVE

Apart from the cost of a good pair of shoes, running is about as basic as it gets. You don't even have to buy fancy clothes. An old pair of shorts, a thick pair of socks, and some running shoes are all you need.

For all of its simplicity, however, running is surprisingly effective at shedding fat. For example, running at a sedate 12-minute-mile pace burns roughly 10 calories a minute. Kick that up to an 8-minute-mile, and you'll burn 15 calories a minute. That's 600 calories burned in a 40-minute run.

Smart running means ignoring people who say that you won't experience any benefits unless you're coughing up your lungs. Even the best runners intersperse hard training with plenty of slow running and outright time off to allow for recovery. Runners who ignore this fact and push too hard generally don't get any fitter. They just get hurt. To get the fitness gains without the pain, here are a few tips that experts recommend.

Move a little, then stretch. "You don't want to stretch muscles that haven't received an increased level of circulation and increased core temperature," says Budd Coates of Emmaus, Pennsylvania, a four-time Olympic Marathon Trials qualifier and a consultant to *Men's Health* and *Runner's World* magazines. "The time to stretch is ei-

TAKE TO THE HIGH COUNTRY

Once you are comfortable with your running regimen and are looking for new challenges, consider heading off-road for some trail running. Trail running—in which you leave the urban jungle and take to meadow, beach, or mountain trails—is like hiking in fifth gear: It can add a substantial amount to your usual running effort, giving you a tougher workout in less time.

"People are realizing that the trails are so much fun," says Nancy Hobbs, race coordinator for the Pikes Peak Ascent and Marathon in Manitou Springs, Colorado. "The visual experience is breathtaking, and they don't get injured as much as road runners—as long as they watch their footing."

In trail running, the "course" can change at a moment's notice, so you have to stay alert. Watch out for tree roots, rocks, uneven ground, and other surprises. It's also a good idea to take water as well as purification tablets, if you think that you'll need a refill. You can also load a fanny pack with a light jacket, sunglasses, and sunscreen, plus an energy bar for added energy.

ther 5 to 10 minutes into your run or after you're done."

You don't have to spend 20 minutes stretching, either. For each major muscle group, about 30 seconds may be all you need, says Coates.

For the hamstrings, for example, he recommends sitting on the floor cross-legged and unfolding one leg in front of you. Slowly reach down that leg toward your ankle and hold for about 30 seconds, then switch legs and do it again. If you can only grab onto your knee, that's okay. Keep doing it and your flexibility will improve.

Get the right shoes. If you're running regularly, don't rely on your all-purpose sneaks to protect your feet. Buy some running shoes instead.

Gone are the days when running shoes meant sneakers. Today, you'll find shoes with features ranging from air soles to dynamic reaction plates and Hydroflow cushioning pads, whatever those are. There are shoes for marathoners and shoes for sprinters. There are even shoes for walkers. And as you move up the price scale, your feet will find shoes loaded with all the high-tech gizmos they could ask for.

It's worth buying quality shoes, which means you're going to spend a minimum of $60 to $70. Shoes should be snug in the backs and flexible at the balls of the feet, and each should have about ½ inch of space between your longest toe and the end of the shoe. The fit and finish of good shoes can make all the difference between running and limping. Spending too much, however, isn't going to make your feet any happier. It will just make the shoemakers happy.

Take the soft route. During a run, every time your foot hits pavement it lands with a force equal to three to four times your body weight, says James M. Rippe, M.D., director of the Center for Clinical and Lifestyle Research and associate professor of medicine at Tufts University School of Medicine in Boston. Concrete is hard and unforgiving; so, you'll discover, are injured feet, ankles, and knees.

To get the joy of running without the jolts, try limiting your strides to a track, dirt trail, or grassy park. Or at least run on blacktop instead of concrete. It has some give and will absorb shocks better.

STYLE COUNTS

It doesn't get much simpler than running. As the old saying goes, you just put one foot in front of the other. But precisely *where* you put that front foot and how you get it there can make all the difference between running injury-free and being hobbled by leg pain.

Hit the right stride. "I hate to be negative, but when people err, they tend to bounce off the ground too high and they tend to overstride," says former U.S. Olympic marathoner Jeff Galloway, author of the bestselling *Galloway's Book on Running*.

When your lead foot strikes the road, it should be directly under your knee. If your foot hits the ground in front of your knee, it's as if you're hitting the brakes with each stride.

You can tell if you're overstriding by taking the sock test, devised by Coates. While running, look down as your lead foot hits the ground. If you can see your sock, you're overstriding. If you're running with the proper form—so that your leg is at a 90-degree angle to the ground when your heel hits the trail—you won't be able to see your sock.

Stay fluid. During your running motion, concentrate on lifting your knee just enough to let your leg swing forward naturally. Again, the idea is to direct your energy into moving forward—not into bouncing up and down.

Keep your lower body loose. Keeping your hips relaxed, your butt tucked, and your pelvis slightly forward will put your center of gravity slightly in front of you, making it easier for your legs to propel your body forward.

It's also important to keep your shoulders and upper arms relaxed, with your shoulders directly above your hips. Your elbows should be close to your body, bent at about 90 degrees through the full range of your arm swing. Your hands should be loose, but not limp.

Keep your body straight. Don't let your upper body twist from side to side while you're running. Remember, the idea is to move forward. Keep your feet pointed basically straight ahead—not twisted to either side.

Heads up. Make a conscious effort to fix your eyes on the horizon. Keeping your head up and your eyes forward will help increase your stride length and will also help you run more efficiently.

SAFE RUNNING

There's something about running that brings out the poetry in people. Rather than focusing on hot feet, chafed thighs, or homicidal cab drivers, they rhapsodize about wind in their hair . . . the echo of falling footsteps . . . the rush of "runner's high." Sounds great—until you hit the streets and realize that there's a real world out there.

To get the joy of running without the mishaps, here's what experts advise.

Face the danger. To avoid becoming roadkill, always run facing oncoming traffic. It makes you more visible to drivers, plus it gives you an extra second or two to dive to safety if you need to. And always wear light-colored reflective clothing, particularly when running after work or at night.

Break in slowly. If you're new to running, don't even run—not at first, says Coates. For about a week, just walk, he advises. Walk about 20 minutes for 4 days in a row. On days 5 through 8, increase the time to 30 minutes. But keep walking.

As your legs (and lungs) start feeling stronger, do about 2 minutes of running followed by 4 minutes of walking, says Coates. Again, do this for about a week, 30 minutes each time. After that, you may feel comfortable going into a full run—30 minutes without stopping. But don't be discouraged if you continue to walk and run. Every step is burning weight and helping you get into shape. The running will follow.

Check your speed. "One of the biggest mistakes most beginning runners make is that they try to run too fast," says Coates.

To keep your pace comfortable, use the talk-sing rule, he suggests. Run slow enough that you can talk without gasping for breath, yet fast enough that you can't sing opera.

Warm up to a winter run. If you live just about anywhere north of Florida, you'll face Old Man Winter eventually. Don't let him keep you home. But do prepare for him.

Wear socks made of polypropylene or acrylic. They're better than cotton or wool at keeping your feet warm and dry. And be sure to wear a hat. This will keep your whole body warm, since a significant amount of body heat escapes through your head.

Beat the heat. To prevent yourself from overheating, drink plenty of fluids, even when you're not thirsty. Direct sun can cause your temperature to rise, so wear light clothing instead of going shirtless. If it's particularly hot, soak your shirt in water before setting out. You'll be wearing portable air-conditioning.

Stop slowly. A lot of runners hurtle around the track like racehorses—then stop. Studies show that a more gradual cooldown can help remove excess lactic acid—a waste product that causes muscle fatigue—from stressed tissues, says David Costill, Ph.D., an exercise physiologist in the human-performance lab at Ball State University in Muncie, Indiana. He recommends ending workouts by slowly jogging until your heart rate returns to normal.

Inline Skating

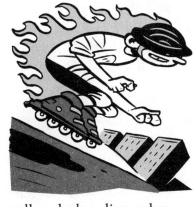

You may remember *Kansas City Bomber*, the 1972 epic film in which a skimpily clad Raquel Welch portrayed a roller-derby diva who exchanged elbow checks and bad dialogue with a rink full of other female four-wheelers.

The movie may have lived up to its title at the box office, but it proved one thing: Roller skating can certainly get your heart rate going. Just ask the guys watching it.

Today, with more scientific data to rely on, researchers have come to the same conclusion as those testosterone-fueled film buffs. Skating, even when it doesn't involve Raquel, can get your pulse rate up as much as running, and it burns even more calories, says Joel Rappelfeld, founder of Roll America Inline Skate School in New York City, a professional inline skater, and author of *The Complete Blader*. Rappelfeld, who also has done a video, *Get Started in Blading*, says that inline skating can torch up to 700 calories in an hour, making it one of the most time-productive workouts there is.

"Many people don't realize just how great of a workout you can get from inline skating," says Rappelfeld. "It gives you a fabulous aerobic workout and works all the major muscle groups, particularly in the lower body."

SKATING THROUGH LIFE

Of course, few guys have the time for the intense daily workouts practiced by Rappelfeld, who has taught Diana Ross, Howard Stern's sidekick Robin Quivers, and other celebrities how to street skate at Roll America. Here are some ways to get the most from real-life inline skating.

Change your approach constantly. The best way to get the most out of your inline skating is to vary your routine. "Too many people get out there and just glide around," Rappelfeld says. "But in order to get good, you need to mix things up in your workout. Once you're comfortable on your inline skates, start with long, low strides and practice that for about 5 minutes. Then sprint for 1 to 2 minutes. By adding intensity, you'll get the most workout in the shortest amount of time."

Think like a skier. "One of the biggest mistakes that most inline skaters make is with their form," Rappelfeld says. "They stand too straight and keep their knees locked, like Frankenstein. Instead, your skating position should be like a skier, with your nose, knees, and toes in alignment with each other."

In proper position, you lean forward from the waist and bend at the knees, so that a slightly diagonal line could be drawn from the tip of your nose down through your knees and your toes. Besides putting more stress on your joints, an incorrect skating position makes it easier to fall. You also have to skate harder to keep moving. "Knees should be flexed at all times to act as shock absorbers," Rappelfeld says. To help lower your position, try skating with your elbows on your knees, which really gives your legs a good workout, lengthens your stride, and helps improve your form.

Do it daily. Maybe you don't have 4 hours a day to devote to inline skating the way that Ryan Jacklone, the 1995 Aggressive Skating Association world champion from New York City, does. "But to be a better skater, you have to make it part of your daily ritual—even if it's only for a few minutes," Jacklone says. "That may mean strapping on your inlines to go to the corner to buy the newspaper or a quart of milk. The people who make the most of their time skating are those who make time for skating every day, even if it's only for 5 minutes."

Use your arms. Swinging your arms from front to back keeps you in better balance and is advised when you're sprinting, says Rappelfeld.

ALL-SEASON SKATING

For serious skaters like Joel Rappelfeld, founder of Roll America Inline Skate School in New York City and a professional inline skater, time isn't always the biggest obstacle. Mother Nature is.

"Basically, inline skating means that you're at the mercy of the weather," he says. "You can't do it when it rains or snows." But even when the weather is bad, you still can use wheels to stay in shape.

"I complement my skating with bicycling and using a horizontal slide board. With bicycling, you use similar muscles as those used in skating, and it definitely has increased my endurance. And whenever the weather is bad, I pull out the horizontal slide board and use it in my home."

A horizontal slide board is a sheet of plastic that can be used to simulate the skating motion. It's available at some sporting goods shops for less than $100. "With a slide board, you do the same routine you would use skating: long, smooth, and easy strokes followed by shorter, more intense, sprinting-type motions," Rappelfeld says.

For a harder workout, he suggests skating with your arms behind your back, like a speed ice-skater. "Start with one arm behind your back, and when you're comfortable in that position, put the other arm behind your back. With both arms behind you, you're working the lower body more and strengthening your leg muscles more quickly." If you feel that you are out of balance with two arms behind your back, practice with just one arm behind you (alternating left and right arms every once in a while to get used to both) until you are comfortable. Eventually, you will be able to skate with both arms behind you.

Use all-wheel drive. The correct way to push off is with all your wheels. "Most people push off on their toes, so their stroke ends with their heel up, which can result in falling," says Rappelfeld. "So make sure that you stroke out to the side using all wheels, and recover letting your foot back in, close to the other foot."

Skate on an incline. Studies show that running and cycling give you a better aerobic workout than inline skating does. The reason is that, with inline skating, you're gliding—in other words, resting—between strokes. But here's a simple way to ratchet up the intensity, provided you're not a flatlander. Find a long, gradual incline and repeatedly skate up it, then rest by walking back down the hill. Inline skating uphill provides an aerobic workout that on flat ground you would only get at dangerously high speeds.

Mix it up. For an innovative full-body workout, Rappelfeld suggests combining skating with other simple exercises. For instance, skate for 10 minutes, then stop and do some crunches. Skate for 10 minutes more, then hit the ground for some pushups. And since each skate weighs 3 to 5 pounds, you can even use them for leg lifts.

Basketball

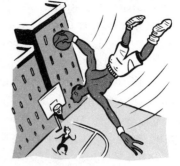

There are good reasons why most of us can't compete with the average NBA player . . . and height, genetics, and talent are just a few of them. The typical pro player earns nearly $1.9 million a year, higher than the salaries in any other team sport.

What does he do to get all that dough? He plays the game you wish you had time to play. Your schedule is filled with meetings, lunches, and conference calls. His schedule is filled with . . . games.

Unless you hit the lottery, you aren't going to be quitting your 9-to-5 job anytime soon to perfect your 3-pointer. So your only real choice is to make the most of the time you do manage to spend on the court. It's worth doing because basketball provides a heck of workout that will burn a lot of calories in a hurry.

COURTING FITNESS

"Unlike professionals, most regular guys play basketball only occasionally—like on Saturday mornings," says Ron Culp, president of the NBA Trainers Association and team trainer for the Miami Heat and the 1996 U.S. Olympic Dream Team. "And that's why they pay the price on Sunday and take about a week to recover."

You may not have time to play more than once or twice a week, but there are ways to turn up the intensity and rebound more quickly. Here are some tips to employ before the next tip-off.

Play full-court. "Most pickup games are played half-court, but if you really want a killer workout, make it full-court," suggests Tom LaGarde, former center with the 1979 NBA champion Seattle Supersonics and a member of the gold medal–winning 1976 U.S. Olympic basketball team.

"One of the hardest things you can do in basketball is play one-on-one full-court, but even a three-on-three full-court game will kick your butt and give you an incredible workout in a small amount of time," says LaGarde. "Anything that makes you run up and down the court continuously will get you in great shape fast."

Focus on defense. Michael Jordan took the art of scoring to new heights, but what *really* made him the greatest player ever was his ferocious defense. "Many recreational players, when they don't have the ball, tend to stand around with their hands on their hips, *waiting* for the ball," LaGarde says. "But if you only have an hour or so and want to get the best workout you can, keep moving all the time in order to keep your heart rate up. Playing defense is a great way to keep moving, but even on offense, always move so that the guy playing defense on you always has to move."

Beat the clock. The NBA uses a 24-second shot clock to keep the game moving. College players have 45 seconds to get a shot off. If you're tired of wasting too much time on the court while some clown puts on a dribbling exhibition, try using a game clock. Set a time limit—24, 30, or 45 seconds—to put up a shot or the ball goes to the other side.

Do laps before layups. If you want to even *survive* that full-court game and ferocious defense, Culp suggests that you run around the perimeter of the court three or four times before hitting the hardwood. "The only way to get the quick energy you need for a better workout and a better game is to run," he says. "You need to warm up your muscles before actually playing in order to prevent injuries and increase your endurance."

Not into laps? "Try walking to the gym instead of riding," suggests Culp. "Or if you're playing on your lunch hour, walk down the stairs instead of taking the elevator." Of course, he also recommends a regular road workout. "If you want to play ball—even for an hour—play on Monday, Wednesday, and Friday, and run sprints on Tuesday, Thursday, and Saturday. The single best thing you can do to get more from your basketball workout is to run."

Stretch. If you have only an hour or so to play, chances are that you don't want to spend 10 minutes of it stretching. But you're making a big mistake.

"As you age, the first thing to go is flexibility, which is why so many guys have sore backs and knees after playing," Culp says. "I can't stress enough how important it is to stretch before and after playing. By stretching, you not only improve your flexibility so that you're less likely to get injured but you also improve your workout because your body will be able to handle the game." He suggests paying particular attention to your lower back, hamstrings, groin, and Achilles tendons.

Jump for power. If you want to increase your vertical leap and build stronger legs, practice this move: Stand with your knees slightly bent and your arms relaxed at your sides. Then, jump forward as if you were doing a broad jump, suggests Mike Brungardt, strength and conditioning coach for the NBA's San Antonio Spurs and coauthor of *The Complete Book of Butt and Legs.*

As soon as you land—with knees bent to absorb the shock—jump again, this time raising your arms over your head to lift you higher. Make the second jump as quickly as possible to increase speed and strength. Do 8 to 10 repetitions.

Skiing

When your goal is fighting fat, put on your parka and strap on skis. Whether you prefer downhill or cross-country, skiing is an exhilarating strategy for strengthening your muscles and burning off calories—and having a great time in the bargain.

"Cross-country skiing rates highest in lab tests for burning the most calories per minute, because you're using your legs, your upper body, and even your torso," says Wayne Westcott, Ph.D., of Quincy, Massachusetts, national strength-training consultant for the YMCA.

You don't need fresh flurries to make skiing part of your fitness plan. With a combination of snowmaking technology and indoor ski machines, it's possible to be on the slopes every day of the year.

DOWN OR ACROSS?

If you're just now thinking about taking up skiing (and buying equipment), there's one decision you have to make up front: whether to go downhill or cross-country. Downhill is typically the favored style for speedmeisters and adrenaline junkies—guys who crave quick thrills. Cross-country, on the other hand, is slower and more contemplative. It's for guys who are into the journey, not the destination.

Cross-country burns up to 660 calories per hour. Downhill is no slouch, either, burning about 570 calories per hour.

THE GREAT OUTDOORS

Whether you opt for downhill or cross-country, take time beforehand to get prepared. Here's what ski pros advise.

Start with warmups. Doing a pre-ski warmup will prime your body for peak performance and at the same time help prevent injuries. Experts advise doing a few light toe touches, hamstring stretches, and shoulder rolls before heading out.

Dress the part. When you're spending all day in the cold and wet, what you wear can determine whether you'll have the time of your life or a miserable experience. Here's what experts recommend.

• Dress warmer than you think is necessary. Try wearing insulated pants over long underwear or spandex tights. Above the waist, start with a zip turtleneck made of a moisture-wicking material such as Capilene or Thermax. Add a fleece pullover if it's below 40°F or a wool sweater if it's below 25°F. Over that, you can wear a waterproof and windproof shell or a parka, but a versatile midweight jacket works best. Don't forget a thick hat or hood.

- Wear shades or goggles. Nothing is brighter than sun on snow.
- Don't wear jeans. They may embody the spirit of the West, but once they get wet and freeze, you'll look more like cardboard than like a cowboy.
- Go easy on the socks. Some people put on multiple pairs of socks to keep their feet warm. Too much bulk, however, can cut off circulation, prevent sweat evaporation, and reduce foot-to-ski sensitivity. One pair of polypropylene socks combined with your boot's insulated lining should be enough.

INDOOR SLOPES

Unless you happen to live in some frosty northern clime or are rich enough to jet-set in search of virgin slopes, skiing is something you can do only a few months out of the year. In addition, while some guys thrill to nature's chill, others would just as soon stay indoors.

No problem. With today's technology, it's easy to get the workout without the cold. Here's how.

Hit your stride. To get the fat-burning power of cross-country skiing without leaving the neighborhood, try walking with a pair of Exerstriders. Essentially, these are aluminum ski poles with rubber bumpers on the bottoms. You mimic the moves of cross-country skiing, except you do it on dry land.

Man the machine. Indoor ski machines work all the major muscle groups, plus you can work out year-round.

There are two types of ski machines. The ones popularized by NordicTrack actually look like skis. The user puts his feet through stirruplike attachments similar to those on cross-country skis and pushes the two long ski-like rails back and forth, while his arms, also swinging back and forth, pull on cables straight out in front. On the other kind, the ski-size tracks remain stationary but have planted-in "platforms" for your feet that do the actual sliding. Your hands, meanwhile, usually pull on poles at the sides rather than on cables. The first type gives you a greater range of motion but generally requires more coordination.

Look for distractions. Only true exercise diehards can ride a ski machine for any length of time without getting bored. To make your workouts more enjoyable, set up the machine in front of the TV. Or listen to music or Books on Tape. Once you get the rhythm going, the time passes quickly.

Swimming

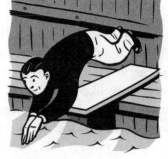

President John Quincy Adams and his steward, Antoine Guista, used to swim across the Potomac River almost every morning, both of them stark naked. The thought of any of our recent presidents reenacting Adams's morning ritual is too horrific to even contemplate.

But if one of the chief executives of the world's most powerful nation could find time for a swim, maybe you can, too.

Swimming has a lot going for it. It's a safe, effective way to boost strength and aerobic capacity. A typical 180-pound guy can burn 630 calories in an hour doing a slow crawl—about the same number he would burn running on hilly terrain or cross-country skiing. This same guy could substantially boost his calorie burn just by swimming faster. The intensity of water sports explains why Olympic swimmers have the sorts of bodies that get the role of Tarzan.

INCREASING INTENSITY, SAVING TIME

The one problem with swimming is that it's not as fast as, say, pulling on some shoes and running around the park. There's the drive to the pool. You have to change into your suit and maybe take a shower first. As if that weren't enough to drown your enthusiasm, the time men spend in the water is generally far from efficient.

"Most recreational swimmers go to a pool and just do the same thing—swim laps in their favorite stroke," says "Spanky" Stephens, head athletic trainer at the University of Texas in Austin. "And that's why they never really improve or get the most from their swimming workouts."

If you want to get more out of your time in the pool, here's what Stephens and other experts recommend.

Put a cap on laps. "If you want to get the best workout in a short time period, probably the worst thing that you can do is to just swim laps at a comfortable pace," says Drury Gallagher, a New York City business executive who holds 10 Masters' swimming records and who, in 1983, set the onetime world record for swimming around Manhattan Island. "To improve your cardiovascular training and overall swimming, you need interval training—mixing up your routine and really going hard at 70 to 85 percent of your maximum speed," says Gallagher. "Push your pulse rate up with the fast pace, then slow down on the rest period."

So instead of swimming, say, 40 laps at the same pace, he recommends breaking it up into 10 4-lap or 20 2-lap swims, with a rest break of 10 to 20 seconds. Start slowly, but with each drill, try to increase your speed. "And mix up your routine. Sometimes, I just kick for one lap and swim one lap, with a 10- to 20-second rest in between," says Gallagher, considered by many to be the best American swimmer over the age of 50. "Or I'll swim 1 set using a pull buoy."

Change your stroke. To be a better swimmer, practice your worst strokes. "I see a lot of guys sticking with their best stroke, usually the crawl," Stephens says. "But when you vary your strokes—do some breaststroke, some butterfly, some backstroke—you'll work muscles that you may normally not be working. And since they are harder for you, you'll get your heart rate

up faster. You always get a better workout practicing your weakest strokes."

Focus on specific muscle groups. Swimming may be an all-body sport, but experts recommend working specific muscles at different times. "One of the best things you can do is tie your legs together so that you just work your arms and shoulders," Stephens says. "You can strengthen your leg muscles by getting a kickboard and just kicking your way across the pool to improve your kick."

By targeting specific muscle areas, Stephens says, you'll get a more intense workout and burn more calories at the same time.

Work on your form. To go faster longer, you need proper technique and form. One of the most common mistakes among recreational swimmers is not using the "S-shaped pull," says Jane Katz, Ed.D., a Masters swim-

WATER RUNS

Swimming pools aren't just for swimming anymore.

"Deep-water running is the closest thing you can do to simulate running without the pounding you get from the road," says Doug Stern, a New York City triathlete, writer for *Triathlete* magazine, and owner of Doug Stern Swimming Clinics. And because water is a lot denser than air, your muscles have to push harder, which burns a lot of calories. "It gives you a great workout and can actually improve your running performance."

In deep-water running, you wear a life preserver, ski belt, or some other flotation device that keeps your head above water. You "run" in place for up to 45 minutes, with your toes pointed downward, your hands below your elbows, and your hips in line with your shoulders.

As you progress, you can practice "hurdle jumping" by reaching forward with your arm to touch your lead foot, or "uphill running" by exaggerating the backswing of your elbows and lifting your knees slightly higher.

ming champion, world-record holder, and author of seven books on swimming technique, including *The All-American Aquatics Handbook.* "With the S pull, you're moving your hands underwater in an 'S' motion during a crawl—your right hand makes a question mark and your left hand makes a reverse question mark," she explains. "If you practice that during your workout, you'll get a better workout because it enhances your swimming technique, it makes swimming more efficient, and you'll be able to go faster and go longer."

Work on your lungs. To improve endurance, some experts suggest that you practice underwater swimming, which trains your body to work on less oxygen. Try this drill, recommended by Jane Cappaert, director of biomechanics with the 1992 and 1996 U.S. Olympic swimming teams. At one side of the pool, take a deep breath, then submerge as you push off the wall with your feet. Hold your arms in front of you, like a torpedo, and move yourself with a dolphin kick, keeping your legs together and outstretched as you move them up and down, just like a dolphin moves its tail. Once you've gotten to the point where you can cross the pool in one breath, try to increase your speed.

SUITING UP

There's not a lot you have to buy when you take up swimming: just a suit and swimming goggles. Almost any goggles will protect your eyes from pool chemicals, but you want to spend some time getting the right suit.

There are two basic choices in suits: a racing suit or your standard beach britches. You might be embarrassed about wearing a racing suit, but it's a good investment. It's light and comfortable, and it offers virtually no drag in the water. Britches, on the other hand, usually have pockets, which tend to fill with water and drag you to the bottom.

Rowing

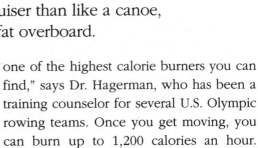

As a member of the U.S. rowing team at the 1984 Olympics—and one of the oldest athletes on the team—Bruce Beall knows the importance of staying trim. But even if you're built more like a cargo cruiser than like a canoe, rowing is an outstanding way to throw fat overboard.

"Your initial response to rowing may be that you feel tired. It takes a lot out of you and your body has to adapt," says Beall, a former rowing coach and fitness trainer, now in his late forties. "But after that initial break-in period, then all of a sudden you'll start feeling more alert and seeing better muscle definition. You'll start noticing the difference rowing makes as a fat-fighting exercise."

A VERY TOUGH WORKOUT

Although rowing has long had the reputation of being a sport for upper-crust collegians, the U.S. Rowing Association estimates that more than 100,000 Americans regularly ply the oars.

Rowing provides more than opportunities for weekend excursions. It's a very efficient fat burner, ranking with cross-country skiing as one of the best aerobic exercises you can do, says Fredrick C. Hagerman, Ph.D., biological-sciences professor at Ohio University in Athens.

"If you look at the energy cost for any given level of exercise, rowing is probably one of the highest calorie burners you can find," says Dr. Hagerman, who has been a training counselor for several U.S. Olympic rowing teams. Once you get moving, you can burn up to 1,200 calories an hour. "Rowing is easy to perform," he adds. "Heck, you're sitting down."

Here's advice for getting started and doing it right.

Get your feet wet. While some land-locked communities are unable to take up oars, most major cities—Philadelphia, Seattle, and Boston, to name a few—boast a number of rowing clubs that are open to the public. You'll probably pay a nominal entry fee to join, plus rental fees when you take a boat on the water.

"Every club's looking for new members—it makes the club more viable," says Beall, who is also executive director of the George Pocock Rowing Foundation in Seattle, an organization that promotes rowing. "The problem is, rowing has this deceptive elitist image. Even though it has been popularized by all the Ivy League schools, anyone can row."

THE RIGHT STROKES

Rowing is a lot like running in that technique—good or bad—spells the difference between beginners and experts. Even if you've been a landlubber all your life, you can learn the basics of rowing very quickly.

According to Bruce Beall, executive director of the George Pocock Rowing Foundation, here's what you need to do.

Phase 1: The catch. With your upper body leaning slightly forward, move forward on the rower, drawing your knees up to your chest. Your back should be firm, your muscles flexed, your head up, and your arms straight. Don't worry, it sounds more complicated than it really is.

Phase 2: The power stroke. With your feet braced on the pedals, push back, exhaling as you go. With your legs fully extended, continue the stroke by leaning backward slightly and drawing your hands to your abdomen. This stroke, which should be fluid and graceful, works muscles in your legs, back, and arms.

Phase 3: The recovery. Push forward with your palms and wrists. This movement, which also works muscles in your arms, back, and legs, completes the cycle.

Get a mentor. While it's not impossible to take up rowing without knowing port from starboard, it's a little more complicated than, say, jogging around the high school track. "Trust me. I'm not sure rowing lends itself well to learning it by reading out of a manual," Beall says. "You're better off learning from an accomplished rower."

Start slowly. If you go out on the water your first day and try to pull a Lewis and Clark—who, you'll recall, canoed through a substantial part of the Northwest—your muscles will feel like they were hit with the oars instead of like they were pulling them. If you're already in pretty good shape, you should be able to row nonstop for about 2 minutes, Dr. Hagerman says.

That's about the limit at first. Row for 2 minutes, then rest for 30 seconds. Then start rowing again, Dr. Hagerman says. Your goal should be to row nonstop for 20 minutes, doing about 20 strokes per minute.

Don't worry about your back. A lot of rowing newcomers worry that the sport is bad for their backs. Not true, says Dr. Hagerman.

"Rowing really works your back, so if you hopped in a boat for the first time and pulled as hard as you could, you might do something to yourself," Beall adds. "But otherwise, it's good exercise."

STAYING HIGH AND DRY

For those who get queasy even in the bathtub or who live in areas where water is in short supply, it's still possible to take up oars. The solution, of course, is to use an indoor rowing machine or an ergometer—

machines that are compact and relatively affordable. Regardless of the weather, they make it possible to get hours of fat-torching workouts.

All too often, however, would-be scullers buy machines in the first flush of enthusiasm, then lose interest and use them thereafter as a catch for dirty laundry. To get the right machine and keep your interest high, here's what experts recommend.

Spend some money. While a number of rowing machines rely on pneumatic pistons to provide resistance—which makes it hard to adjust to various fitness levels—more expensive models deliver their power via a weighted flywheel coupled to a drivechain and fins. When you pull on the "oars," the fins catch air, creating drag much like water does. "If you look at most rowing machines, they put too much resistance on you—they're not ergonomically sound," says Dr. Hagerman.

Watch your form. Since good form is critical, not only to get the most out of your workout but also to prevent injury, it's a good idea to set your machine in front of a mirror so you can see what you're doing. "Rowing is like anything else you do quickly and repetitively," says Beall. "You can pick up bad habits, and it can take a lifetime to correct the mistakes."

Confront the competition. If you think that indoor rowing is strictly a solitary activity, think again. Every February, more than 1,000 competitors arrive in Boston for the Crash B Sprint World Indoor Rowing Championship. Just be warned that the world record for the 2,500-meter "course" is 7 minutes, 11 seconds. For many of us, covering the course in double that time would mean a week's worth of physical rehabilitation just to regain use of our arms. For serious rowers, however, it's all in a day's work.

Martial Arts

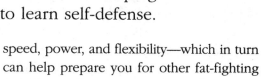

More than 3.6 million Americans age 7 and older have tried their hands—and feet—at martial arts. While some weekend warriors dream of combat, most participants have little interest in developing fists of fury. Most begin martial arts study to learn self-defense.

They stay because, along with the meditative aspects, martial arts provide a very intense workout that burns fat and increases muscle and speed.

"Not everybody likes martial arts, but they really are great training. They can be very aerobic, depending on your style," says Richard Carrera, Ph.D., a psychologist at the University of Miami who has studied the psychological effects of karate.

A WHOLE-BODY WORKOUT

Martial arts are specialized training techniques and strategies originally used in war—hence the term *martial*. The original purpose of karate, kung fu, judo, and other styles of fighting was to make the practitioners more formidable on the field of battle.

While some guys still gravitate to the dojo—the workout area where martial arts are practiced—to get in fighting trim, many others swear by the total-body workout provided by martial arts. An hour on the mats several times a week combines serious aerobics with strength training. You gain speed, power, and flexibility—which in turn can help prepare you for other fat-fighting activities such as running or aerobics.

"Particularly for older guys, a lack of flexibility can lead to injuries," says black belt Dan Millman, author of *The Way of the Peaceful Warrior* and founder of Peaceful Warrior Services in San Rafael, California. "There are some wonderful things that come with flexibility, and martial arts definitely are one way to gain them.

"There's a martial art form for anyone and everyone, no matter what level of fitness they're at," adds Millman.

Some people fear martial arts as muscular, macho sports that force you to break boards and bricks with your head. If you're one of those people, you should know that there are also soft arts such as tai chi that emphasize coordination and suppleness, more like dance, Millman says.

GO TO THE MATS

If you think that martial arts would be a kick, here are some tips on getting started.

Find your form. Martial arts are like cars: All will get you where you're going, but they come in a wide variety of makes and models. In martial arts, these differences are called styles.

Two of the best-known styles—tae kwon do and Shotokan karate—are Asian. There are also martial arts that are indigenous to India, Israel, France, and Brazil.

"Some martial arts don't offer as much aerobic training, while others offer supplementary training, like weight training or meditation," Millman says. "In terms of someone wanting to lose weight, you're going to want a more active type of training." Any style of karate will provide a good aerobic burn. So will styles such as tae kwon do, kung fu, and judo.

Keep in mind, however, that virtually any martial art, done vigorously, will help get your heart rate up and your weight down, Millman adds.

Pick your teacher wisely. "It takes more than skill and a black belt to be a compassionate teacher," says Millman. "As in many fields, quality of instruction varies, but most teachers are sincerely interested in the progress and development of their students."

Before signing up for a program, visit for a few hours. Many instructors encourage newcomers to attend a few classes for free to see whether the program is right for them. Being in a hurry and choosing the wrong instructor or school could turn you off to what could otherwise be a lifetime avocation.

Go for comfort. A *gi* (pronounced GEE) is the most common karate uniform: baggy white pants and a jacketlike white top cinched with a belt. Don't buy it yet. "Most

A MENU OF STYLES

Just as life on Earth is classified by kingdom, class, and species, the broad term *martial arts* can also be subdivided. In this country, there are dozens of martial arts styles to choose from. Among the more popular are:

Aikido. This stresses flips, throws, and joint locks, yet at the same time is graceful and dancelike. It requires tremendous discipline and concentration.

Judo. More like wrestling, it stresses flips and throws, with some emphasis on low kicks.

Karate. Originating in Japan, karate is known for its hard punches, blocks, and no-nonsense kicks. Shotokan karate is considered one of the most rugged and demanding of all the martial arts.

Tae kwon do. Now an Olympic sport, tae kwon do originated in Korea. Known for airborne, breathtaking kicks, it requires great flexibility to manage the fancy footwork.

Tai chi. This is a very slow and relaxed martial art, stressing coordination and grace. It is probably the softest of the martial arts and emphasizes mental concentration instead of physically demanding moves.

beginners start with sweatpants and T-shirts. Comfort and utility are the most important things," Millman says. That way, if martial arts aren't for you, you don't get stuck with an expensive pair of white pajamas.

Tame the beast within. Guys are raised to be competitive and to win at all costs. While this attitude may work on the basketball or tennis court, it has no place in martial arts training, where unchecked aggression can get you or someone else hurt.

Discover positive control. With martial arts, perhaps more than with any other physical activity, you can develop a strong sense of confidence and physical control. Dr. Carrera studied aggression in male karate students. He found that, compared with other men, the martial artists were better able to turn their aggression on or off.

"Karate devalues impulsive violence," he explains. "Because of its emphasis on discipline, a martial art tends to increase one's self-control." And just as martial arts can channel your aggression to resist wily opponents, they can also give you the control to resist everyday enemies—like second helpings or third beers.

Explore your options. Depending on where you live and where the local instructors trained, each martial art can be subdivided into potentially dozens of styles.

"I myself explored a number of different styles of martial arts," Millman says. "In my own view, especially for beginners, it's important to make a point of exploring different styles so you find one that works best for you."

Mic Rodgers, Stuntman

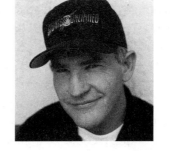

For a decade, he has been *the* stunt double for Mel Gibson, and *the* guy all the studios call when they need serious movie magic. In one of his biggest challenges, he personally managed the painfully realistic battle scenes that helped win *Braveheart* an Academy Award.

And if all goes as planned, he'll be the man directing a few of the blockbusters coming soon to a theater near you.

But to hear Mic Rodgers talk, none of that is quite as important as what his father told him before dying of cancer. It was a message that has been reinforced time and again on television and movie sets from Hollywood and Miami to London and Israel: Be there for your brothers in the business. And be willing to give it all back.

"I am a high school graduate, the son of a truck driver," says Rodgers. "And I stumbled into this almost by accident. Now, I've done my part to get where I'm at on the physical and mental level, but a lot of guys have taken the time to help me out. They said, 'You have potential. I'm going to help you.' And now that's what I'm trying to do."

BREAKING IN

Growing up in the Los Angeles suburb of San Gabriel, Rodgers never even thought about working in Hollywood. But because he was dyslexic, any time his teachers allowed the class to work on a student play or film instead of turning in an English paper, Rodgers was game—especially since a friend's father who owned a camera shop made it so convenient. "Every time a 16-millimeter camera came in, he would hold it for an extra week so we could use it," Rodgers says.

When the teens tried to perform more daring stunts for their films, it occurred to Rodgers to ask a pro how it was really done. And that led him to his first mentor in the business, Paul Stader. "He ran sort of a stunt school, but it was more like you became part of his entourage, one of his protégés," Rodgers says.

Soon after, Stader took Rodgers to the set of the blockbuster disaster film *The Towering Inferno*. "Paul was the stunt coordinator for the show. One minute, I'm just standing around watching what's going on; and the next minute, I have a fire extinguisher in my hand. Then Steve McQueen, one of my heroes, walks by and I'm like, 'I can't believe this!'"

Although Rodgers already had a full-time job as a mechanic's helper at a tractor dealership, he slowly took on more stunt work. "I came in at a good time," says Rodgers. "There were tons of TV action series on . . . *The Dukes of Hazzard, Wonder Woman, Baa Baa Black Sheep.* So someone my age, 23 or 24, could be a guard or a soldier, if that's what they needed. I'd cut my hair. It didn't matter."

Before long, Rodgers found himself running from Universal and Warner Brothers to Twentieth Century Fox, performing stunts 5 days a week. But it wasn't just the thrill of steady work at something he loved that made it great. "Every day, we were learning something new. How to coordinate stunts—without any prep time or money. So when I broke into features, it was easy. They give you so much time and so much money and you think, Wow, I could have done this with $1.95 and a roll of masking tape."

Since his first 2 years in the business, Rodgers has never worked fewer than 300 days a year. And it shows. His seven-page résumé includes appearances in everything from *Baywatch* and *The Bionic Woman* to *Matt Houston* and *M*A*S*H* as well as dozens of others shows, miniseries, and made-for-TV movies. And—oh yeah—more than 150 feature films.

LEARNING HIS CRAFT

If it was Stader who got Rodgers into the business and taught the 6-foot-tall 185-pounder how to get flattened without breaking too many bones, it was a director named Richard Donner who became like a father to him. Not only did Donner hire Rodgers for stunts on the first *Lethal Weapon* movie but the veteran producer also seemed to be grooming him for even bigger things.

On the set of films such as *Scrooged, Lethal Weapon 2, Lethal Weapon 3*, and *Maverick*, Donner mentored his younger, soft-spoken friend. "I'd stand around the set and watch them shoot dialogue scenes. And he'd say, 'What would you do with these actors?' And I'd say, 'I would do this or that.' Then he'd say, 'Go tell them. It's a good idea.' He was semitraining me to express myself, to speak up about things that I thought weren't my domain. It was good stuff."

Rodgers's training continued in earnest after Mel Gibson tapped him to be second unit director on *Braveheart*. His first responsibility on the film: whipping 1,500 regulars from Ireland's version of the national guard into shape for the climactic battle scene.

After 2 weeks of training—just moments before Gibson was to arrive to inspect the troops—Rodgers gave a pep talk that sounds like it would have done William Wallace proud.

"I went to one side and told them Mel was coming to see the test battle, and they were the Scots. And those guys on the other end of the field were the English. And so they were booing them and making all kinds of noise. And then we walked down to the other side, and I said, 'Okay, you guys down here, *you* are the Scots and those guys over there are the English.' They were all freakin' out."

When the two celluloid armies clashed, Gibson's mouth fell open. "It was unreal," says Rodgers. "It took 3 minutes to stop them. And everyone was screaming and using bullhorns going, 'Cut, cut, cut.' And they were still going at it. Broke every sword we had."

While Rodgers's movie life is certainly full of action and glamour, those things pale in comparison to the friendships, trust, and respect that he has developed for his fellow stunt performers over the years. "When you're asked to join Stunts Unlimited (a fraternal stunt organization), you take the oath to be a brother to the other members. Now, you may have a personality problem along the way with some other member, but you have to put that aside and hire him if he is the right guy for the job," Rodgers says.

And that brotherhood extends to both good times and bad. Members who are hurt or disabled often have their bills paid or are given money by the other members. In one such situation, a stunt performer who de-veloped cancer and couldn't work for a year had his mortgage paid by the group.

Such generosity is hard to imagine—until you remember that stuntmen and stuntwomen routinely risk their lives for one another. "Respect to us is that if I say I'm going to be somewhere at a certain time, I'm there. Or if you say, 'I have to light myself on fire for this scene,' I'll promise you that I will put you out before you get burned, no matter what. I'll do that. I'll sacrifice my body or my life to keep a guy from getting hurt. That's what commands respect."

And in the same way that Stader and Donner and Gibson mentored Rodgers, he's giving back now to a young man named Chris Tuck. "When Chris got out of high school, he came out here to live with my wife and me," says Rodgers. "He's 25 now and on the verge of becoming a great stunt guy. He doubled for Bill Paxton in *Twister*—did all the car driving. In 10 years, he might find someone to pass it on to. Who knows? He might pass it along to my son, Cooper. You have to pass it on. You have to replace yourself. If you don't, it's like bad mojo."

Jack LaLanne, Fitness Icon

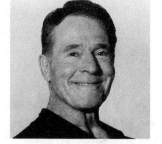

At age 45, Jack LaLanne completed 1,000 pushups and 1,000 chinups in 1 hour and 22 minutes. At age 61, he swam the length of the Golden Gate Strait, handcuffed, shackled, and towing a 2,000-pound boat against the tide.

At age 70, again handcuffed and shackled, he towed 70 boats with 70 people from Queen's Way Bridge in Long Beach Harbor to the Queen Mary, 1½ miles away.

And that's just to name a few famous feats.

Is he mad? Perhaps. But more than that, LaLanne has a higher purpose. "I take my lead from Jesus," says LaLanne. "Not that I would *ever* compare myself to Him, but Jesus performed wonderful miracles to call attention to His message. I wanted to do that, too."

Now in his mideighties, he still does. LaLanne admits that some folks find him a tad fanatical. But what they don't understand is that he's a man with a mission. And he's not leaving this Earth until he's through. "I haven't done a thing yet," says LaLanne. "I can't think about dying. I have so much to do. And though my message is more accepted today than it used to be, there are millions of people whom I still need to reach."

BELIEVE, BELIEVE

It's hard to believe, now that everyone and his grandmother is hoisting free weights, but in the 1930s when LaLanne first started making a name for himself as a paragon of health and fitness, he had more than his share of doubting Thomases trying to run him out of town.

One reason was that when LaLanne first started preaching the benefits of nutrition and exercise, he was practically all alone. It started when he was 15. With his father already dead by his midforties, LaLanne was, by his own admission, one sickly adolescent. "I was 30 pounds underweight. I lived off junk food. I had pimples, boils, glasses, arch supports, and one sickness after another," recalls LaLanne. Things got so bad that he left school for 6 months due to ill health and began a downward spiral. "I was thinking about suicide. It just seemed hopeless. Then, our next-door neighbor Mrs. Joy told my mother to take me to hear a health lecture by this man named Paul Bragg. He saved my life that night," says LaLanne. "He said that it didn't matter what condition you were in or how old you were. If you followed nature's laws, you could be reborn. And man, did I want to be reborn."

LaLanne wasted no time. "I gave up white flour and white sugar. I joined the local YMCA. I became a vegetarian. And I bought *Gray's Anatomy* and read it cover to cover. I started working out and became captain of the football team and state wrestling champion. Then, in 1931, while I was still at Berkeley, California, High School, I bought dumbbells and opened my first gym in my backyard. I would train local police officers and firemen and sell seeds, dates, honey, and other health foods. My fellow students shunned me. Lots of people thought I was nuts," he says. And that was before he went public.

After graduating from chiropractic college, LaLanne opened his first real gym, complete with carpeted floors and mirrored walls. At a time when gyms were dark, dank places called sweat boxes, where only boxers went, no one had ever seen anything like it. "Doctors would actually tell their patients not to see me because I was a 'dumb nut,' a 'cheat', and a 'crook,'" LaLanne says. "They would tell women not to lift weights because they'd look like men. They would actually tell athletes not to lift weights be-cause they would get so muscle-bound that they wouldn't be able to perform. That's when I started doing all those swimming events to show them they were wrong."

Thirty-four years of syndicated workout shows and a half-dozen books later, LaLanne has been vindicated. In fact, there's talk of LaLanne putting together a new television show, once again showing millions of Americans the benefits of nutrition and exercise.

BUILT WITH PRIDE

Sure, you say. It's easy for Jack LaLanne to swim lots of miles, lift lots of weights, and keep in shape. That's what he gets paid for. But LaLanne begs to differ. "C'mon, guys. Be honest with yourselves. How many hours do you waste watching TV? Yeah, if you want to perform amazing feats, you have to work out more. But for the average person, investing ½ hour to an hour, three or four times a week, is plenty."

Good health, no matter what your age, simply takes pride and discipline, says LaLanne. "You think I like to leave a hot woman and a warm bed to get up at 5:00 A.M. and go to a cold gym? Absolutely not. But I love the results. We all hate to train. But it doesn't take much to reap huge benefits. Get up. Stretch. Do some pushups. Go for a vigorous walk. Live with enthusiasm and energy. Don't be like so many millions of Americans and start dying from your own bad habits and lack of enthusiasm as soon as you hit 30. Your body is the only machine that gets better the more you use it."

Besides hard work and discipline, what

has kept Jack LaLanne's biceps bulging against his spandex sleeves all these decades? "I keep aiming higher," he says. Here are a few tips on how the quintessential Mr. America got and stayed where he is today.

- No rest. "I see these guys waiting minutes between sets at the gym. You should lift to fatigue and rest only 10 seconds between sets for maximum strength and endurance," he says.

- Write it down and shake it up. "Write down exactly what you're doing. Do it for 3 weeks. Then change it," advises LaLanne. "If you've been lifting low weight at high repetitions, start lifting more weight fewer times. Do that for 3 weeks, and change again. That keeps your muscles developing and your mind from getting bored."

- Pop those pills. No matter how good your diet is, you should consider vitamin and mineral supplements to put back what is taken from your food during processing and cooking, says LaLanne.

- Push the envelope. Complacency is your enemy. Always strive for a higher goal and a new challenge. "I'd swim from Alcatraz to San Francisco in handcuffs one year. Then the next year,

I'd do it again, only I'd pull a boat, too. Now that people are saying I'm too old for those stunts, I'd like to swim the 26 miles from Catalina Island to Los Angeles underwater—with oxygen provided from a boat above. You just can't stop."

Well, let him amend that. If you're going to stop anything, stop filling your body with junk, says LaLanne. "Society has gone so far awry with its eating habits. Turn on your television right now and all you'll see are advertisements telling you to drink sugar-filled soft drinks and eat foods loaded with butter, cream, and cheese. That's not to mention all the magazines telling you to smoke cigarettes and drink booze. People get addicted to all of these things. And they drag the country down, leaving millions of people feeling lousy."

In the final analysis, that's why LaLanne believes he's here: to help us save ourselves. "I can't leave this planet yet. There are millions of people out there drowning in that lake of bad health and lack of enthusiasm. The biggest measure of the quality and success in life is how many people you can help. And I have a lot yet to do."

Galen Rowell, Adventure Photographer

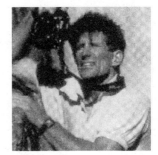

Galen Rowell is one of the nation's premier adventure photographers and an expert mountain climber whose commitment to health has helped him conquer some of the world's most challenging peaks and rock faces. Now in his fifties, Rowell has led an expedition to Mount Everest and made the first 1-day ascent of Mount McKinley in Alaska.

Nearer to home, he has made more than 1,000 climbs on the rock faces of Yosemite National Park and the High Sierra.

His photos have graced the pages of *National Geographic, Life, Outside,* and numerous calendars. His work is also featured in a dozen of his own books, including *My Tibet,* written with the Dalai Lama.

"I've always had a high degree of personal energy that empowers my work as well as my play," Rowell says. "When I stay fit, I can do things that others do and record them on film without getting left in the dust."

Rowell realized the advantages of being fit in 1974 during a 16-day, 80-mile cross-country ski trip through the White Mountains of California. Rowell, who was 33 at the time and a bit out of shape, set up camp with three friends in wind-packed snow at 13,000 feet. To his surprise, his 43-year-old campmate got up in the morning and took off running to see how it felt. The older man had been consistently stronger than Rowell on the trail. He told Rowell that he ran daily in the city and offered to take him out sometime.

"When he later took me on a 9-mile hill run, I made it, but I was completely whipped," Rowell says. "I began running regularly then and dropped from a high of 185 pounds to 145 a year later at the end of a hard expedition. I eventually put on 10 pounds and have stayed about the same ever since."

Once a week, he runs up to 10 miles at full race pace. Other weekly workouts include 9-milers on Tuesday mornings and mountain biking on Fridays. He also does extensive rock climbing, for which he trains by climbing on local boulders or using a home climbing simulator in his garage.

Rowell prefers doing several high-intensity workouts a few times a week to daily workouts of lower intensity. He limits fat and avoids red meat, but he never keeps a food journal or counts calories or grams of fat. "Moderation is key here," he says. "When I'm on the road, I'll sometimes eat a hamburger or slab of prime rib, and I'll have a beer or two with dinner, but rarely more."

And although he's at an age where most men start slowing down, relaxing and taking it easy isn't Rowell's style.

"When I'm in the mountains or on a long run, I rarely feel any different than I did at 30 or even 25," Rowell says. "For me, keeping fit is simply the best investment I can make in my future."

Part 7

LIFTING WEIGHTS, LOSING WEIGHT

Strength Training for Instant Results

There's no question that aerobic workouts are a great way to burn fat. But they're not the only way. In fact, the fastest, most efficient way to lose weight and get in shape is to combine aerobic exercise with weight training.

"Resistance training builds muscle much more quickly than aerobic activity, which mainly improves the cardiovascular system," Morris B. Mellion, M.D., clinical associate professor of family practice and orthopedic surgery at the University of Nebraska Medical Center in Omaha. "And muscles are a major source of metabolic activity. More muscle mass means more metabolic activity."

Put another way, the more muscle you have, the more efficient your body is at burning fat. Men who start weight-training programs report feeling toned after the first sessions. And in a study at the University of Maryland, men who lifted weights for 4 months shed 4 pounds of fat and added about 4 pounds of muscle. Better yet, almost half the fat lost was from their guts.

There can also be more intangible, but infinitely more satisfying, benefits. Like having larger biceps. A bigger chest. Stronger thighs. In other words, self-confidence and satisfaction—and with it the desire to keep coming back for more.

GETTING STARTED

One of the great things about lifting weights is that anyone can do it. You don't have to be athletically inclined. You don't even have to talk with a heavy Austrian accent. But there are some strategies that can make your entry into the weight world a little bit easier.

Pick your place. These days, it's possible to set up a tidy home gym in the garage or spare bedroom without spending more than a few hundred bucks for some free weights and perhaps a bench. It's convenient, parking is easy, and you don't have to wait for some monster with 32-inch arms to step aside and let you work in.

On the other hand, you probably don't have amenities such as a whirlpool or snack bar in the basement. It can be lonely and boring to work out alone. Plus, you don't have more experienced people milling around to answer your questions or to just hang out with.

Combine machines with free weights. There has been much debate about which type of lifting gives the better workout: barbell-style free weights or the machines popularized in upscale clubs.

In fact, both can provide an excellent workout. Bodybuilders typically prefer free weights because they can confer bigger improvements at a faster rate. The machines, however, are safer to use and easier to set up. Plus, you can work out on your own without depending on a partner to spot for you. Try both to see which you're more comfortable with.

GET FIT FAST

Although lifting is good for cardiovascular fitness, stress relief, and weight loss, what good are those things if you don't also look better in a T-shirt and jeans? To get the most gain from your strain, here's what experts recommend.

Don't forget to breathe. When lifting, a lot of guys literally forget to breathe—a trick that can send blood pressure skyrocketing and starve your brain of oxygen. Proper breathing means exhaling when you push, thrust, or lift. Then, inhale when you release.

Set reasonable goals. Unless you're moving to Muscle Beach or trying for a role in the next Stallone flick, a standard lifting regimen is 10 repetitions of each exercise—curls, bench presses, whatever. The goal is always to keep your muscles challenged but

WEIGHT-LIFTING LINGO

Every hobby has a specialized vocabulary, and weight lifting is no exception. Here are the basics you'll want to know.

Rep. Short for repetition, this means one completed exercise.

Set. This refers to a completed number of reps. For example, doing 3 sets of 8 arm curls means you did 24 curls.

Overload principle. Muscles must be taxed beyond what they are accustomed to in order to achieve strength and endurance gains. If your workout seems too easy, it probably is.

Concentric phase. When you're lifting, your muscles contract—the concentric phase. When doing a biceps curl, for example, the concentric phase is when you lift the dumbbell.

Eccentric phase. Also called the negative phase, this is when the muscle lengthens. With the biceps curl, the eccentric phase is when you slowly lower the weight.

not overly stressed. Not only will you get stronger, you'll also have the muscle definition to prove it.

Start light. Men are competitive, which is why the most common sight in any gym is the weight-room warrior—the guy who piles so much weight on the bar that he's woofing like a walrus and his head looks like it's going to explode.

When it comes to lifting, good form counts more than sheer weight. As a rule of thumb, limit the amount you lift to about 70 percent of your ability. In other words, if you're capable of lifting 100 pounds, put 70 pounds on the bar. You're going to be lifting it more than once, and that last lift will feel a heck of a lot heavier than the first.

Lift less—more often. If your goal is to get stronger rather than to add muscle mass, consider lifting light weights at high repetitions. In one preliminary study, Australian researchers got good results by having people lift at only 20 percent of their max-

imal capacity and do multiple sets with a high number of repetitions.

Add weight to bulk up. If you're less interested in getting strong than in building a mighty chest or massive thighs, forget the strategy of high repetitions and low weights. Go for higher weights and lower repetitions.

If, for example, you would normally do several sets of 10 repetitions using about 70 percent of your maximum weight, try doing sets of only 5 repetitions using 85 percent of your max. Tool around a bit to find what works for you, and don't overdo it.

Muscle in on the big guys. Going to a gym can be intimidating at first. You may feel as though you're Ichabod Crane at a Mr. Universe competition. But most gym rats are nice guys, even the ones who look like Godzilla. They're happy to give beginners a hand when it comes to the finer points of pumping iron. Just observe commonsense etiquette—like saying "sir" to the big guys.

The Gear You Need

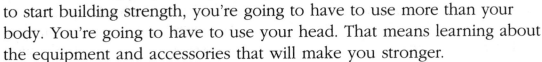

Pushups, crunches, and calisthenics are all well and good, but if you truly want to start building strength, you're going to have to use more than your body. You're going to have to use your head. That means learning about the equipment and accessories that will make you stronger.

And they run the gamut, from simple tools with one function to massive contraptions so elaborate you'd think Rube Goldberg designed them. But believe it: Every equipment or accessory choice you make, from the shoes on your feet to the weights you heft, can have a direct impact on your fitness. Here's an overview of the gear you must have as well as what you might want.

FREE WEIGHTS

Perhaps more than any other items, free weights are the weapons of choice in your quest for strength and weight loss. And well they should be—nothing will make you fit faster.

"The fact is, you can get a more complete workout with free weights than with machine weights. Machine weights are supported by the machine. Free weights are supported only by your muscles," says Steven McCaw, Ph.D., associate professor of biomechanics at Illinois State University in Normal. Dr. McCaw and his colleague, Jeff

Friday, a strength and conditioning coach at Northwestern University in Evanston, Illinois, studied the differences between machine and free weights and found that exercisers actually used more muscles when they exercised with free weights. "There are a lot of secondary muscles that get exercised with free weights that you just don't use on a machine," Dr. McCaw says.

All free weights are not necessarily created equal. There may be vast differences between the ones in the gym, those on sale in the sporting goods store, and the plastic, sand-filled barbell set you left in your parents' basement. We asked exercise experts and equipment designers for their insights. Here's what they recommend.

Olympic weights. In the world of free weights, experts agree that the gold medal goes to the cast-iron Olympic weight set.

"It's a nice, basic design, very straightforward, and easy to use. And if you're buying weights for a home gym, you can get a completely affordable package of weights that will let you do a lot of different exercises," says Tim Krivanek, an equipment designer for National Barbell Supply in Cleveland. A basic Olympic set includes 255 pounds of weight plates, a 45-pound straight bar, and two spring clips. Prices for the basic set range from $100 to $300, so shop around. "Then, you can always buy additional weight plates to augment your workout—they'll run you about 40 to 50 cents a pound," Krivanek says. That's cheaper than hamburger, and not nearly as fattening.

Spring-loaded collars. To keep those weight plates from sliding off the bar, make sure that you use spring-loaded collars. "The screw-on clamps are a pain to remove. That makes it harder to change weights for different exercises," says Krivanek. With a spring-loaded collar, you just squeeze it, slip it on the bar, and let go. Most basic weight sets come with two clamps; replacements can cost $10 to $20.

A bench. Don't even bother buying weights unless you're going to buy a bench. "A free-weight barbell set isn't much good without a bench. You can't do a good workout unless you have one," says John Amberge, a certified strength and conditioning specialist and director of corporate programs for the Sports Training Institute in New York City. Plus, there's a safety aspect to think about. If you're all alone in the basement and you suddenly need to set that barbell somewhere, where do you put it? Experts recommend an Olympic power bench, which has safety catches—vertical posts with several brackets to rack the weight off at various points if you're unable to complete the full range of motion. By it-

self, an Olympic bench with safety standards will set you back about $400 to $500, but Krivanek says that you can save money on a total weight-and-bench system if you negotiate a package deal.

"Some stores have a regular deal where, if you buy a bench, they'll give you the weights for, say, $99. If the place where you're shopping doesn't advertise a deal like that, ask the salesperson anyway—most stores will give you a break," he says.

Dumbbells. Even after they've invested in the Olympic weight set and bench, smart lifters add a few dumbbells.

"What's nice about dumbbells is that they give you a little more range of motion than the basic weight set. When you're doing a flat bench press with a barbell, for example, you can only come down so far before the bar hits you in the chest," says Krivanek. "With dumbbells, you can go down just a little bit more, getting that greater range, that greater stretch." Plus, you can exercise each arm individually, which keeps your dominant hand from doing most of the work. Start with four dumbbells: two 15-pounders and two 25-pounders. All four will run you about $50 total.

MACHINES

Although free weights offer a superb way to lose weight and tone your midsection, machine weights—circuit-training machines and home gym systems—do have their place in a workout.

"If you belong to a club and you have access to circuit machines, or you already own a home gym, there's no reason not to incorporate it into your workout," Dr.

McCaw says. Although you work more muscles on free weights, machine weights allow you to work safely with heavier weights. The machine prevents the loaded bar from falling and crushing your body.

In the home-gym arena, there's a raft of styles, technologies, and prices. Here's a look at the different systems.

Weight-stack systems. Weight stacks are as close as you'll come at home to the machines at health clubs. They give a very professional workout. "Some are just as good as what you'll find in a fitness club, and, again, a machine-weight system like that ensures a smooth, stable, safe lift," says Krivanek. But you get what you pay for: Weight-stack systems start at around $700.

Body-weight systems. The least expensive systems—running $300 to $500—often don't involve weights at all. "Some low-end ones rely on your body weight," explains Krivanek. You sit on a bench, lift the bar, and suddenly the bench—and you—are moving up and down. You can change the resistance by adjusting the fulcrum that seesaws your body up and down. These aren't your best choice. It's cheaper and just as easy to do situps and pushups.

Other resistance systems. Because weight stacks are so expensive and because less costly body-weight systems may not give you enough of a workout, some manufacturers hit a happy medium with home gyms that rely on some type of resistance-applying device, such as flexible rods, rubber weight straps, or hydraulic cylinders. The main difference among these systems, says Krivanek, is the feel of the motion. "The disadvantage to the resistance-type home gym is the lack of durability. Component parts will wear out faster," he says. On the other hand, these midrange systems are convenient and relatively affordable—$500 to $1,000—and are fine if you're looking for a modest, maintenance workout.

OUTFITTING FOR FITNESS

Clothes make the man, but they can also help you make the most of your workout. With the proper clothes, you can keep your body temperature consistent, preventing overheating. Plus, the gear you choose for your hands and feet can help you keep a grip on workout surfaces.

"The more comfortable and appropriate the clothing, the better you'll feel when you're exercising," says Budd Coates of Emmaus, Pennsylvania, a four-time Olympic Marathon Trials qualifier and a consultant to *Men's Health* and *Runner's World* magazines. And, as Coates points out, some apparel is absolutely essential for a safe workout.

Wear sweats for comfort. Heavy cotton sweatshirts, shorts, and pants are perennial favorites. Nice and loose, they also soak up sweat, which keeps you from feeling too funky. You have to be sensible with what you wear, though. It doesn't help to bundle up in a futile attempt to sweat off weight. "You'll just overheat yourself," Coates says.

Give Lycra a try. The latest synthetic fabrics—nonabsorbent polyesters such as Lycra—do a great job at wicking away moisture from your body. That's important—it helps to regulate your body temperature. The drawback is that if you're not used to it, this high-tech clothing can seem constricting or, worse, make you feel like a refugee from a Richard Simmons video. But it's worth trying. Just get a pair of Lycra shorts and wear a T-shirt or sweatshirt to cover them. No one's looking at you—trust us.

Make life easy with cotton. If you can't get used to the feel of Lycra, Coates recommends wearing the tried-and-true cotton-shorts-and-T-shirt wardrobe. "Cotton is really the best material for absorbing perspiration during workouts," says Coates, "and it's cooler."

Get a grip. When you're lifting weights, get yourself a pair of padded, fingerless, leather weight-lifting gloves (about $12 to $20 a pair). Besides saving your hands from countless blisters, they'll help you keep a tight grip on the bar.

Get the right shoes. Obviously, you need different foot gear depending on which sport you play: high-tops for hard-on-the-ankle sports like basketball, for example, or shoes with a balance of cushioning and support for running. For weight workouts, you may want to look at a good pair of cross-trainers.

"Midcut cross-trainers provide a good base of support, which is important when you're lifting weights. Plus, you have cushioning for those dynamic activities in the weight room," says Tom Brunick, director of the Athlete's Foot Weartest Center at North Central College in Naperville, Illinois, and footwear editor for *Runner's World* magazine. "You can do a little bit of everything with a shoe like that. You can do weights, then jump on the stairclimbing machine, for example."

COMBINING WEIGHTS AND AEROBICS

As beneficial as weight lifting is, you're going to have to devote some time to get-

WHEN TO WEAR A BELT

According to Norse mythology, the thunder god Thor owned a magic belt. Whenever he strapped it on, he was endowed with fantastic strength, which came in pretty handy against trolls and frost giants.

Today, weight lifters like to think they also have magic belts, ones that make them stronger. They're called weight belts—big slabs of leather that lifters wrap around their lower backs. For decades, bodybuilders have sworn by them, but now some experts are saying that you should give them up. Just like Thor and his magic belt, the reputation of weight belts is based more on myth than on fact.

"They may protect the back in certain exercises if worn correctly," says Steven McCaw, Ph.D., associate professor of biomechanics at Illinois State University in Normal. The problem is that many lifters end up using belts as crutches, relying on them to help them lift weights when what they really should be doing is strengthening the muscles around their spines. Wearing weight belts regularly is controversial, but exercise physiologists do recommend their use for lifting while recovering from lower-back strains.

SLIDE AND STEP AEROBICS

Way over on the other side of the club, you may have noticed those Lycra-clad bodies hopping up and down or sliding side to side and wondered: What the heck are they doing?

Those exercises are called slide and step aerobics. They use very simple equipment and they burn a lot of calories in a hurry. They may be worth adding to your workout.

"Steps work like stairclimbing machines, only they're not as mechanical," says John Amberge, a certified strength and conditioning specialist and director of corporate programs for the Sports Training Institute in New York City. You step up and down at varying rhythms on the steps, which usually come in adjustable heights.

Slides, meanwhile, are rectangular plastic or vinyl strips on which you slide from side to side, mimicking the motions of skating. "Slides are good because they enhance your balance skills and improve leg strength," Amberge says. "Both are great for improving heart and lung capacity and are great warmup exercises before weight training."

ting your heart pumping. And if weather conditions or time constraints keep you indoors, that means exercising with devices that look like they're doing all the work for you—aerobic machines and accessories.

"These machines help to train your cardiovascular system, which is as important as—if not more important than—just weight training," Amberge says. Weight training may get your heart beating faster and make your breathing heavier, but it doesn't get your heart rate up to the consistent, higher training level that's so important for losing weight and keeping your cardiovascular system healthy.

Treadmill. Experts say that this is one of the most popular machines, especially for men. This might be because of the collective memory of watching the Six Million Dollar Man hit 60 miles an hour every week on *his* treadmill. Granted, you won't need the mile-a-minute setting on the average

treadmill, but you can see how fast and how far you're running, which is nice. Plus, you can increase or decrease the pace or the incline of the treadmill so you can have an uphill or downhill workout. Best of all, some of these devices feature handy emergency shutoff switches so you won't end up like another TV icon, George Jetson, yelling for Jane to stop this crazy thing.

A basic treadmill—nothing more than a conveyor belt with handles—costs a couple of hundred bucks. You don't need to be a Six Million Dollar Man to afford higher-end models with inclines, digital readouts, and built-in heart-rate monitors. But they are selling briskly above the $1,300 mark.

Stairclimber. This one is easy to learn and doesn't require a ton of coordination. You can program it for different levels of difficulty, and some models even monitor calorie burn off and heart rate. Prices range from about $1,000 to more than $2,000. You may find one that's significantly less expensive, but try it before you buy it. Many of the smaller steppers don't have a wide support base. The result is that they're unstable and have been known to flip over in the heat of a furious workout.

Stationary cycle. This device is great for times when your schedule or the weather forbids a bike ride. Newer cycling machines even have heart-rate monitors built in: Grip the handles and you'll get a reading. If you're not up for the expense—cycles with heart-rate monitors and other bells and whistles will run you around $1,000 or more—Amberge suggests checking your local bike or sporting goods shop for a wind trainer or a turbo trainer. Many stores also sell a roller wheel that positions the rear wheel of your road bike off the floor, converting it into a stationary bike for a little more than $100.

Rower. This machine provides a powerful workout not just for your heart and lungs but also for your arms, legs, and back. Some models feature built-in screens that allow you to race against an onscreen opponent. Prices range from $200 for a basic model to well over $1,000 for the built-in arcade game.

Cross-country skier. One of the most aerobic machines around, a cross-country skier can also be one of the most finicky. "They're great because they mimic the actions of cross-country skiing," a sport that is tremendously aerobic, Amberge says. But the machines, like the sport, take some getting used to, since your feet are sliding backward at the same time that your arms are swinging forward. Expect to spend around $600 to $800.

EXERCISE EXTRAS

Some exercise equipment isn't vital to your fitness, but it sure makes life easier. And easy is good. After all, exercising with weights is hard, sweaty work. Having some convenient and helpful extras handy will make it more enjoyable. Here's a sampling of items you may be glad to have.

Mats. Experts agree that you shouldn't do any floor exercises on a hard, unyielding surface. Instead, use an exercise mat. Inexpensive (some cost about $10), convenient, and easy on the body, exercise mats are great for doing crunches, stretches, and other calisthenics. And you can roll them up and stash them in a duffel bag.

Rope. Another take-anywhere bit of equipment is a jump rope. It can improve your balance when you're weight training and give you explosive power for your favorite sports. As if that's not enough, rope jumping also makes a great exercise for your heart and lungs and will burn tremendous numbers of calories. But watch the surface you're jumping on, Dr. McCaw cautions. Look for soft flooring, not concrete.

Ankle and wrist weights. Priced at $10 to $15 a pair, ankle and wrist weights can turn a minor exercise into a major calorie burner. Doing moderate exercises with slow motion is the key. "Swing around too much while you're wearing weights—say, while you're running or doing jumping jacks—and you can damage muscles and joints," warns Dr. McCaw. On the other hand, wearing weights while doing chinups can magnify your workout so that you're lifting more than just body weight.

Flexing and Flexibility

Behind any successful team is an accomplished coach. Coaches work behind the scenes. They don't get the headlines or make the dazzling shots, but without them the best teams would grind to a halt. Muscular flexibility is like that. Strength and endurance get all the glory.

Men want to hoist hundreds of pounds or cycle up mountains or make the winning shot. Flexibility doesn't get much attention.

That's too bad, because flexibility is what keeps you in the game. It allows for better physical performance by making it possible to use your muscles more fully. It helps prevent debilitating injuries. It will even make you look stronger and leaner by improving your posture.

"Flexibility is one of the key components of a balanced fitness program. When you're talking balanced fitness, you're talking strength training, cardiovascular training, and flexibility training," says Ed Burke, Ph.D., associate professor at the University of Colorado at Colorado Springs and vice president of the National Strength and Conditioning Association.

Flexibility is simply the ability to get the full range of motion out of a joint. If you can no longer serve tennis balls as well as you used to or, more practically, if you find

it more difficult to twist in the driver's seat to glance behind you, you could have a flexibility problem.

The improved range of motion that comes with flexibility will help with any of the activities men use to lose weight, Dr. Burke says. When you're running or bicycling, it will help you go farther with more comfort. When you're lifting weights, it will help your muscles grow evenly and thoroughly.

And speaking of strength training, forget the notion that more muscle means less flexibility. "There is absolutely no evidence that strength gains come at the expense of flexibility," asserts Wade A. Lillegard, M.D., director of the primary-care sports medicine fellowship at the Uniformed Services University of the Health Sciences in Bethesda, Maryland. "You can have a bodybuilder or power-lifter who's just as flexible as a dancer if they include stretching as part of their exercise routine."

ARE YOU FLEXIBLE?

Here are some easy ways to test your flexibility. If you have back, hip, or hamstring problems, check with your doctor before proceeding.

Hamstrings. Lie on your back with your butt against a wall and your legs extended up. Your knees should be bent, with your heels against the wall.

Slide your heels up the wall as you slowly straighten your knees. Don't force the stretch. Move your butt away from the wall a few inches until you can find a position that you can hold for 30 or more seconds. If you can straighten your knees comfortably without moving your rear away from the wall, your hamstrings are flexible. If you had to move your rear more than 2 inches away from the wall, they aren't.

Shoulders. Raise one arm like you're asking a question in class. Bend that elbow and reach down your back. Put the back of your other hand against your middle back and move it up. If your fingers meet, your shoulder is flexible. Then, try it on the other side.

Hips. Find a sturdy, knee-high surface, like a weight-room bench. With your feet flat on the floor, lie back on the bench with your thighs parallel to the floor. Pull one knee up to your chest. If you can comfortably keep the other foot flat on the floor, your hip is flexible. Switch legs to test the other side.

A JOINT APPROACH

The motion of a joint is affected by three things: the shape of the bones that meet in the joint, the surrounding ligaments, and the elasticity of the tendons and muscles involved. That last factor is one you can control: You make a joint more flexible by regularly stretching the muscles and tendons surrounding it.

Muscles that are not stretched frequently become shorter and tighter—particularly muscles that are kept strong through regular activity. Stretching is thought to lengthen small parts of the muscle fiber called sarcomeres. When a muscle is first stretched, the nerves get, well, nervous. They send messages to the muscle, telling it to contract to protect itself

from overstretching. When you hold the stretch for 20 seconds or more, the nerve impulses fade and allow a more thorough, more comfortable stretch.

Stretching routines are usually simple. They should be part of any training program, whether that includes walking, running, swimming, or lifting.

EASY STRETCHING

"Stretching is very important before a workout so you don't go into it with really tight, cold muscles," says Wayne W. Campbell, Ph.D., an applied physiologist at Noll Physiological Research Center at Pennsylvania State University in University Park. "It's equally important to do stretching after a workout so that your body's had a chance to relax while it's still doing things, as opposed to just abruptly stopping it."

Warm up before stretching. To stretch safely, you need to first prime your body, says Dr. Lillegard. Do 5 to 10 minutes of light aerobic exercise to get your blood moving and your muscles warm. Stretch, then work out. Cool down with light activity for 5 to 10 minutes more, and include more stretches. This method will help prevent pulled muscles and reduce muscle and joint soreness.

Stretch slowly. Ease the joint to the limit of its movement, until you feel resistance but not any pain. Don't stretch with jerking or twisting motions. You can injure yourself that way.

Hold the stretch. Fitness experts generally recommend holding a stretch for 20 seconds or more. In fact, researchers at the University of Central Arkansas in Conway found that a 30-second stretch was ideal for improving hamstring flexibility. They divided 57 people into groups and assigned them to do stretches 5 days a week for 6 weeks. One group stretched for 15 seconds, another for 30 seconds, and the third for 60 seconds. The people who stretched for 30 seconds acquired substantially more flexibility than those who stretched for 15 seconds. Those who stretched for 60 seconds improved no more than the 30-second bunch.

Work into it slowly. If you're just starting out, you may need to gradually increase your stretching time. Hold each stretch briefly and repeat it four times, with short rest periods in between. Do your stretches daily, including on weekends. It will take a little time, but you'll gradually notice that you're feeling more limber.

The Core Weight Workout

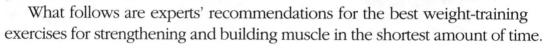

Any activity more vigorous than hefting a beer can is going to burn calories. When you're serious about losing weight, however, you have to do more than that.

What follows are experts' recommendations for the best weight-training exercises for strengthening and building muscle in the shortest amount of time.

To find out which weight-lifting exercises belong on the can't-miss list, we talked to John Abdo, certified strength and conditioning specialist and host of the syndicated fitness television show *Training and Nutrition 2000.*

We also talked to Bob Lefavi, Ph.D., a sports-nutrition and strength-training specialist at Armstrong Atlantic State University in Savannah, Georgia, and the bantamweight bodybuilding champion of the 1990 International Federation of Bodybuilding North American.

Most of the exercises they recommended allow you to work several muscle groups at once, providing more muscular bang for your workout buck. And remember that apart from the calorie burning that occurs while you lift weights, the extra muscle you gain will help burn fat even when you're not exercising.

You'll get the best muscle-building gains

if you can perform 3 sets of 8 to 12 repetitions. But if you're pinched for time, performing 1 set with a moderately heavy weight for 12 to 20 repetitions is a solid alternative. Under this 1-set scenario, if it takes you about a minute to perform each exercise and you rest and shoot the breeze for a minute between sets, you'll be hitting the showers in just 20 minutes.

INSTRUCTIONS

1. Train three times a week. Allow sufficient recovery by waiting at least 48 hours between sessions of training the same body area.
2. Vary your routines. You may train more frequently if you wish, say 4 or 5 days per week, but to do so you must rotate through different body areas in order to allow each area 48 hours of recovery time. This type of rotation is called a split routine. Another variation

is to do supersets—two exercises in succession without a rest. (It is possible to do any two exercises this way.) Supersets increase the intensity of a workout, create some variety, and can shorten a workout session. Don't do these as a beginner; supersets are for intermediate and advanced lifters. Yet another variation is to use a lighter load than usual and do 15 to 20 repetitions. Or increase the load on successive sets and reduce the number of repetitions (this last technique is called reverse pyramids). So, for example, in set 1, you might do 10 repetitions with 200 pounds; in set 2, you might do 7 repetitions with 250 pounds; and in set 3, you might do 4 repetitions with 300 pounds.

3. Always do a warmup set by performing 1 set of 6 to 10 repetitions with a light to moderate load. This minimizes the chances of a muscle strain or pull during the subsequent training period.

4. Your standard intermediate routine is 3 sets of 8 to 12 repetitions for each exercise listed below. The starting load after the warmup set should be one that is difficult to lift eight times. As your strength increases, increase repetitions per set until you can do 12 repetitions while maintaining proper form. Then, for your next session, increase the load and drop back to 8 repetitions.

Chest, Shoulders, Triceps, Biceps

Bench Press

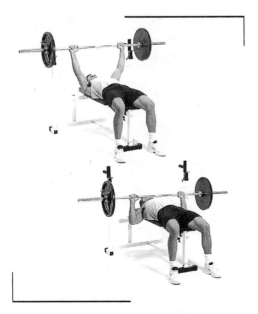

■ Lie on your back on a bench-press bench, holding a barbell above your chest with your palms up in a wider-than-shoulder-width grip. Keep your feet flat on the floor. Keep your back straight and against the bench.

■ Slowly lower the barbell to your nipple line. Don't arch your back or bounce the bar off your chest. Raise to the starting position.

Upper Chest, Shoulders, Triceps
Incline Bench Press

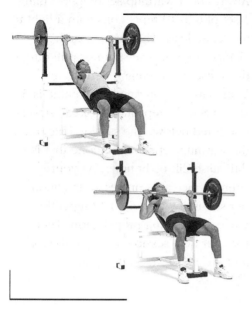

■ Lie on your back on an incline bench-press apparatus set at an angle of 15 to 35 degrees. Grasp a barbell with your palms up and your hands slightly farther than shoulder-width apart. Take the weight off the rack so that your arms are perpendicular to the floor.

■ Lower the bar to a point on your chest 2 inches below the clavicle, or collarbone, area of your upper chest. Try to keep your elbows away from your torso. Raise to the starting point, hold briefly, and repeat.

Upper Back, Rear Shoulders, Biceps
Bent-Over Row

■ With a barbell on the floor in front of you and your feet roughly shoulder-width apart, bend over at the waist and grasp the bar palms-down so that your hands are about 24 to 26 inches from each other. Keep a slight bend in your knees, and maintain a natural curve in your lower back. Raise your torso so that your upper body is parallel to the floor, and keep your arms straight. The weight should come off the floor and shouldn't touch the floor again until the set is over.

■ Pull the bar upward so that it touches your lower chest. Your elbows should point toward the ceiling. Hold briefly, then lower to the starting position.

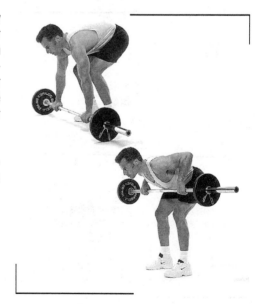

Front Lat Pulldown

■ Sit at a lat pulldown machine (unless it doesn't have a seat, in which case you can kneel underneath it). Grasp the handle overhead with a moderately wide grip. Look up slightly to tilt your head back.

■ Pull the bar down to your collarbone. Resist the weight as it goes back up. For the best gains, concentrate on squeezing your shoulder blades together as you perform the movement. Raise to the starting position.

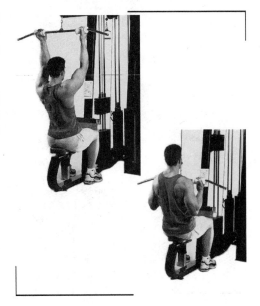

Triceps
Seated Overhead Triceps Extension

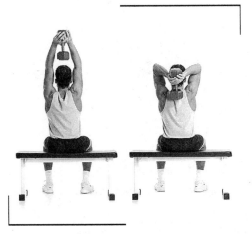

■ Sit on a bench with your feet flat on the floor and a dumbbell held overhead, your palms facing up. Your upper torso should be erect and facing forward, with a slight natural forward lean in your lower back.

■ Keeping your upper body in place, lower the dumbbell behind your head. Keep your upper arms close to your head, and lower the dumbbell in a semicircular motion until your forearms are as close to your biceps as possible. You may lean slightly forward to help offset the weight, but don't sway or arch your back. Your elbows should be facing forward. Raise to the starting position.

Seated Dumbbell Curl

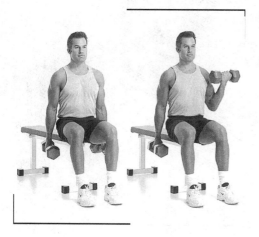

- Sit on the end of a bench, holding a dumbbell in each hand. Your back should be upright and your palms facing in.

- Slowly curl the weight in your left hand. As the dumbbell passes your thigh, twist your hand and wrist, rotating your thumb outward. For added benefit, flex your biceps at the top. Lower the weight slowly, reversing the rotation on the way down, and repeat with your right arm.

Shoulders, Triceps

Seated Military Press

- Sit on the end of a bench with your feet flat on the floor. Hold a barbell across the fronts of your shoulders with your palms facing out, your hands slightly farther than shoulder-width apart. Sit up straight, with your shoulders, back, and chest slightly out.

- Without rocking or swaying to gain momentum, push the barbell above your head until your arms are fully extended. Lower to the starting position.

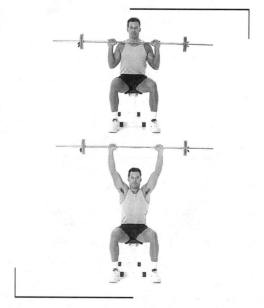

Upright Row

- Stand upright, holding a barbell with your palms down in a narrow grip, a few inches from the center of the bar. Your arms should be fully extended in front of you, the barbell at your upper thighs. Allow your shoulders to relax slightly, but keep your back straight, with a slight forward lean to your lower back.

- Pull the barbell straight up and tuck it under your chin. Your elbows should be pointing up and out. Don't sway or rock for momentum. Hold briefly, then lower to the starting position.

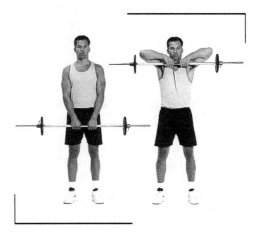

Quadriceps, Hips, Butt, Back, Calves
Back Squat

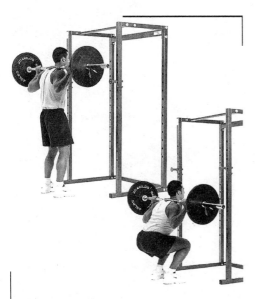

- Lay a two-by-four two steps in front of a barbell on a squat rack. Stand facing the squat rack, grasping the bar palms-down. Dip your head and step under the bar until it rests just below your neck and across your upper back. Lift the bar by straightening your legs, and carefully step backward until your heels rest shoulder-width apart on the two-by-four.

- With your head up, your back straight, your feet shoulder-width apart, and your toes facing slightly outward, squat until your thighs are parallel to the floor. Exhale as you press your body up. Do not lean forward.

Note: Wear a weight belt for this exercise to support your lower back.

Stiff-Legged Deadlift

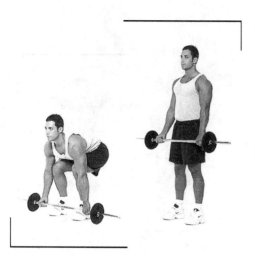

- Stand with your feet shoulder-width apart, with a barbell on the floor in front of you (the bar should be over your feet and close to your shins). Keeping your back straight, your head up, and your shoulders directly over or a little ahead of the bar, squat down and grasp the bar with your arms extended and positioned just outside your knees. One palm should face out, the other palm in.

- Stand up holding the bar, raising it straight up off the floor by straightening your thighs and back. Keep your arms extended and your back straight. Once upright, lower to the starting position.

The Core Weightless Workout

You don't have to invest in a gym membership or an Olympic weight set to build muscle and lose weight. All you need is some rubber exercise tubing, common office furniture, and determination.

"For guys out there who are thinking, There's no rubber band out there that can challenge me! I can tell you that we've done studies that show that these work for even the strongest of men," says Alan Mikesky, Ph.D., an exercise physiologist and director of the Human Performance and Biochemistry Laboratory at Indiana University–Purdue University in Indianapolis. "And the great part is that they weigh next to nothing and take virtually no space. You can throw them in your suitcase and take them on the road."

The weightless exercises that follow are recommended by John Abdo, certified strength and conditioning specialist and host of the syndicated fitness television show *Training and Nutrition 2000*, and Bob Lefavi, Ph.D., a sports-nutrition and strength-training specialist at Armstrong Atlantic State University in Savannah, Georgia, and the bantamweight bodybuilding champion of the 1990 International Federation of Bodybuilding North American.

Weightless workouts go against conventional thinking in some ways, Abdo says. Men have always believed that they have to go into a gym and lift weights to gain muscle and lose substantial amounts of fat. "But if you look at skaters or swimmers or rowers or boxers, who do hundreds of sports-specific movements, most people would agree that they have well-built physiques. Whatever exercise you are doing, if you take that muscle past its normal rep range and push beyond that—even without weights—you are going to see increases in muscular development."

The weightless exercises that follow should be performed as many times as possible until you experience muscular fatigue, Abdo says.

"You push until you can't do any more. Then, you stop," he says.

"You don't sit there for 3 seconds and then try to squeeze out more repetitions. If you have to pause 3 or more seconds, the set is over. The muscle has failed at that point, and that was the objective—to bring the muscle to failure."

Chest, Shoulders, Triceps
Pushup between Chairs

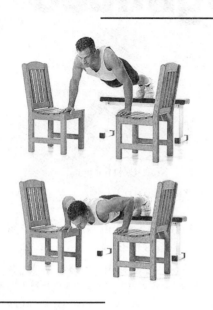

■ Position two sturdy chairs far enough from a bench or bed so that you can place your feet on the bench and each hand on one of the two chairs so that your hands are shoulder-width apart. The chairs must be far enough apart for your chest to fit between them. Get into the starting position with your legs and back rigid and your arms perpendicular to the floor.

■ Slowly bend your elbows, lowering your chest until it descends below the level of your hands on the two chairs. Pause, then press back to the starting position.

Chest, Shoulders, Triceps
Decline Pushup

■ Kneel on the floor facing away from a bench or table with your hands shoulder-width apart and under your chest. Place your feet on the bench or table behind you.

■ With your back straight and your head up, slowly bend your elbows until your chest slightly touches the floor. Pause, then press back to the starting position.

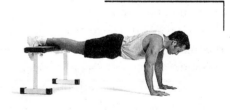

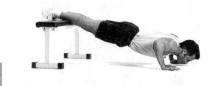

- Place your hands slightly farther than shoulder-width apart on the front edge of a sturdy desk. Straighten your arms and step back until your body forms a 45-degree angle with the floor. Your weight should rest on your hands and the balls of your feet.

- Keeping your legs and back rigid, slowly bend your elbows until your chest slightly touches the desk. Press back to the starting position.

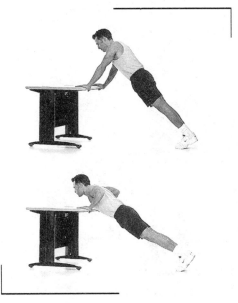

Upper Back, Rear Shoulders, Biceps, Lower Back
Seated Row with Tubing

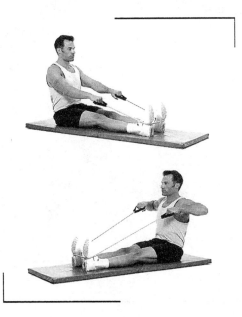

- Sit on the floor with your legs straight in front of you and your feet pointing up. Place rubber exercise tubing around your feet and grasp it by the handles. Your arms should be extended straight in front of you, and your back should be upright.

- Pull the tubing toward your chest, squeezing your shoulder blades together as you move. Return to the starting position.

Desk Dip

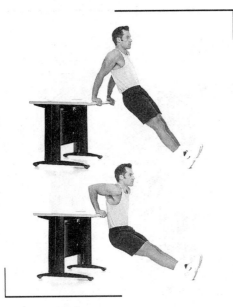

■ Stand with your back toward a sturdy desk and your palms braced on the edge, just outside the width of your butt. Move your feet forward until your butt just clears the edge of the desk. Support your weight on your heels.

■ Slowly bend your elbows, lowering your rear end toward the floor until your elbows are bent at 90 degrees. Press back to the starting position.

Biceps

Biceps Curl with Tubing

■ With your feet spread shoulder-width apart, hook rubber exercise tubing under your feet and grasp the handles.

■ With your arms at your sides and your palms facing in, slowly curl your right arm up, keeping your right elbow against your side. As your right hand passes your thigh, twist your wrist so that your palm faces up. Continue curling until your hand reaches shoulder height. Slowly lower, then repeat with your left hand.

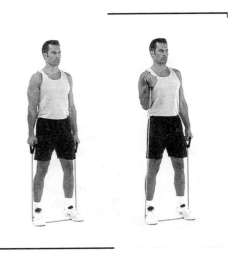

- Hook rubber exercise tubing under your feet and grasp the handles with your palms facing toward your body.

- Pull the tubing up, leading with your elbows, until your hands are tucked under your chin. (Keep your elbows out as you perform the movement.) Return to the starting position.

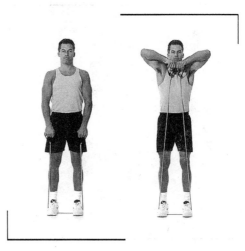

Quadriceps, Hamstrings, Butt, Hips, Back
Squat

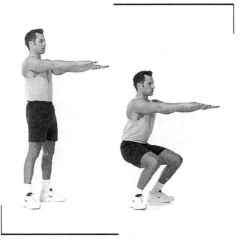

- Stand upright with your feet shoulder-width apart and your toes pointed slightly outward. Your arms should be straight out in front of you for balance, with your palms facing down. Keep your back straight.

- Squat down until your thighs are parallel to the floor. Keep your back straight through the motion, using your arms for balance. Press back to the starting position. Don't pause between repetitions; you should look like a piston pumping up and down. Feel free to shift your feet to a wider or narrower stance to isolate different portions of your leg muscles and reduce fatigue on others.

Quadriceps, Hips, Hamstrings, Inner Thighs, Butt, Calves

Front Lunge

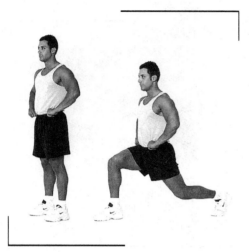

■ Stand upright with your hands on your hips or clasped behind your head.

■ Keeping your back straight, step forward with your right foot until your right thigh is parallel to the floor. Press back to the starting position, then repeat with your left leg.

Calves, Achilles Tendons

One-Leg Heel Raise

■ Stand upright with the ball of your right foot on the edge of a step or a raised object a few inches off the ground. Wrap your left foot around and behind your right ankle.

■ With your back straight, raise your right heel as high as possible, pushing down with your toes. Hold that position for 2 seconds, then slowly lower to the starting position. Repeat with your left leg.

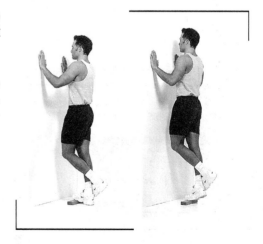

The Ultimate Fat-Burning Workout

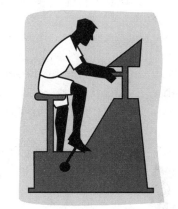

Like Tim Allen's classic character from *Home Improvement*, constantly looking to turbo-charge the vacuum, lawn mower, and toaster oven, guys naturally believe that more power is always better. Well, that's not always so, especially when it comes to fitness. Sometimes, making like an iron man isn't the best course of action—especially if your goal is to burn fat.

That's because research indicates that working harder might actually leave you fatter. "One study found that walking at about 3.8 miles per hour for ½ hour burned 240 calories, 40 percent of which was fat," says Wayne Westcott, Ph.D., of Quincy, Massachusetts, national strength-training consultant for the YMCA. "Running at 6.5 miles per hour for that same ½ hour burned 450 calories . . . however, only 25 percent of them were from fat."

Slow, easy, and relaxed is effective. The reason is that the harder you exercise, the faster you need energy. And the high-carbohydrate snack that you ate before exercising is far more easily metabolized than the layers of burgers and lager that you've been carrying around for years. To burn those off, you have to retrofit your fat incinerator.

INCREASE INTENSITY

The key to burning fat is interval training. Consider a study conducted at Laval University in Sainte Foy, Quebec, where researchers measured differences in fat loss between two groups of exercisers following two different workout programs. The first group pedaled stationary bikes four or five times a week for a moderate burn of 300 to 400 calories per 30- to 45-minute session.

The second group did the same, but only one or two times a week, and they filled in the rest of their sessions with short intervals of high-intensity cycling: They hopped on their stationary bikes and pedaled as quickly as they could for 30 to 90 seconds, rested, and then repeated the process several times per exercise session.

As a result, these slackers burned only about 225 to 250 calories while cycling. But they also burned more fat by the end of the study than the hard workers in the other group did. In fact, their fat loss was *nine times greater.*

Researchers offer a theory about what happened to the second group. "It's true that during the actual workout, the harder you exercise, the more likely it is that your body will preferentially burn carbohydrates over fat," says study leader Angelo Tremblay, Ph.D., professor of physiology and nutrition at Laval University. "But eventually, after the workout is over, your body has to replace the calories that it used. We think that the fat-reduction effect occurs after the exercise."

High-intensity interval training, anyone?

While the jury is still out pending additional research, Dr. Tremblay suggests that short-term, high-intensity training may encourage the body to find lost calories by pillaging fat stores to a greater degree than it would after moderate exercise. And your body does it long after the last wind sprint is over.

"There are studies that show that the metabolism stays elevated for 15 hours after high-intensity strength training," says Dr. Westcott. So if you open your throttle for several 60- to 90-second intervals over the course of your workout, your fat burners may be turned up for nearly two-thirds of

the day. And this is an exchange rate we can all live with.

But before you get started, you need to understand what *high-intensity* really means. Exercise is really intense if you're pedaling, running, or stairclimbing fast enough to make conversation difficult. To test yourself, try chanting the first three lines of your favorite song at about the 60-second mark. If you can't make it to line two, you're in the target zone. If you can get through the first verse of "Layla" (acoustic version), you need to work harder.

And you have to go hard for as long as you can, with 90 seconds as your goal. If you lower the intensity to last longer, your fat-burning inferno will die down to Zippo-lighter strength.

A WINNING COMBINATION

Okay, next it's time to up the ante. In addition to using the interval method, try doing it at the same time as you're weight training.

There are two reasons. First, while the high-intensity interval trainers in the Laval University study did rest between their short bursts of activity, their heart rates never dropped below 120 beats per minute. Some light resistance training will make sure that yours doesn't either. Second, you'll add muscle, another fat burner.

"Muscle is more metabolically active than fat, so each pound of lean tissue you add means that you burn an extra 35 calories a day whether you are sitting, sleeping, or watching TV," explains Dr. Westcott. "Add 3 pounds of muscle to your frame and you can figure in about an extra pound of fat burned each month, without even trying."

GET WITH THE PROGRAM

To make the principle of interval training work for you, take whatever kind of aerobic exercise machine you have—a treadmill, a stairclimber, a stationary bike—and stick it in one room. Then, pick up your resistance-training equipment—whether it's dumbbells, barbells, a machine, or just exercise tubing—and put it in an adjoining room. Of course, if you work out at a gym, they already have things set up for you. The idea here is to move back and forth between the two forms of exercise so that you get a brief—maybe 10-second—cooling-off period between each activity.

Here's the program recommended by Bob Lefavi, Ph.D., a sports-nutrition and strength-training specialist at Armstrong Atlantic State University in Savannah, Georgia, and the bantamweight bodybuilding champion of the 1990 International Federation of Bodybuilding North American.

Warm up. This is a strenuous workout, and the worst way to go about it is to explode from the starting block at top speed. Spend 3 to 5 minutes on a treadmill, bike,

or steps, moving at a slow to moderate pace. The same advice applies when you're cooling down at the end of your workout.

Run like hell. After you've warmed up, continue treading, pedaling, or stepping, but pick up the pace to heart-pounding levels. You've just started the workout proper. Do this for 30, 60, or 90 seconds, whatever you can manage initially.

Walk this way. Stop, walk down the hall (permission to pant granted), and pick up the dumbbells for a round of resistance exercise.

Lift. Do 1 set of one resistance exercise. Then, drop the weights, head back up the hall, and do the aerobics for another 90 seconds. Then, go back down the hall. Get the picture?

The circuit should include seven resistance moves and eight aerobic bouts, using your workouts of choice. It will take you about 20 minutes. Try to go around twice, for a 40-minute workout. But be prudent. Do what you can.

If 20 minutes seems to be your limit, use the remaining 20 for moderate aerobic activity—light walking or comfortable stationary biking. Eventually, you'll find yourself extending the heavy-duty workout and cutting back on the light to moderate.

Part 8

THE BEST WORKOUTS FOR YOUR MIDSECTION

Why You Need a Strong Stomach

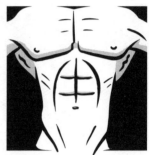

In the 1994 comedy *Junior*, audiences were treated to the spectacle of Arnold Schwarzenegger waddling around on-screen with a bulging belly. Thanks to the magic of movies, the former Mr. Universe was pregnant.

That's a better excuse than most guys have for their potbellies. But it may provide some solace that, at least in his film role, Schwarzenegger got to experience what men with extra weight around their midsections are forced to live with—aching backs, sore legs, and waddling walks.

"It's important to keep your lower back in mind if you carry excess weight around your midsection," says Richard T. Cotton, editor-in-chief of the American Council on Exercise's publication *ACE Fitness Matters*. "That added weight forces your lower back to arch, and this increases your risk for back pain and injury."

A SIX-PACK TO GO

Your abs are actually several muscle groups, all located in the midsection from just below your chest to past your waistline.

- The stomach muscle that gets the most attention is the *rectus abdominis*, the one responsible for the defined "six-pack" look that men admire. The rectus starts near the middle of your sternum and runs vertically to the lower part of your pelvis.
- The *transversus abdominis* is a deep muscle and the only abdominal muscle whose fibers run horizontally. It runs around your body much like a girdle and, in fact, has a similar function: It helps compress and support your internal organs.
- Then there are the *obliques*, which are the stomach muscles that make up your waist.

Achieving a rock-hard stomach isn't easy. It takes effort and dedication. But it isn't impossible. And the benefits are twofold: Not only will your abs look better, the rest of your body—including your back—will feel better.

A word on the exercises: Abs are about the only muscles you can work every day, so don't feel that you need to take it easy on them. Keep in mind that some experts have found that the upper ab muscles work 90 to 100 percent of their maximum ability in crunch exercises, but only about 30 percent in pelvic lift exercises. In contrast, pelvic lifts work the lower abs at about 80 percent, but the upper abs at only 30 percent. Knowing this will help you target which exercises to use for each muscle.

Despite what your gym teacher told you, don't lock your hands behind your head when doing ab work. Yanking your head up may hurt your neck or back. Instead, cup your fingertips behind your ears. Or, if you find that too difficult, try folding your hands across your chest.

Finally, keep in mind that abdominal exercises will give you definition only when they're part of a *lifestyle* fitness plan. Crunches and other midsection workouts will make the muscles stronger, but the muscles won't come into view unless you also burn calories—and weight—throughout your body. That means combining these exercises with a low-fat diet and aerobic and weight-lifting workouts.

Upper Abdominals
Crunch

The crunch is the cornerstone of many abdominal workouts. Despite the simplicity of this exercise, it puts a lot of pressure on your abs without stressing muscles in your lower back.

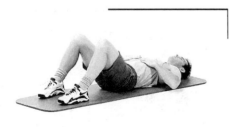

- Lie flat on your back with your knees bent, your feet flat on the floor, and your hands touching your upper abs.

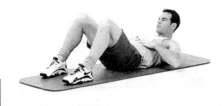

- Using only your upper abdominal muscles, curl your chest up a few inches until your shoulder blades are slightly off the floor. Hold briefly, then lower to the starting position.

Upper and Lower Abdominals
Curl-Up

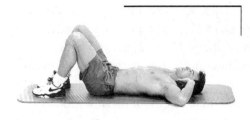

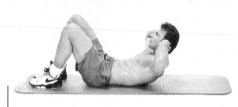

This exercise involves curling your torso into your body (as opposed to a crunch, in which you're pushing your upper body more or less straight up). You may find this bent-knee version easier than the straight-leg variety, since bringing your knees up naturally pulls your lower back to the floor.

- Lie flat on your back with your knees bent at about a 45-degree angle and your legs slightly apart. Keep your feet together, flat on the floor and about 6 inches from your butt. Cup your fingertips behind your ears.

- Without moving your lower body, curl your upper torso up and in toward your knees until your shoulder blades are as high off the floor as you can get them. Only your shoulders should lift—not your back. Hold the contraction for a second, then lower to the starting position. Repeat without relaxing between repetitions.

Upper and Lower Abdominals
Frog-Leg Crunch

The crunch has eclipsed the situp as the most widely recommended exercise for the abs. The reason is that crunches put less strain on your back than situps, and at the same time they do a good job of isolating your upper and lower abdominal muscles.

- Lie flat on your back with your knees spread and the soles of your feet together. Your knees should be as close to the floor as you comfortably can get them. Cup your fingertips behind your ears.

- Lift your shoulder blades and upper back off the floor. At the same time, slightly curl your pelvis up and in, but don't lift your lower back off the floor. Concentrate on your ab contraction. Hold the contraction for a second, then lower to the starting position. Repeat without relaxing between repetitions, keeping your abs tight.

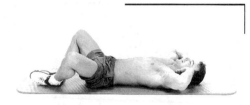

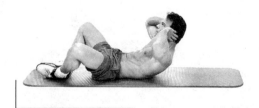

Many "twisting" sports such as golf, basketball, and tennis require intense rotations of your trunk. The muscles involved in twisting movements are the oblique (side) abdominals as well as the upper and lower abs. When doing this exercise, you should feel tension in all these muscles throughout the entire range of motion.

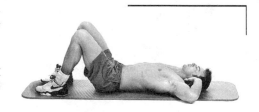

- Lie flat on your back with your knees bent. Keep your feet about hip-width apart and flat on the floor. Cup your fingertips behind your ears.

- Raise your trunk, lifting your shoulders and shoulder blades off the floor. But instead of pausing at the top, slightly twist toward your left knee. Hold the contraction for a second, then lower to the starting position. Repeat, but this time twist to your right knee. Don't relax between repetitions.

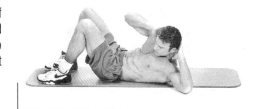

Upper and Lower Abdominals
Seated Ab Crunch

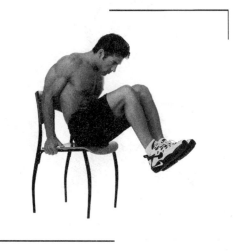

Any abdominal exercise that involves curling your upper torso works your upper abs. This exercise also uses your legs to work your lower abs.

- Sit on the edge of a stable chair. Place your hands behind your butt and grip the sides of the seat. Lean back slightly and extend your legs down and away, keeping your heels 4 to 6 inches off the floor. To begin the exercise, bend your knees and slowly raise your legs toward your chest. At the same time, lean forward with your upper body, allowing your chest to approach your thighs. Slowly return to the starting position. Do 15 to 20 repetitions, keeping your abs tight.

Upper and Lower Abdominals
Raised-Leg Crunch

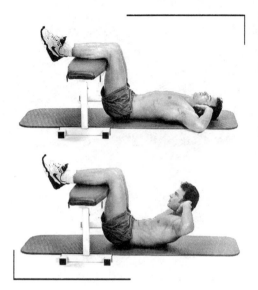

One of the quickest ways to develop the "six-pack" look is to work your upper abs. This exercise isolates these muscles, which are usually the first ones to develop fully.

■ Lie flat on your back with your knees bent and your legs up on a bench or chair. Your thighs should be perpendicular to the floor and your fingertips cupped behind your ears.

■ Lift your torso up and in toward your knees, lifting your shoulders and shoulder blades off the floor. Hold the contraction for a second, then lower to the starting position. Repeat without relaxing between repetitions.

Upper and Lower Abdominals
Decline Crunch

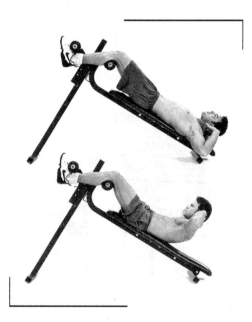

Any time you change the angle at which you do an exercise, the stresses also change. This exercise works both your upper and lower abs. And because you're working against gravity, you get a very effective workout in a short time.

■ Lie on your back on a decline board, with your ankles locked under the padded support bars and your fingertips cupped behind your ears.

■ Lift your shoulder blades up off the bench, keeping your lower back flat. Don't jerk your body to build momentum. Hold the contraction for a second, then lower to the starting position. Repeat without relaxing between repetitions.

Vacuum

The great thing about abdominal workouts is that they generally don't require a lot of fancy gear. This exercise, which requires nothing more than pulling your stomach in, is deceptively simple: You'll feel the burn almost instantly.

■ Sit in a kneeling position with your hands on your thighs. Keep your upper body upright. Breathe out, then immediately suck your stomach up and in as far as it will go. Hold for 10 seconds. Repeat.

Note: You can increase the "vacuum" time to up to 30 seconds as your stomach gets stronger. You can also do this exercise from a standing position.

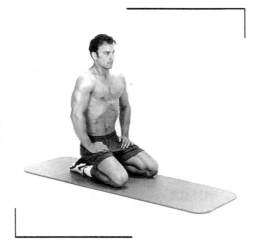

Raised-Leg Knee-In

By raising your legs, you contract, or shorten, your abdominal muscles and produce muscle tension. Lowering your legs creates an eccentric action—that is, it allows the muscles to lengthen while still remaining tense. It's the constant tension that makes this exercise so effective.

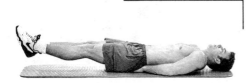

■ Lie on your back. Your arms should be close to your sides, with your hands palms-down and just under your lower back and butt. Press the small of your back against the floor and extend your legs outward with your heels about 3 inches above the floor.

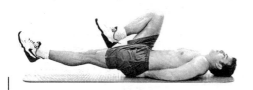

■ Keeping your lower back against the floor, lift your right knee toward your chest. Your left leg should remain hovering above the floor. Hold, then straighten your right leg to the starting position and repeat with your left leg. Keep your abs tight throughout the exercise.

Upper and Lower Abdominals
V-Spread Toe Touch

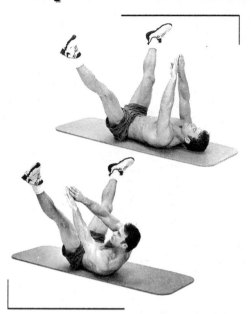

This exercise is superb for isolating your abdominal muscles while also providing a good hip stretch.

■ Lie flat on your back with your legs straight up in a V position; don't lock your knees. Raise your arms to the ceiling.

■ Curl your shoulder blades up and reach toward your left foot. Hold the contraction for a second, concentrating on your abs, then lower to the starting position. Repeat, this time reaching for your right foot. Don't pause at the lower position. Keep your abs tight.

Obliques
Oblique Crunch

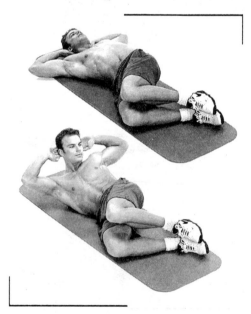

Also known as a side crunch, this exercise works your external and internal obliques, muscles that run along the sides of your upper and lower abs. Strong obliques do more than make you look good; they can also add power to your golf swing.

■ Lie flat on your back with your knees bent. Let your legs fall as far as they can to your right side so that your upper body is flat on the floor and your lower body is on its side. Cup your finger-tips behind your ears.

■ Keeping your shoulders as close to parallel to the floor as possible, lift your upper body up until your shoulder blades clear the floor. Hold the contraction for a second, concentrating on your obliques. Then, lower to the starting position. Repeat without relaxing between repetitions. Keep your abs tight. After 1 set on your right side, switch to your left and continue.

This exercise seems almost too easy—all you do is twist. But the twisting hits your oblique (side) muscles and also helps to work your abs.

- Stand upright with your feet about shoulder-width apart and your knees unlocked. Hold a broomstick across your shoulders, behind your neck, so that it's resting on your trapezius and upper deltoid muscles. Your hands should be grasping the ends of the broomstick or as close to the ends as you can reach.

- Keeping your hips still and facing forward, twist to your left as far as you can go. Then, twist to your right. Keep a slow, steady pace and concentrate on working your obliques.

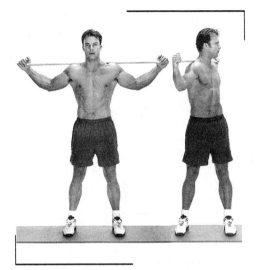

Upper and Lower Abdominals, Obliques
Hanging Single-Knee Raise

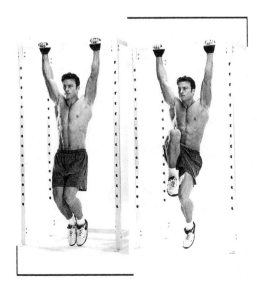

This multipurpose exercise strengthens your upper, lower, and oblique abdominal muscles as well as your hip flexor (front hip) muscles. In addition, you get a great stretch for your back and shoulders. You may want to use a pair of lifting gloves; the better grip will prolong the hanging time.

- Hang fully extended from a chinning bar with your palms facing out and your hands a little farther than shoulder-width apart. Your feet should lightly touch the floor.

- Without swinging to pick up momentum, raise your right knee toward your left shoulder as far as you can, using your abs for power. Slightly thrust your pelvis forward to help, but don't rock. Hold for a second, then lower to the starting position and repeat with your left leg, raising toward your right shoulder.

Hanging Knee-Raise Crossover

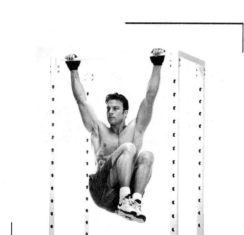

As with the hanging single-knee raise, this exercise hits all of your abdominal muscles. Because of the twisting motion, it's especially effective for strengthening and stretching your obliques.

■ Hang fully extended from a chinning bar with your palms facing out and your hands a little farther than shoulder-width apart. Your feet should lightly touch the floor. Keeping your legs together, slowly lift your knees toward your left shoulder as far as you can. Slightly thrust your pelvis forward, but don't rock or sway for momentum. Hold for a second, then lower to the starting position and repeat on your right side without relaxing between repetitions. Keep your abs tight.

Hanging Leg-Raise Crossover

When you're first starting an ab workout program, this isn't the exercise to start with—it's difficult. Once your midsection has gotten stronger, however, this provides a very effective workout for both your abs and your obliques.

■ Hang fully extended from a chinning bar with your palms facing out and your hands a little farther than shoulder-width apart. Your feet should lightly touch the floor. Keeping your feet together, slowly lift your legs toward your left shoulder as far as you can, so that your legs are at roughly a 45-degree angle to your body. You'll need to slightly thrust your pelvis forward. Lower to the starting position and repeat on your right side without relaxing between repetitions. Keep your abs tight.

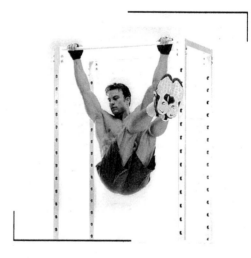

Dumbbell Sidebend

The simplicity of this exercise has made it a favorite of beginning and experienced lifters alike. Unlike many exercises targeting your side muscles, this one doesn't share the stress with your abs—it's very focused.

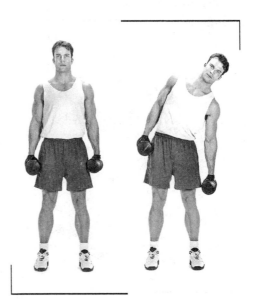

■ Stand upright, holding a dumbbell in each hand, your arms resting at your sides with your palms facing in. Your feet should be about shoulder-width apart.

■ Bend to your left side, allowing the dumbbell to drop down your left leg until you feel your obliques working. Keep your body facing front in the same plane—don't turn your torso into the sidebend. Once you've gone as low as you can, slowly bring yourself upright to the starting position, then repeat without relaxing between repetitions. Keep your abs and obliques tight. When you're done with your left side, work your right side.

Upper and Lower Abdominals, Obliques
Weighted Trunk Curl

The traditional curl provides a very effective workout, but there may be diminishing returns: For some men, it gets too easy after a while. Here's a way to keep curling at a muscle- and fat-burning pitch.

■ Lie on your back with your knees bent at a 40-degree angle. Keep your feet flat on the floor and about 6 inches from your butt. Clutch a 5-pound weight plate to your chest. Keep your lower back pressed to the floor. With your chin close to your chest, curl up until your shoulder blades are about 6 inches off the floor. Hold for a second, then lower to the starting position.

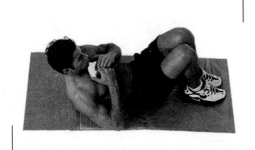

Russian Twist

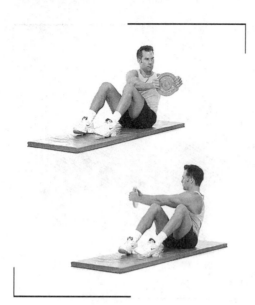

Almost any twisting motion will stretch and strengthen your obliques, but to build size and definition, it helps to add some weight to the exercise.

■ Grab a 10-pound weight plate with both hands and sit on the floor with your knees bent at about a 90-degree angle, your feet flat on the floor. Sit so that your back is at a 45-degree angle to the floor. Your body should be shaped like a Z.

■ Holding the plate with your arms extended, slowly twist as far to your right as possible. Then slowly twist to your left. Do 20 repetitions.

The Ultimate 10-Minute Ab Workout

They're the Holy Grail of fitness: washboard abs. But with your schedule, you're lucky to find time to get your wash done, let alone to try to deflate a bulging belly. We sympathize with your dilemma, friend. That's why, with the help of certified strength and conditioning specialist John Abdo, we've created this 10-minute, foolproof, gut-busting plan.

It's an exercise routine that, performed daily, will not only strengthen your waist but also carve in those cuts.

"I take an athletic approach to abdominal training," says Abdo, host of the syndicated fitness television show *Training and Nutrition 2000.* "So many athletes need to bend, twist, pivot, and rotate their torsos during their sports. These exercises and those that I've developed for my exercise video *Waste to Waist* were initially designed to improve the functionality of your torso, which includes your abdominals, obliques, and lower back. But these sports-training principles also manifest themselves as cosmetic benefits. That means that not only can you perform or function better but also your entire midsection starts looking terrific."

Before you begin, however, keep a couple of things in mind. You'll get the best burn if you do these exercises in sequence. And forget counting repetitions. Simply perform each for 30 seconds and, after a brief rest, move to the next. (That goes for all but the oblique crunch and the arm-and-leg reach; these should be performed for 30 seconds on each side.) After working through all the exercises, go back and select four favorites that train your upper abs, lower abs, obliques, and lower back.

Unless you're in great shape, chances are good that you'll have trouble performing these exercises for 10 minutes. But stay with it—that's the goal.

Go slowly if you've never exercised before or if you have had lower-back or other health problems.

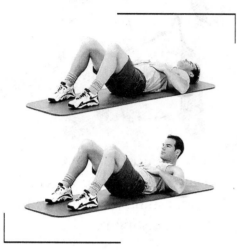

- Lie flat on your back with your knees bent, your feet flat on the floor, and your hands touching your upper abs.

- Using only your upper abdominal muscles, curl your chest up a few inches until your shoulder blades are slightly off the floor. Hold briefly, then lower to the starting position.

Lower Abdominals, Hips
V-Sit

- Sit on the edge of a bench with your knees bent, and hold on to the sides.

- Slowly pull your knees toward your chest, contracting your lower abdominals. Hold briefly, then lower to the starting position.

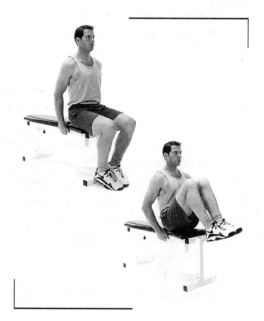

- Lie flat on your back with your knees bent. Let your legs fall as far as they can to your right side so that your upper body is flat on the floor and your lower body is on its side. Cup your fingertips behind your ears.

- Lift your shoulders and chest only a few inches off the floor, squeezing your left oblique muscles as you move. Then, lower to the starting position. Repeat without relaxing between repetitions. Keep your abs tight. After 1 set on your right side, switch to your left side.

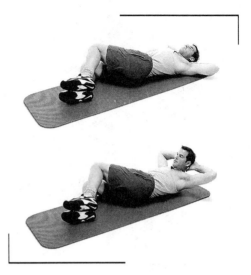

Lower Abdominals, Hips
Reverse Crunch

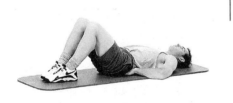

- Lie on your back with your knees bent, your feet flat on the floor, and your hands palms-down under your lower back for support.

- Slowly pull your knees toward your chest and shoulders, curling your midsection and lifting your pelvis and butt off the floor. Your mid- to upper back should stay pressed against the floor. Slowly lower to the starting position.

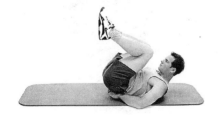

Seated Sidebend

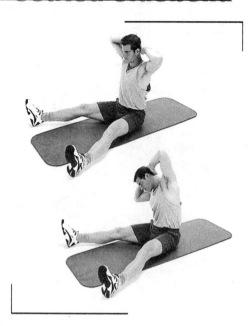

■ Sit upright on the floor with your legs spread as far apart as possible. Lift your chest up so that your back is straight, and lock your arms behind your head.

■ Lean a few inches to your right side, then swing over to the left. Continue pivoting like a pendulum while trying to tense your stomach muscles.

Jackknife Situp

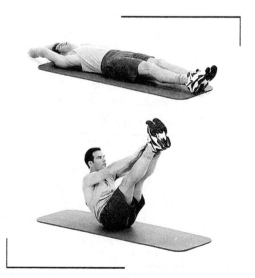

■ Lie flat on your back, placing your arms on the floor, straight over your head.

■ Bending at the waist and balancing on your buttocks, simultaneously raise your arms and legs until your hands and feet meet like a jackknife. Lower to the starting position.

Caution: Do not attempt this exercise if you have back problems.

Oblique Twist

- Sit upright on the floor with your knees bent. Your chin and chest should both be up.

- Lean back slightly, then twist your torso from right to left with short pivots as if you were performing a slow jog with your upper body. Use your arms to set a good tempo.

Caution: Do not attempt this exercise if you have back problems.

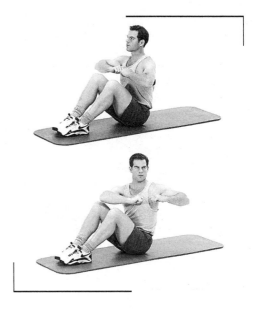

Lower to Middle Abdominals, Hips
Vertical Leg Lift

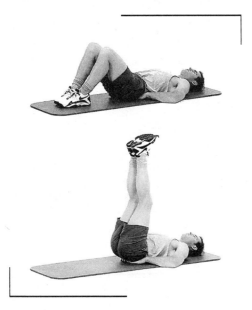

- Lie on your back with your knees bent, your feet flat on the floor, and your hands palms-down under your lower back for support.

- Pull your knees toward your chest until your thighs are perpendicular to the floor, then straighten your lower legs by lifting your feet toward the sky. For added benefit, lift your butt and lower back off the ground as if you were pressing your toes into the air. Slowly lower your butt, legs, and feet until you make contact with the floor, then repeat.

Arm-and-Leg Reach

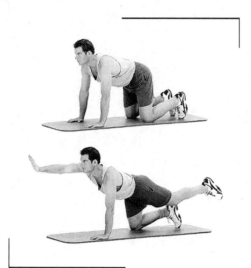

- This exercise is necessary to isolate the rear portion of your lower back, a significant and often overlooked part of your midsection. To start, get down on the floor on all fours.

- Reach with your right arm while simultaneously pushing your left leg back. Momentarily hold your arm and leg in their upright positions, tensing all of your back and butt muscles, focusing mostly on your lower back, your spinal muscles, and the rear portion of your midsection. Perform this action without touching your right hand or left knee to the floor. Relax and return to starting position. Repeat until you have completed all the repetitions for that side. Rest only a few seconds, then repeat with your left arm and right leg.

Part 9

14 EXERCISES FOR YOUR CHEST, BACK, AND ARMS

Build Your Upper Body

W hen you stand in front of the mirror, what do you see? Do you check your belly first, then your chest and shoulders? Vanity may play a role, but there are great reasons to keep your upper body in good shape.

Nearly all of the things you do, from hobbies to weekend sports, call on upper-body strength and fitness.

YOUR CHEST

Researchers once asked college-age men what they disliked most about their appearance, and a small chest ranked right up there with waist size. "If you have a large chest, it helps to de-emphasize an overly fed stomach," adds Thomas R. Baechle, Ed.D., professor of exercise science at Creighton University in Omaha, Nebraska, and executive director of certification for the National Strength and Conditioning Association.

The chest muscles are called the pectorals, or pecs. The largest of the pectorals is the *pectoralis major*. This thick, fan-shaped muscle spans most of your clavicle and sternum and attaches to your upper arm. There's also the *pectoralis minor*, a thin triangular muscle located beneath its big brother.

Men have a tendency to focus too much on their chests and ignore other upper-body muscles, says James E. Graves, Ph.D., associate professor and chair of the department of health and education at Syracuse University in New York. This is a mistake. The chest emphasis leads some guys to show off. They try to bench-press too much weight, for instance, and they don't use a spotter—a dangerous combination. And an obsession with your chest gives you an unbalanced physique, which just plain looks funny. If you want to stay safe and look great (and who doesn't?), use a spotter for heavy weights, and work all your upper-body muscles equally.

YOUR BACK

The only way to achieve the V-shaped look that men admire is to exercise your back. The main back muscles, the *latissimi dorsi*, or lats, run along your sides. Other back muscles are the *rhomboidei*, or rhomboids—compact muscles located a few inches down from your neck. The *erector spinae* run along your spine.

Whether you're starting a lifting program to lose weight or to enhance your overall fitness, you neglect your back at your peril. These muscles—and the bones they support—play a huge role in everything you do, from swinging a golf club to picking weeds.

YOUR ARMS

If there's one set of muscles that men don't need encouragement to exercise, it's the muscles in their arms. It's fairly easy to build bigger arms, especially the biceps. The triceps—the muscles on the backs of your arms—require more effort.

The biceps, incidentally, are actually two muscles: the *biceps brachii* and the *brachialis*. Both muscles help you bend your elbow, though the biceps brachii also comes into play when you move your shoulder. The triceps oppose the biceps. They extend your arm after it has been bent at the elbow.

Because the arms develop quickly, men have a bad habit of adding weights before they should—or before they need to. "It's better to grab something that's too light than to try to pick 100 pounds right off the bat," says John Skowron, a physical therapist at Raleigh Community Sports Medicine and Physical Therapy in Raleigh, North Carolina. In a standard workout, you should do 10 repetitions of each exercise with a barbell or dumbbells that are 70 percent of the maximum weight that you are capable of lifting.

Lower and Outer Pectorals
Dip

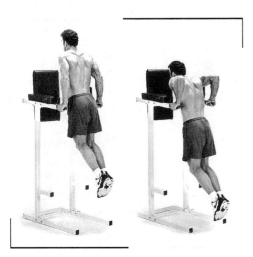

Dips are hard to do at first. If you aren't able to lift your body weight, use a step to help you get into the raised position, then maintain proper form while lowering your body. The downward motion builds a lot of strength, and you'll find that it will help get you in shape to do the complete exercise.

■ Raise yourself off the ground and onto parallel dip bars. Your hands should be gripping the bar handles with your fingers on the outsides, facing away from your body. Keep your elbows close to your sides, and slightly bend your legs if your feet are dragging on the floor.

■ Lower yourself to the point where your upper arms are parallel to the floor. Keep your elbows close to your sides, and slightly bend your legs if your feet are touching the floor. Raise to the starting position.

Bench Press

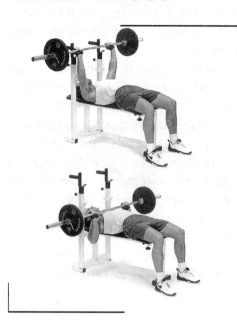

Of all the chest exercises, the bench press is probably the most widely used—and for good reason. It works several major muscles, and most men will progress rapidly.

- Lie on your back on a bench-press bench, holding a barbell above your chest with your palms up in a medium grip (hands about shoulder-width apart) or a slightly wider grip. Keep your feet flat on the floor. Keep your back straight and against the bench.

- Slowly lower the barbell to your nipple line. Don't arch your back or bounce the bar off your chest. Raise to the starting position.

Narrow-Grip Bench Press

This variation on the basic bench press involves using a narrower grip when holding the bar. Using this grip works more of the lower and inner pecs.

- Do a normal bench press with the proper form, but hold the barbell with a narrow grip. Your hands should be equidistant from the center of the bar, 6 to 8 inches apart. Decrease the weight for this exercise since it will stress your pecs from a different angle and you'll find it harder than a standard bench press.

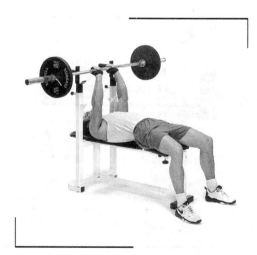

Wide-Grip Bench Press

This is another variation on the basic bench press, one that puts more of the tension on your upper and outer pecs.

■ Do a normal bench press with the proper form, but hold the barbell with a wide grip. Your hands should be equidistant from the center of the bar, a few inches farther than shoulder-width apart. Decrease the weight for this exercise since you'll find it harder than a standard bench press.

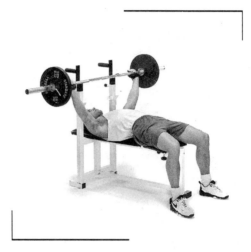

Dumbbell Fly

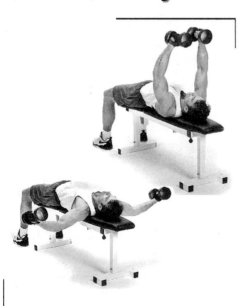

This exercise is superb for developing the middle of the large pectoralis major muscles in your chest. It also works your pectoralis minor muscles as well as your shoulders, your inner upper arms, and the muscles along your upper and outer rib cage.

■ Lie on your back on a bench with your legs parted and your feet flat on the floor. Hold two dumbbells above you with your palms facing in. The dumbbells should nearly touch each other above your chest. Your back should be straight and firm against the bench, and your elbows should be unlocked.

■ Slowly lower the dumbbells out and away from each other in a semicircular motion. Keep your wrists locked. Lower until the dumbbells are at chest level. Your elbows should be bent at roughly a 45-degree angle, while your back is straight. Raise to the starting position.

One-Arm Dumbbell Row

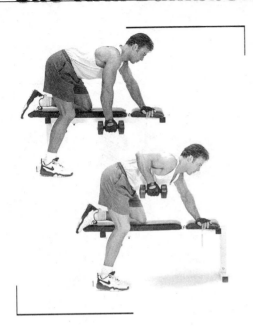

This exercise gets its name from the fact that it helps strengthen the latissimus dorsi, or lats, which are used in rowing. It will also help work your shoulder and chest muscles.

■ Stand partly over a bench, with your body weight resting on your bent left leg and your left hand, both of which should be on the center of the padded portion of the bench. With your right foot flat on the floor, hold a dumbbell in your right hand with your palm facing in toward your body. Keep your back straight, eyes facing the ground. Extend your right arm toward the ground, elbow unlocked.

■ Pull the dumbbell up and in toward your torso. Raise it as high as you can, bringing it in to your lower chest muscles. Your right elbow should point up toward the ceiling as you lift. Lower to the starting position. Finish your repetitions with your right arm, then reverse position and work your left arm.

Latissimi Dorsi
Lat Pulldown

Men tend to neglect their backs when they work out, which doesn't make much sense when you consider that nearly everyone will eventually lose time from work—or worse—because of lower-back problems. This exercise will help strengthen your back and help prevent injuries later on.

■ Sit at a lat pulldown machine (unless it doesn't have a seat, in which case you can kneel underneath it). Grasp the handle overhead with as wide a grip as is comfortable, or at least wider than shoulder-width. Your palms should face away from your body, your upper body should be straight, and your eyes should be forward.

■ Pull the bar down to your body, behind your neck. Your upper body should stay in the same upright position, but your elbows should point to the ground and slightly outward. Raise to the starting position.

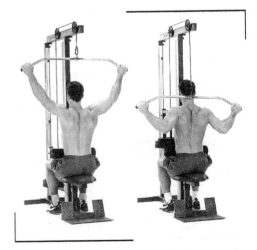

Bent-Over Row

This exercise puts quite a bit of stress on your lower back, so you don't want to do it if you're just starting out or if you've had back problems in the past. Once you're in decent shape, however, it will hit back muscles that other exercises miss.

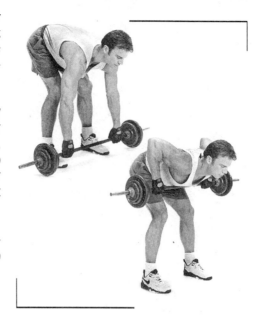

■ With a barbell on the floor in front of you and your feet roughly shoulder-width apart, bend over at the waist and grasp the bar palms-down in a wide grip. Keep a slight bend in your knees, and maintain a natural curve in your lower back. Raise your torso so that your upper body is parallel to the floor, and keep your arms straight. The weight should come off the floor and shouldn't touch the floor again until the set is over.

■ Pull the bar upward so that it touches your lower chest. Your elbows should point toward the ceiling. Hold briefly, then lower to the starting position.

Lower Back
Back Extension

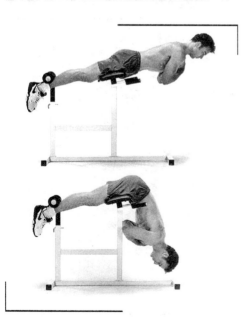

Strengthening the muscles of your lower back is one of the best ways to prevent back problems later. Your spine needs a lot of support, and strong muscles essentially anchor it in place, reducing your risk of back pain as well as of more serious problems such as herniated disks.

■ Lie on your stomach in a back extension machine with your ankles locked under the padded support bars and your groin area and upper thighs resting on the padded platform. Your hips should be over the edge of the platform and your body bent over until your back is parallel to the floor. Fold your arms across your chest.

■ Bend over at the waist, with your upper torso lowered to the point where it's just a few inches above being perpendicular to the floor. Your arms should still be crossed over your chest and the rest of your body should stay in the starting position. Raise to the starting position.

Barbell Curl

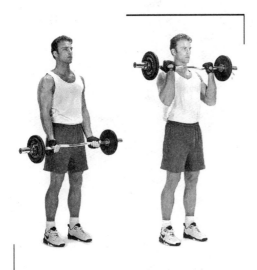

If your goal is to develop large, well-defined arms, this exercise is a must. It concentrates all of its force on the biceps, allowing these muscles to get a maximum workout in a short time.

■ Stand upright, holding a barbell with your palms up and your hands about shoulder-width apart. Your arms should be fully extended in front of you, the barbell at your upper thighs. Your knees should be unlocked.

■ Keeping your elbows close to your body, use your biceps to curl the bar slowly up toward your chin. Keep your wrists straight throughout the curl, and don't sway your back or rock your body for momentum. Lower to the starting position.

Alternating Incline Dumbbell Curl

The relaxed reclining position makes this exercise look easy, but it puts intense strain on your biceps. And because it provides good back support, you're less likely to strain a back muscle than when doing standing curls.

■ Lie on an incline bench with a dumbbell in each hand and your arms down at your sides. Hold the dumbbells with your palms facing in toward your body.

■ Curl the weight in your left hand toward your biceps. Keep your wrist straight, and don't sway your shoulder for momentum. As you curl, slowly twist your wrist out so that your palm faces up toward the ceiling at the apex of the curl. Lower to the starting position and repeat with your right arm.

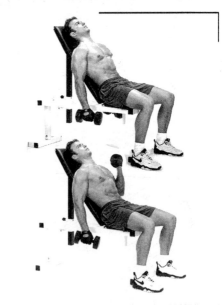

True to its name, this exercise is very effective at isolating the biceps because it prevents other muscles from coming into play. Since it works one arm at a time, both arms get an equal workout.

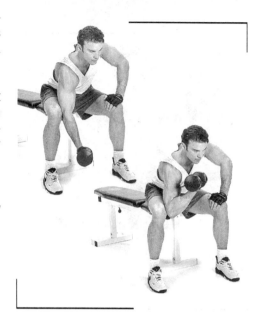

- Straddle the end of a bench, holding a dumbbell in your right hand with your palm up. Your feet should be farther than shoulder-width apart and your knees should be bent. Bend forward and extend your right arm between your legs so that your elbow and upper arm are braced against the inside of your thigh. Lean slightly to the right. Rest your left hand on your left knee.

- Curl the dumbbell toward your shoulder, bracing your elbow against your thigh and leaning on your other hand for support. Hold the curl, then lower to the starting position with control. Finish your repetitions with your right arm, then reverse position and work your left arm.

Triceps
Triceps Pulldown

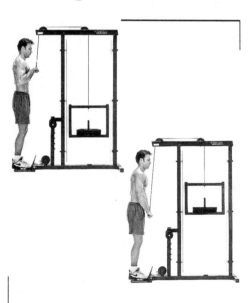

Triceps exercises are a great preliminary to chest workouts because these muscles work with your chest when you're lifting weights on the bench. This is a very effective workout that exercises your triceps at all of its attachment points.

- Stand facing a triceps pulldown machine, gripping the bar with both hands, palms facing away from you in a narrow grip. Your hands should grip the bar as high as you comfortably can while keeping your elbows in by your sides and your upper arms perpendicular to the floor.

- In a smooth motion, pull down on the bar until you've straightened out both arms and they're pointing toward the floor. Your elbows should remain close to your body, and you should feel the contraction in your triceps. Your wrists should be locked and straight. Raise the bar to the starting position with control.

Triceps
Dumbbell Kickback

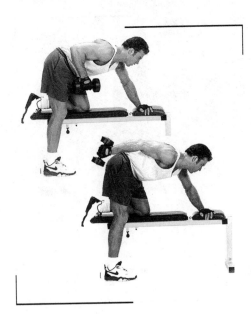

This exercise looks easy—until you try it. It focuses a tremendous amount of stress on your triceps without allowing much help from other muscles. As long as you maintain good form and control, you don't need to use a lot of weight.

■ Stand partly over a bench, with your body weight resting on your bent left leg and your left hand, both of which should be on the center of the padded portion of the bench. With your right foot firmly on the floor, hold a dumbbell in your right hand with your palm facing in toward your body. Pull the dumbbell up and in toward your torso, close to your lower chest muscles. Your right arm should be close to your rib cage, with your elbow pointing up toward the ceiling. Your back should be straight and roughly parallel to the floor.

■ Resting on your left knee and hand, extend the dumbbell out and behind your body with your right arm. You should feel the contraction in your triceps. Extend your arm until it's straight and your triceps are fully contracted. Don't lean or sway or arch your back. Finish your repetitions with your right arm, then reverse position and work your left arm.

Part 10

6 EXERCISES FOR YOUR SHOULDERS AND NECK

Command Attention with Your Strong Shoulders and Neck

It's easy to admire the posture of military men. They carry themselves with an alert energy, like peacocks in uniform. "There's something about standing tall with your shoulders back and your chest out that says power," says Sergeant Larry Brown, a retired U.S. Army and Air Force officer living in New Tripoli, Pennsylvania.

One way of getting this power posture—short of 6 weeks' basic training—is to build the muscles in your upper body, says Thomas R. Baechle, Ed.D., professor of exercise science at Creighton University in Omaha, Nebraska, and executive director of certification for the National Strength and Conditioning Association.

"Your upper-body development affects your image," he says. "When you walk into a room, you command respect by the way you carry yourself. You don't want to look like you're peeping down a dark hole."

Serious lifters spend a lot of time working their shoulders. The shoulder mus-

cles are called the deltoids. The name is descriptive, deriving from the Latin word for "triangular in outline." Weight lifters talk about the anterior, lateral, and posterior parts of the delts, meaning the front, side, and back "heads" of the muscles. Each receives specific attention from various exercises for a well-rounded appearance.

Even if you're not interested in getting that specific in your workouts, you'll see results in your shoulders fairly quickly. Almost every upper-body exercise works the shoulders to some extent, so you'll see muscle growth even when you're not doing shoulder-specific exercises. For the fastest results, however, it's worth incorporating at least a few shoulder-only exercises into your workouts.

While working your shoulders, don't be discouraged if you tire halfway through your second set. "The shoulder muscles are not designed for endurance; they're designed for strength. If you've ever tried painting a ceiling with a paint roller, you know that it doesn't take long before your shoulders wear out," says James E. Graves, Ph.D., associate professor and chair of the department of health and education at Syracuse University in New York.

Most men don't think about strength-ening their neck muscles, but they should. If your neck muscles are weak, they're likely to be injured when stress is put on your shoulders. Of course, they'll also be at risk when you're doing things that involve the neck, such as twisting your head while driving or following through on a golf swing.

There's really only one neck muscle you need to know: It's the *trapezius*. It slopes down each side of your neck, from the base of your skull to the middle of your back. The trapeziuses raise your shoulders and rotate your shoulder blades.

Trapeziuses
Shoulder Shrug

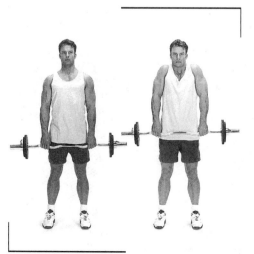

This exercise is deceptively simple. It works more than just your shoulders. It also hits major muscles in your back, including the rhomboids and the levator scapulae—muscles beneath the trapeziuses.

■ Stand upright, holding a lightly weighted barbell with your palms down in a medium grip. Your arms should be fully extended in front of you, the barbell at your upper thighs. Your feet should be shoulder-width apart, with your shoulders back but drooped down as far as they naturally will go. Your chest should be out and your lower back should be straight, with a slight forward lean.

■ Lift the barbell up and out by raising both shoulders to the front of your body. At the highest point, rotate your shoulders toward your ears, lifting them higher. Lower to the starting position.

Behind-the-Neck Press

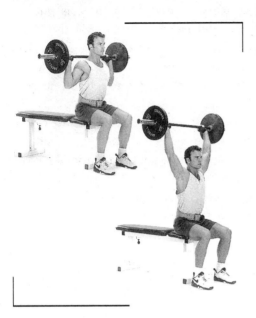

This is an excellent exercise that works many muscles—not only in your shoulders but also in your upper back, neck, and rib cage. It's difficult to control the bar at first, so begin with lighter-than-usual weights.

- Straddle the end of a bench with your feet a little farther than shoulder-width apart. Hold a barbell behind your neck and across your deltoids and trapeziuses, with your palms out, your hands shoulder-width apart, and your elbows pointing down. Your back should be perpendicular to the ground, with your shoulders back, your chest out, and a slight forward lean to your lower back.

- Lift the barbell above your head with your arms fully extended and your elbows unlocked. Don't sway or arch your upper body for momentum. Lower to the starting position.

Note: Wear a weight belt for this exercise to support your lower back.

Upright Row

It takes some getting used to, but the upright row is a good, all-around exercise that works the front of your shoulders as well as your upper back and neck. Muscles in your forearms and chest also get a workout.

- Stand upright, holding a barbell with your palms down in a narrow grip, a few inches from the center of the bar. Your arms should be fully extended in front of you, the barbell at your upper thighs. Allow your shoulders to relax slightly, but keep your back straight, with a slight forward lean to your lower back.

- Pull the barbell straight up and tuck it under your chin. Your elbows should be pointing up and out. Don't sway or rock for momentum. Hold briefly, then lower to the starting position.

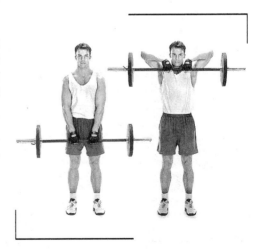

Side Lateral Raise

This simple but effective exercise focuses a lot of stress on the sides of your shoulder muscles. Men who use their shoulders a lot, for golfing, baseball, or swimming, will want to do it regularly.

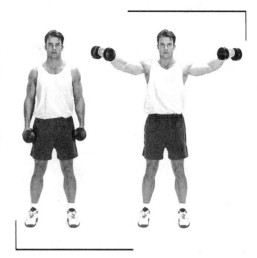

- Stand upright with your arms at your sides, holding a dumbbell in each hand, with your palms in and your elbows slightly bent. Keep your shoulders back, your chest out, and your lower back straight with a slight forward lean. Your feet should be shoulder-width apart.

- Raise both dumbbells in unison in a straight line until they're at shoulder level. Make sure your elbows are slightly bent, and keep your arms in the same plane as your torso. Lower to the starting position.

Posterior Deltoids
Bent-Over Lateral Raise

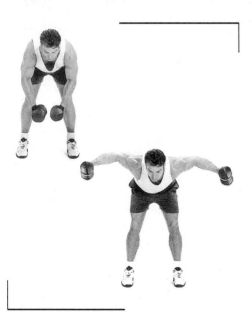

Similar to the side lateral raise, this exercise hits an even broader range of muscle targets. As with any exercise that requires you to bend over, be cautious if you have a history of lower-back problems.

- Bend over at the waist, a dumbbell in each hand. Your palms should face in, and your arms should be in front of you, elbows slightly bent. Position your feet slightly wider than shoulder-width apart, with your back straight and roughly parallel to the floor.

- Raise both dumbbells in unison out toward your sides as if you were flapping your arms. Raise your arms until they're parallel to the floor. Keep your back straight. Lower to the starting position.

Deltoids
Alternating Seated Dumbbell Press

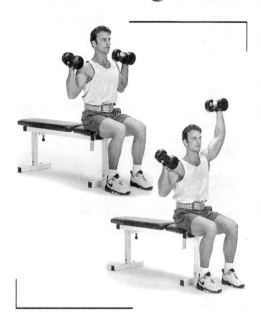

The advantage of working with dumbbells is that muscles on both sides of your body get an equal workout. Make it a point to maintain good form; there's a tendency when using dumbbells to drop the weight too quickly, which reduces the benefits.

■ Grasp two dumbbells and straddle a bench with your legs slightly parted, your feet flat on the floor, and your arms raised. Hold the dumbbells about shoulder-width apart at shoulder level, your palms facing in. Keep your shoulders back, your chest out, and your lower back straight with a slight forward lean.

■ Raise the left dumbbell up until your arm is straight, but don't lock your elbow. Lower to the starting position; then repeat with your right arm.

Note: Wear a weight belt for this exercise to support your lower back.

Part 11

10 EXERCISES FOR YOUR BUTT AND LEGS

Butt and Legs: Your Body's Secret Power Station

Whether they're working out in a gym or looking at themselves in a mirror, men tend to focus first on their upper bodies, then give some cursory attention to their legs and butts. That's why a lot of serious lifters have that carrot look—a strong torso supported by spindly legs.

One reason for this is that a man's lower half isn't as hot of a commodity in our upper-body-focused media culture. More practically, the leg and butt muscles are the largest, and they're farther away from your heart than your chest and arms are. So your body has to work harder to keep them supplied with blood and oxygen during exercise. In other words, men often neglect their legs because not neglecting them is such hard work. Most guys would just as soon spend an hour on the bench press as spend 10 minutes doing leg workouts, says Ed Burke, Ph.D., associate professor at the University of Colorado at Colorado Springs and

vice president of the National Strength and Conditioning Association.

MOBILITY AND LOOKS

When you're trying to lose weight, it's crazy to ignore your leg and butt muscles. Because they're so large, they're capable of burning tremendous numbers of calories. Any increase in size will increase your body's metabolism significantly.

Even apart from weight loss, a strong lower half makes it possible for you to do all the other things you need to do to stay in shape—walking, biking, swimming, and climbing stairs.

Here's a quick look at what these muscles are.

- The butt muscles come in three sizes: the *gluteus maximus*, *gluteus medius*, and *gluteus minimus*. The maximus, as you can guess by its name, is the biggest and most noticeable of the three. The medius and the minimus aren't as eye-catching.

  Although no one wants a weather balloon for a butt, size isn't really the issue. You should be more concerned with how toned your butt is. A strong butt helps build explosive power in your lower body, Dr. Burke says. Plus, research shows that strong glutes can alleviate back pain. So if you're among the 80 per-cent of American men who suffer from an aching lower back, working these muscles could take you off the disabled list.

- Your legs are hosts to the foot-long thigh muscles, called the quadriceps. Bringing up the rear are the hamstring muscles. Farther down, behind your shins, are your calf muscles, which enable you to walk, jump, or sprint.

  It takes patience to work your lower body. Results are nowhere near as dramatic as when you work your chest or biceps. But the payoff for fitness—and for weight loss—is considerable, so it's worth spending some time making sure that it's as strong as it can be.

Gluteal Muscles
Pelvic Lift

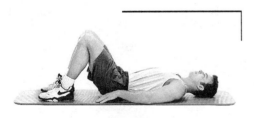
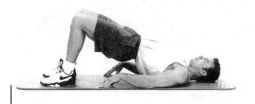

Exercises don't get any simpler than this: Lie on your back and arch your pelvis. That's it. Yet this exercise will quickly strengthen muscles in your butt. In addition, it's often the first exercise recommended for relieving back pain.

- Lie on your back with your knees bent and your feet slightly apart, flat on the floor. Your arms should be at your sides, with your hands palms-down on the floor.

- Lift your pelvis up toward the ceiling. Squeeze your buttocks together as you lift until your back is straight. Don't arch your back. Lower to the starting position.

Bent-Kick Cross

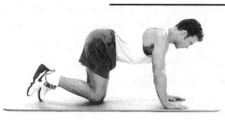

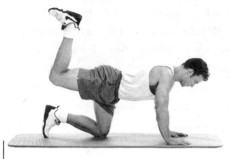

This exercise stretches and strengthens your glutes, and it's recommended for men who are just starting to get themselves into shape.

■ Get down on the floor on all fours. Raise your right leg several inches off the floor and bend it at roughly a 90-degree angle.

■ Push your right leg up and back, reaching your heel toward the ceiling. You should feel your butt contract as you push up. Your thigh should not go beyond being parallel with the floor and your leg should remain bent at a 90-degree angle. Lower to the starting position. Finish your repetitions with your right leg, then work your left leg.

Raised-Leg Curl

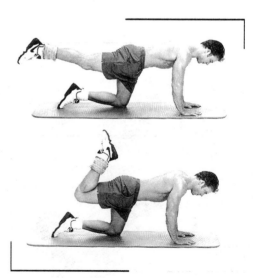

This exercise is usually combined with the bent-kick cross because both begin in the same starting position, down on all fours. It's important to maintain proper form in order to keep full tension on the muscles through the complete range of motion.

■ Get down on the floor on all fours, wearing an ankle weight on your right leg. Raise your right leg to about butt level and extend it so that it's straight, away from your body and roughly parallel to the floor.

■ Curl your heel toward your butt, keeping your thigh level and parallel to the ground. Your thigh shouldn't move much—all the movement is done below the knee. Don't sway your body or arch your back; concentrate on the contraction in your butt. Return to the starting position. Finish your repetitions with your right leg, then switch the ankle weight to your left leg and work that leg.

Standing Kickback

This exercise requires your muscles to work against resistance, which adds definition and also builds endurance.

■ Stand facing a wall, lightly holding on with your hands for balance. You should be wearing an ankle weight on your right leg and leaning slightly forward so that your whole body is in a straight line. Your weight should be shifted onto your left leg.

■ Move your right leg back as far as you can, feeling the contraction in your butt. Your knee should be slightly bent. Don't arch your back or overextend yourself. Hold, then lower to the starting position. Finish your repetitions with your right leg, then switch the ankle weight to your left leg and work that leg.

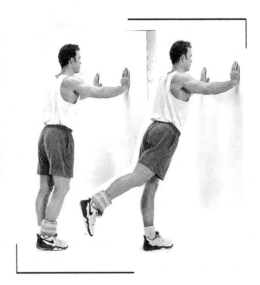

Quadriceps
Leg Extension

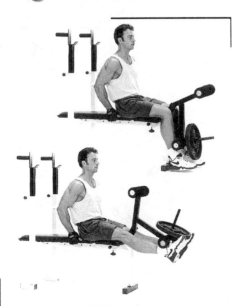

This is probably the most popular exercise for building the muscles in the fronts of the thighs as well as for working the ligaments and tendons of the knees. It's often recommended for men who do sports in which knee injuries are common, such as skiing or running.

■ Sit in a leg extension machine with your legs under the padded lifting bars and your hands grasping the machine's handles or the sides of the bench. Your knees should be bent at 90 degrees or slightly more, with your toes pointing in front of you.

■ Using the machine's handles or the sides of the bench for support, straighten your legs by lifting with your ankles and contracting your quads. Don't lock your knees at full extension, but rather keep a slight bend. Your toes should point up and out at about a 45-degree angle. Lower to the starting position.

Variations: Foot positioning changes the way your muscles are worked. Try pointing your toes back or straight to work different parts of your quads.

Hamstrings
Leg Curl

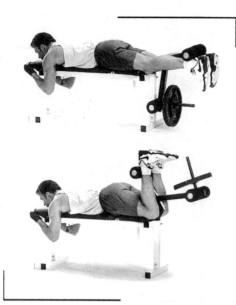

This exercise works those long muscles in the backs of your thighs. Don't expect fast results: Hamstrings take time to develop, which is why injuries are common.

■ Lie on your stomach in a leg curl machine with your ankles locked under the padded lifting bars and your knees just over the bench's edge. Hold on to the machine's handles, if any, for support. Your legs should be fully extended with some natural flex at the knee, and your toes should be pointing down.

■ Keeping your pelvis flush against the bench, curl your heels up toward your butt so that your legs bend to about a 90-degree angle. Use the handles for support, and keep your feet pointing away from your body. Lower to the starting position.

Note: Some leg curl machines are bent slightly at the end to relieve pressure from your pelvis. If yours is not, consider placing a small pillow under your pelvis. Also, your hamstrings are weaker than your quads. Use less weight for leg curls than you would for leg extensions.

Hamstrings
Leg Curl with Ankle Weights

Leg curls are easiest when you're using a machine made just for that, but you can also do them on an exercise bench by strapping ankle weights to your ankles.

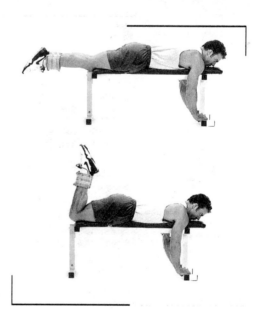

■ Lie on your stomach on a bench with both legs straight out and an ankle weight on each ankle. Your knees should be just past the bench's edge so you can bend your legs up. Your hands can be holding on to the bench's legs for support.

■ Keeping your feet together and pointed out, curl your heels in a semicircular motion up toward your butt so that your legs bend to about a 90-degree angle. Point your toes up, and don't arch your pelvis or back. Your body should remain flush with the bench. Lower to the starting position.

This is one of those exercises that looks as though any dweeb could do it all day—until you try it for yourself and discover that your calves are burning before you've completed a full set. It's faster to work both calves at once. Doing each leg separately, however, will help ensure that the calf muscles develop evenly.

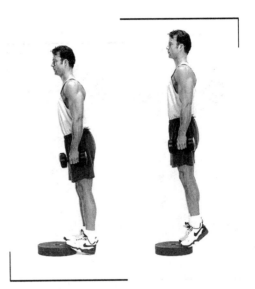

- Stand with your feet hip-width apart, with your toes on a platform raised a couple of inches off the ground. Your heels should be on the floor, and your weight should be on the balls of your feet so that you're leaning forward slightly. Hold a dumbbell in each hand, palms in, with your arms extended down.

- Rise all the way up onto your toes. Feel the contraction in your calves and pause briefly at the top. Your arms should remain in position, though your body will probably be more upright. Lower to the starting position.

Quadriceps
Leg Press

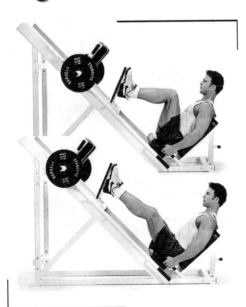

Squats are one of the best exercises for building the thighs, but they're hard for men who have back problems or who don't have a lot of flexibility. Leg presses provide nearly the same benefits, with the bonus of having a machine to support your back.

- Sit in a leg press machine with your feet on the pedals in front of you. The seat should be adjusted so that your knees are bent at about a 90-degree angle or a little straighter. Grasp the handles at your sides and hold your upper body upright but relaxed.

- Push forward on the pedals and straighten your legs until they're fully extended in front of you. Keep your knees slightly bent. Your upper body should remain upright and relaxed, and your hands should hold the handles for support. Return to the starting position.

Quadriceps
Barbell Stepup

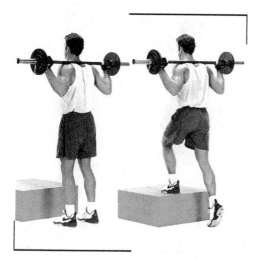

This is a good dual-purpose exercise that provides a tough aerobic workout while also increasing the strength of your quadriceps along with your hamstrings, hip flexors, and glutes.

■ Hold a barbell behind your neck with your palms out. The bar should be even across your shoulders. Stand upright with your shoulders back, your chest out, and a slight forward lean in your lower back. Face a box that's 12 to 18 inches high; stand about a foot away. Make sure it's on a nonslip surface. The box should be high enough that your knee bends at about a 90-degree angle when you step on it.

■ Place your left foot in the center of the box. Your body should be erect, and the barbell should remain in position behind your neck.

■ Your weight should be shifted to your left leg as your right foot steps up, bringing you to a standing position on top of the box with your feet together in the center.

■ Step backward so that the foot of your right leg is near the starting position, then step down with your left foot. Repeat, stepping up first with your right leg.

Note: This exercise also can be done with dumbbells.

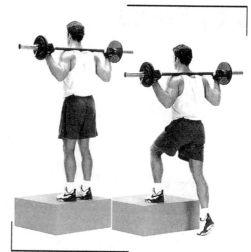

Part 12

FINDING TIME, SAVING TIME

Your Personal Time Zone

Your body follows a daily rhythm. It's called a circadian rhythm. It's an internal clock that governs most of the bodily functions you take for granted—what times you go to sleep and wake up, when you feel most alert, and when you're most susceptible or resistant to pain or illness.

Your body's clock even determines when you're at the peak of physical ability. Aeons of evolution, coupled with your unique chemistry and daily routine, set your clock at its daily rhythm.

"The more you understand how your clock works, the more you can work with it for better physical health, and the less you'll do something to disrupt it," says Phyllis Zee, M.D., Ph.D., director of the sleep disorders program at Northwestern University Medical School in Chicago and an expert on biological rhythms.

When you're trying to adopt a healthier lifestyle, it's worth paying attention to this internal clock because it determines when your motivation is high and when it's flagging, when you're feeling strong and confident and when you're a little weaker. "The things we do or don't do during the day can alter our circadian rhythms, and that can have ramifications on all our body functions—from heart rhythms to bowel func-

tion to athletic performance," Dr. Zee says.

Here are a few items that, for better or worse, may change your body clock.

Drugs. Caffeine, antihistamines, alcohol, sleeping pills, and numerous other drugs can affect your circadian rhythm. "I wouldn't advise taking these an hour before bed, for example," Dr. Zee says. "They can all disrupt sleep patterns, which, in turn, will cause problems with your circadian rhythms." Yes, that goes for sleeping pills, too. "Unless your doctor has prescribed them, I would avoid sleeping aids," she says.

Stress. This is one of the most common causes of body-clock disruption, especially where your sleep cycle is concerned. "And it's not just the stress, but also stress-relieving medications that we might take," Dr. Zee says. All the more reason to adopt a regular workout routine—nothing reduces stress like exercise.

Sex. Luckily, sex isn't detrimental to your body rhythms. In fact, as most men know and most women lament, a little sex can make you drowsy after the fact. Having sex before bedtime is one of the surest ways to get to sleep quickly and soundly.

Travel. Few factors are more vexing to your body's cycle than travel. "It's a frequent cause of body-rhythm disruption, especially when traveling through a couple different time zones," Dr. Zee says. Suddenly, it's light when it should be dark, and you're eating when you should be sleeping. The best way to minimize jet lag is to try to get up and go to bed as close to your home time as possible when you're away, says Adele Pace, M.D., a fitness consultant in Ashland, Kentucky, and author of *The Busy Executive's Guide to Total Fitness.*

WORKING WITH THE CLOCK

Once you understand your biological rhythms—and for every man they'll be a little different—you can work with them to help strengthen your weight-loss plan.

"There are certain times of the day where you're going to be better equipped to perform certain tasks," says Dr. Zee. For example, there are periods throughout the day when your eyesight is sharper and your ability to handle complex mental problems is increased—and times when your body is most receptive to different types of exercise.

The best time to work out is not entirely at the whim of your body clock, says Dr. Pace. "Attitude plays a big role. You may have spent your whole life thinking that you're an evening person, and nothing on Earth could get you out of bed for a 6:00 A.M. run. But until you try it, you'll never know. It may be the perfect thing to wake

you up, clear the mental cobwebs, and get you ready for the day," she says.

So experiment a little. Whatever type of exercise you want to do, there's a perfect time of day for it. Here's how to find that time and make the most of it.

Exercise early. "If you're looking to have a regular, consistent routine, you're better off adopting a morning program," says John Amberge, a certified strength and conditioning specialist and director of corporate programs for the Sports Training Institute in New York City. As Amberge explains, you can get your exercise in first thing, before you are distracted or tired later in the day and get thrown off your schedule.

Biologically, this isn't when your body is at its most powerful, but it's still pretty well-equipped to deal with exercise. Dr. Zee says that in the morning, a man's body is naturally firing off bursts of testosterone, which help maintain muscle mass. It's also pumping cortisol, a hormone that helps us deal with mental and physical stress. Plus, our temperatures are rising from an evening of sleep, priming the pump for physical activity.

Perform in the afternoon. If you are preparing for an endurance event or doing serious weight training where you're trying to push the envelope or break out of a weight-training plateau, then you'll probably want to find time to exercise in the afternoon.

"Several studies show that we tend to be stronger and perform better in the afternoon," Dr. Zee says. "Our grip strength is stronger and muscle tone improves."

Lighten up in the evening. If you are in reasonably good shape or just beginning an

(continued on page 262)

CLOCK WISE

Are you a night owl, a lark (morning type), or something in between? To find out, read each of the following questions, then circle the number that follows the response that best describes you. Add up the numbers to get your score and compare it with the scale at the end of the quiz.

1. If you were completely free to plan your day, when would you get up and when would you go to bed?

Get Up (A.M.)		Go to Bed (P.M.)	
5:00 to 6:30 A.M.	5	8:00 to 9:00 P.M.	5
6:31 to 7:45 A.M.	4	9:01 to 10:15 P.M.	4
7:46 to 9:45 A.M.	3	10:16 P.M. to 12:30 A.M.	3
9:46 to 11:00 A.M.	2	12:31 to 1:45 A.M.	2
11:01 A.M. to noon	1	1:46 to 3:00 A.M.	1

2. If you have to get up at a specific time, how dependent are you on the alarm clock to wake you?

Not at all	4	Fairly	2
Slightly	3	Very	1

3. How easy is getting up in the morning?

Not at all	1	Fairly	3
Slightly	2	Very	4

4. During the first ½ hour after waking up . . .
How alert are you?

Not at all	1	Fairly	3
Slightly	2	Very	4

How tired are you?

Not at all	4	Fairly	2
Slightly	3	Very	1

How hungry are you?

Not at all	1	Fairly	3
Slightly	2	Very	4

5. If you have no commitments the next day, when do you go to bed compared with your usual bedtime?

Seldom or never later	4	1 to 2 hours later	2
Less than 1 hour later	3	More than 2 hours later	1

6. Some friends want you to exercise hard with them. How would you perform . . .

From 7:00 to 8:00 A.M.?		From 10:00 to 11:00 P.M.?	
Quite well	4	Quite well	1
Reasonably well	3	Reasonably well	2
Poorly	2	Poorly	3
Very poorly	1	Very poorly	4

7. When in the evening are you tired and ready for bed?

8:00 to 9:00 P.M.	5	12:46 to 2:00 A.M.	2
9:01 to 10:15 P.M.	4	2:01 to 3:00 A.M.	1
10:16 P.M. to 12:45 A.M.	3		

8. When would you be at your peak for . . .
A grueling 2-hour quiz?

8:00 to 10:00 A.M.	6	3:00 to 5:00 P.M.	2
11:00 A.M. to 1:00 P.M.	4	7:00 to 9:00 P.M.	0

Two hours of exhausting physical work?

8:00 to 10:00 A.M.	4	3:00 to 5:00 P.M.	2
11:00 A.M. to 1:00 P.M.	3	7:00 to 9:00 P.M.	1

9. You've gone to bed several hours later than usual, but you can wake up when you wish to. What is most likely to happen?

You'll wake up at the usual time and stay awake	4
You'll wake up at the usual time and doze lightly	3
You'll wake up at the usual time but fall back asleep	2
You'll wake up later than usual	1

10. One morning, you must be on watch from 4:00 to 6:00 A.M. You have no commitments the rest of the day. Which of the following would you do?

Not go to sleep until watch was over	1
Take a nap before watch and sleep after	2
Have a good sleep before watch and nap after	3
Take all sleep before watch	4

Scoring

Add up your score and compare it with this scale.

14–23:	night owl
24–31:	almost an owl
32–44:	intermediate type
45–52:	almost a lark
53–65:	lark

exercise program, your needs may be lighter, in which case you can do your workout in the evening.

"Evening is probably the time when you'll best respond to light exercise," says Amberge. It'll minimize the impact of a heavy dinner, and light exercise can actually help you rest easier. "It might be just enough to tire you out so that you'll sleep like a baby."

MAKING THE RIGHT TIME

Beyond the biological imperatives, there are ways that you can actively nail down the best time for you to exercise.

"To some degree, it's not a question of finding time but of making time," says Virginia Bass, time-management consultant for Day-Timers in Exton, Pennsylvania. "That's when you have to take a hard look at the daily routine that you—not Mother Nature—have established for yourself. Then, you have to find a way to insert exercise into that routine." Here's how to do it.

Check your appointment book. The first, most obvious step is to review your schedule over the course of the average week.

"Take note of the times you consistently have open. Typically, those are going to be in the morning, at lunch, or after work, but a lot of men have other gaps in their daily schedules," Bass says. For example, you may never have anything going on from 11:00 A.M. to 12:00 noon or from 2:45 P.M. to 3:30 P.M. That's time that you might be able to devote to getting some exercise.

Work on flextime. Many businesses offer flextime hours. As long as you work your 40 hours a week and are working during core

business hours (typically 10:00 A.M. to 4:00 P.M.), when you arrive and leave can be a gray area worth exploring.

"If you've been working 9:00 A.M. to 5:00 P.M. all your life and you haven't found time for exercise, maybe what you need to do is alter your schedule. See if you can work from 7:30 A.M. to 3:30 P.M. or from 10:00 A.M. to 6:00 P.M. All of a sudden, you have extra time in the morning or evening that you can devote entirely to a workout," Bass says. "It never hurts to check with your manager or personnel office to see if this is possible."

Exercise morning, noon, and night. For the moment, forget what your body clock tells you and what your schedule demands of you. Never mind whether you think you're a morning person or a night person. If you're just getting started on an exercise program, the first thing that you should do is exercise at different times of the day.

"Everyone's different. And if you've never exercised regularly before, you really have no idea what time will feel right for you to exercise," says Amberge.

For the first couple of weeks, try getting up earlier and exercising before you go to work. Then, try exercising at lunch. Then, try working out after work. If at any point you find a time that really works for you—where you really feel on top of it, or you reach the point where you enjoy exercise—then stick with it.

If none of these three time periods works, try working out at odd, alternating times—10:30 A.M., 2:00 P.M., 8:00 P.M. "Sooner or later, you'll hit on the right combination," Amberge says.

Commuter Calisthenics

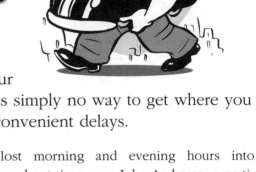

Commuting is one of life's necessary wastes of time, like waiting in a doctor's office or number-punching your way through a voice-mail maze. There's simply no way to get where you need to be without unenviable and inconvenient delays.

In the world of commuting, that delay is pretty significant. According to government estimates, the average worker traveling by car spends nearly 40 minutes a day commuting. If he takes a bus, he's looking at more than an hour round-trip; and if he rides the rails, the commute averages more than 2 hours a day.

To those of us trying to make time for exercise, these statistics certainly seem daunting. Until someone invents a *Star Trek*–style transporter, it seems that the chances for turning commuting time into exercise time are slim. This is unfortunate because losing weight always requires commitment, and commitments take time. How can a man commit time and energy to shopping, exercise, and other lifestyle changes when he's always stuck in traffic?

TRAINING IN TRANSIT

It doesn't have to be an either-or scenario. Whether you're commuting by car, bus, or train, there are ways to turn some of those lost morning and evening hours into workout time, says John Amberge, a certified strength and conditioning specialist and director of corporate programs for the Sports Training Institute in New York City.

"It won't be anything like a good workout in the gym, of course. But if you can steal 5 minutes a day for exercise, that's almost an extra ½ hour of exercise a week," he says. Commuter workouts make great supplements to a man's regular exercise routines.

Take a look at the gaps in your commuting time, says Sandra Lotz Fisher, exercise physiologist and president of New York City's Fitness by Fisher, a fitness and stress-management consulting firm. "When you're waiting for your ride, anytime you're a passenger in a vehicle, when you're at a stoplight, while you're in a traffic jam—these are all times that you can devote to a variety of exercises without endangering yourself or your fellow commuters," she says.

THE FREEWAY TO FITNESS

For those who commute by car, doing anything more strenuous than fidgeting seems impossible without ending up on the eye-in-the-sky traffic report as the accident that's blocking the left lane.

"Not so," says Fisher, who developed an audiotape for drivers called "Freeway Flex: Stretch and Tone Exercises to Do While You Drive." "You absolutely shouldn't do it at any point where it's going to take your attention off the road," she adds.

That said, if you drive in light to moderate conditions, there's plenty of time during your morning or evening drive that you can convert to exercise time.

"Gridlock can be your friend," says Charles Kuntzleman, Ed.D., professor of kinesiology at the University of Michigan in Ann Arbor and director of Blue Cross and Blue Shield of Michigan Fitness for Youth Program, also at the University of Michigan. Any time that traffic is at a standstill, that's time you can spend doing a few simple exercises—burning calories instead of brain cells.

Here are a few in-car exercises that you can do while waiting in traffic—not while driving—that will help make your morning and evening commutes an integral part of your weight-loss plan.

Shrug your shoulders. This is a very simple exercise that works out the large trapezius muscles in your back and neck. Hold on to the steering wheel at the 9 and 3 o'clock positions. Push back against the seat until your arms are straight, and raise your shoulders up toward your ears.

Do 10, 20, or however many you have time for before traffic starts moving, Dr. Kuntzleman says.

Squeeze the wheel. Grabbing the steering wheel in a death grip loosens muscles in your hands and forearms. If you really go after it, it will build hand strength as well. Hold for a count of five, then relax. "Really focus on the release part," Dr. Kuntzleman says. "That stimulates a relaxation response in the body, which will help you be more loose and limber when you get to work."

Vacuum off flab. Similar to crunches, vacuums are abdominal exercises that you can do while sitting up, Dr. Kuntzleman says. Sit up straight in your seat. Suck in your stomach as though you were on a beach and the Swedish Bikini Team were strolling by. Hold for a count of 10, then relax. Vacuums are harder than they sound. Try to do 5 at first, then work up to 10.

Work the "off" leg. Between brake pumping and gas stomping, your right leg gets a pretty good workout in the car. You can work your left leg by doing a simple toning exercise. Tighten it as much as you can for 3 seconds. Feel the tightness in your quadriceps and hamstring. Then release. You can do a similar thing with your ankle and toes. "You won't have nearly the cramps and sore-leg problems a lot of drivers complain about," Fisher says.

POWER ON THE PLATFORM

Transportation schedules being what they are—that is to say, inaccurate—you probably find yourself waiting for your ride a few times a week. The time you currently spend reading can be time spent exercising. Here are a few quick workouts you may want to try. They'll burn just as many calories as the exercise that you'd do in a gym, and you're doing them in your "free" time.

Pace. "If it's a bus stop, walk up to the corner and back to the stop. Try to do 10 laps before the bus arrives. If it's a train station, try to do as many brisk, walking laps around the station as you can before your train pulls in," suggests Amberge.

Do the bus-stop stretch. Every man needs to stretch, and it's especially important for men who are working out. Dr. Kunt-zleman recommends using waiting time to get in some quick stretches. See that chain-link fence near the bus stop? Stand facing away from it. Stretch your arms out behind you, hook your hands into the fence at about chest level, and lean forward. This gives a solid stretch to your arms and shoulders.

Work your calves. Another exercise you can do on any city street is a heel raise. Stand on a curb with your heels hanging off the edge. Slowly rise up on your toes, then lower your weight so that your heels are as low as they'll go. This exercise looks simple, but you'll start feeling the burn after doing

WORKOUTS FOR DRIVERS

So driving isn't how you get to work: It *is* your work. Here are three exercises, suggested by Marge Rodgers, a physical therapist and rehabilitation-services coordinator for Genesis Rehabilitation Services in Baltimore, that will loosen you up, tighten your gut, and burn some calories at the same time.

Stretch your hamstrings. The main muscle in the back of your leg, called the hamstring, always tends to be tight, causing knee and back pain. It pays to keep it loose—even if you're sitting behind the wheel of a tractor trailer all day. Before you climb into the cab, stand by the side of your truck, facing the door. Lift your foot up and rest your heel on the step. Your knee should be straight, not bent. Hold for a few seconds, then relax.

Roll with it. Crunches are among the best abdominal exercises, but you can't do them when you're driving. Here's a gut workout that you can do. Slump in the seat, lift your chest, and push your stomach muscles out. Find the place of maximum tension, then hold the stretch for a few seconds. Relax, then do it again. This exercise is surprisingly effective at stretching and strengthening your abs. "These muscles need to be strong to help support your spine," Rodgers says.

Bend over backward. "Every time you get out of the cab, step to the side of the truck, put your hands on your hips, and bend backward, keeping your knees straight," says Rodgers. This will help relax all the muscles in your back, which can help prevent tension backaches from getting started.

two or three. It's very effective for strengthening your calves and stretching your toes and ankles. It may be hard to keep your balance, however, so it's good to do it near a parking meter or signpost.

Hurry to catch the train. If you commute by train or subway, you probably stand right where you think the doors are going to open. "When you think about it, that's really pretty lazy," says Fisher. She recommends waiting a lot farther away. As the train comes to a complete stop, walk briskly toward the front or back of the train, whichever is farther away. You'll get a quick aerobic hit, and you may even get on faster than if you tried to squeeze your way in with the throng.

WORKING OUT EN ROUTE

If you take public transportation, there's no reason to stay locked in your seat. "If you're not doing the driving and you're not packed in like sardines, then you have time and space to do some exercise," Fisher says. Here are some ideas to get you started.

Get off early. Probably the easiest way to convert commute time into exercise time is to get off the train or bus one or two stops shy of your destination and walk or run the rest of the way, Dr. Kuntzleman says. "The way traffic is in most cities, you'll probably get there faster on foot." Just remember to wear walking or running shoes—those executive wing tips won't do you any favors out on the streets.

Stand whenever you can. Men who take trains and buses always head for the first free seat. That's fine when you're reading the paper, but you can burn some additional calories just by being a strap-hanger, says Dr. Kuntzleman.

"Unless you have some back problems or a condition that prevents you from standing for long periods of time, you'll get more exercise from simply standing," he says. The swaying of buses and trains causes muscles to fire in your legs, back, torso, and arms. "It's not a lot, but it's better than sitting and doing nothing," Dr. Kuntzleman says.

The Real Power Lunch

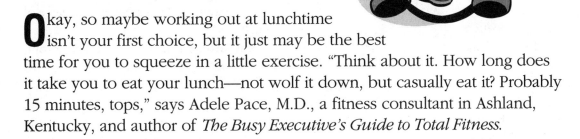

Okay, so maybe working out at lunchtime isn't your first choice, but it just may be the best time for you to squeeze in a little exercise. "Think about it. How long does it take you to eat your lunch—not wolf it down, but casually eat it? Probably 15 minutes, tops," says Adele Pace, M.D., a fitness consultant in Ashland, Kentucky, and author of *The Busy Executive's Guide to Total Fitness*.

Assuming that you get an hour for lunch, that leaves 45 minutes for exercise.

Men who are busy naturally gravitate to lunchtime workouts, adds John Amberge, a certified strength and conditioning specialist and director of corporate programs for the Sports Training Institute in New York City. "It's a great way to recharge your batteries after a hard morning, and that pick-me-up can carry through the rest of the day."

MAKING IT WORK

Cramming a lunchtime workout into your schedule is eminently doable, says Amberge.

"If your exercise facilities are within 10 minutes of your office, you have plenty of time to work out and eat lunch," he says. "We get a lot of executives in here at around 11:30 A.M. They work out for ½ hour to 45 minutes, then they grab lunch on the way back to the office."

Maybe that's not an option for you. Maybe your office is miles from a club, or perhaps your job demands that you be close by, just in case. Well, you can always work out in the office. That's better in some ways. Since you don't have to go anywhere, you'll have even more time to exercise.

"Of course, if you exercise around the office, you'll probably want to modify your workout a little bit. You'll want to do enough so that you feel like you're getting some benefit from the activity, but not so much that you end up all sweaty going into your afternoon meetings," says Amberge.

Whatever type of exercise you have time for, heed the following advice. These tips will help you make the most of your midday plan.

Drink before noon. Even before the lunch whistle blows, you can start preparing for exercise by making sure that you have plenty of fluids in your system.

"If you're not well-hydrated, it may adversely affect your performance," says Barry Franklin, Ph.D., director of cardiac rehabilitation and exercise laboratories at William Beaumont Hospital Rehabilitation and Health Center in Birmingham, Michigan. "You won't be able to make the most of your workout time. I definitely recommend getting some fluids into you." That means water, not coffee.

The caffeine in coffee will actually cause your body to get rid of more fluids, not to mention the fact that caffeine can increase stress on your heart, Dr. Franklin says. "A couple of cups in the morning is fine. But after that, switch to water."

Eat at midmorning. Roughly an hour before you exercise, start fueling for your workout. "If you're doing any kind of serious weight training or heavy exercise, do not eat lunch before you do it. You'll be too loaded down with food—you'll feel awful," Amberge says. But you have to have some fuel, so he recommends eating something that's high in carbohydrates and easy to digest, such as a bagel or a piece of fruit.

Eat afterward. After your workout, your body will practically be starving for more fuel. So go get some lunch—but wait until your heart rate has dropped down out of the aerobic zone, says Joanne Curran-Celentano, R.D., Ph.D., associate professor of nutrition and food science

MEET YOU AT THE CLUB

For years, you've wined and dined your clients. How about slimming and toning them instead?

John Amberge, a certified strength and conditioning specialist and director of corporate programs for the Sports Training Institute in New York City, has found some creative ways to mix business and exercise.

Schedule meetings at the gym. If you have an in-house exercise facility or company memberships at a local club, skip the conference room and head straight to the gym.

"If it's just two or three of you and you all work out on a semiregular basis, just meet there," Amberge says. "You can have a discussion on the stairclimbing machines as easily as you can sitting around a conference table. Then, you can all go out for lunch afterward."

Play your client's game. So your weeks of cold calls have finally snagged you a meeting with the executive vice president of purchasing for ThingamaBob Inc. Instead of stupefying him with a big lunch, join him in an activity that he enjoys. "It's no different than meeting someone for golf and conducting business that way," Amberge says. Besides playing golf, you can meet for racquetball or tennis, whatever his favorite game is. Even if he's not into exercise, chances are that your approach will stand out from the pile of business-lunch invitations that he gets all the time.

at the University of New Hampshire in Durham.

Take a walk. Men who go to gyms at midday usually rush back to the office without allowing much time for a cooldown period. To help your body make the transition from exercise to rest, walk an easy lap or two around the parking lot.

"It'll be a lot easier on your body—especially your heart and the muscles you just worked out—if you go for a walk or do some light stretching in your office than if you go back upstairs and sit still for the next 4 to 5 hours," says Dr. Pace.

Consolidate your efforts. Even if the gym is across the street, you may find yourself crunched for time, between changing, exercising, changing back, showering, *and* eating lunch. So cut some corners. When you work out, stick to a 5-minute warmup and do only the lifts that work compound muscle groups—squats, for example, which work several muscles at once, says Amberge.

Bring your own gear. If you get serious about working out where you work, bring in a pair of 10- to 15-pound dumbbells and keep them in your office. "There's any number of arm, shoulder, and chest exercises that you can do right in your own office chair," Amberge says. These range from basic curls to overhead presses.

THE OFFICE CIRCUIT

Even men who find time to get to a gym and exercise at lunch don't always have enough time for a serious workout. That's okay. It doesn't mean that you can't fit in some decent exercise at lunch anyway. And you don't need equipment to do it.

"There are a number of exercises that you can do at lunch right around your office, if you want to be creative about it," Amberge says. The idea is to get your heart working and your metabolism up, but without getting so hot and sweaty that your aroma precedes you into afternoon meetings. Amberge, who helps corporations set up in-house exercise programs, recommends the following office plan.

The Warmup

Even when you're doing low-intensity exercises, you need to get your muscles primed and ready. You won't have time for a lengthy stretching regimen, but here are a few ways to warm up quickly.

Visit your vehicle. When you get to work in the morning, make it a point to park your car in the farthest reaches of the parking lot. Before you work out, find an excuse to walk out there. Maybe carry some papers that you know you'll be taking home. Walk quickly, swinging your arms. From your desk chair to the driver's seat and back is one lap. Do at least two laps.

Walk the halls. Do one circuit around the perimeter of the floor on which your office is located. "You can even mix it up with some interval training," Amberge says. Walk quickly for a minute, then sprint, then slow back to a walk. If you're truly creative, you can time the sprints so that they always occur in front of the boss's office—you'll look like you're

WORKING AROUND THE WORKING LUNCH

Sooner or later, it's going to happen: Your boss will come into your office and announce that the department will be having a "working lunch" in the dungeon conference room. Your lunchtime plans for a workout will be shot, and there will be no way that you can make it up earlier or later. So how will you keep on schedule?

Double up. It's rare for companies to schedule business meetings during lunch without giving some sort of notice. When you know that something is coming up, you can make up for the lost time, says Adele Pace, M.D., a fitness consultant in Ashland, Kentucky, and author of *The Busy Executive's Guide to Total Fitness.*

"Spend a few extra minutes the day before and the day after on your workout. Or make the day before a high-tempo day when you're going to push yourself. Set the stairclimbing machine at a higher level than you normally do for a few intervals. Add on an extra set to some of your lifts," she says. "This way, missing a workout the next day gives you the rest you need to recover. You've gained, not lost."

Cut your losses. Just because you can't exercise doesn't mean that you can't treat your body well at the restaurant, if that's where your working lunch happens to be. Make smart choices. Order a big salad, and avoid the heavy slabs of meat. Or, when you're working through lunch at the office, plan on brown-bagging it. This allows you to participate fully in the group without eating the pizzas or sub sandwiches that seem to be the staple of working lunches.

Don't beat yourself up. If you miss a workout once in a while, remember that your body is resilient and that there's no reason to be a fanatic. Enjoy the day off. "Just resolve to stick with the workout tomorrow and you won't get sidetracked," says Dr. Pace.

rushing to an important meeting, at lunch no less!

The Workout

Once you're warmed up, you're ready to get down to business. Try these exercises.

Climb the corporate ladder. You don't want to look as though you're roaming the floor with nothing to do, so don't do multiple laps around the floor where you work. Instead, expand to other floors of your building. For this part of the workout, do a lap around your floor, then take the stairs up to the next floor, walk the perimeter, then hit the stairs again for the floor above that. Do three to five floors, then come back down, taking the steps as fast as you can.

Toe-climb the stairs. Find an isolated stairwell and work on your calves for a few minutes. Putting your weight on one foot, slowly raise your heel as high as it will go. Then, step up with the other foot, raising that heel. Basically, you're climbing the stairs on your toes and the balls of your feet. You'll feel an intense burn in your calves, proof that a lot of muscle work is happening.

Find a place to lie down. If your work life revolves around a cubicle, you'll need to find a place where you can have some privacy. "Conference rooms make excellent exercise rooms," says Amberge. "There's plenty of room to maneuver, and they're usually empty at lunch."

Once the door is closed, do some pushups and crunches, as many as you can. You can also do lunges and squats.

The Cooldown

You don't want to head straight back to work after your workout. It's hard on your heart and, if you're sweating enough, it could be hard on your career. Take a few minutes to recover and prepare yourself for the rest of the workday.

Drink a lot of water. If you've been exercising at a brisk pace, you need to replenish the fluids that the exercise took out of you. "It's always a good idea to rehydrate after any exercise," says Amberge.

Refuel. Nearly everyone experiences an after-lunch slump, and it can be intense if you don't replenish your body with the necessary nutrients. You don't need to eat a lot—many men, in fact, eat less when they're working out. But you do need something, Amberge says.

Workday Workouts

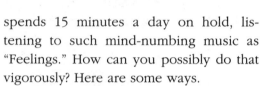

Researchers at Tufts University measured daylong energy expenditures among men and came to the conclusion that—hold on to your hats here, fellas—active guys were significantly leaner than sofa spuds.

Actually, there was something truly surprising about their findings.

The kinds of activities in which the lean men engaged were not necessarily traditional exercise. They included such things as shifting in your chair, pacing around the office, even getting excited about good ideas. All of these things added to the total daily calories burned. In fact, in the course of 16 hours, men doing nonexercise activities burned more calories than they would have in 30 minutes of sweating at the gym.

In other words, little things do indeed add up. You can take advantage of this by consciously doing everything a little more vigorously, says Susan Roberts, Ph.D., chief of the energy metabolism laboratory at the Jean Mayer USDA Human Nutrition Research Center on Aging at Tufts University in Boston.

CALL WEIGHTING

Men who work in offices spend inordinate amounts of time on the telephone. It's estimated, in fact, that the average executive spends 15 minutes a day on hold, listening to such mind-numbing music as "Feelings." How can you possibly do that vigorously? Here are some ways.

Keep your hands busy. One of the first things that men learn is the importance of a firm handshake. So why not work on it while you're on the phone? Many executives have begun keeping small exercise balls, designed for building hand strength, on their desks. While you're talking, squeeze the ball with everything you have. Relax for a second, then repeat.

Do some curls. Buy some rubber exercise tubing, available at sporting goods stores. Stand on one end of the tubing with your right foot, and grab the free end with your right hand. Curl your hand, palm-up, toward your armpit. Repeat 10 times, then repeat with the other arm. You can easily do this exercise when you're on the phone or between meetings.

Work your calves. Another exercise you

can do while talking on the phone is calf raises. Stand up—assuming the phone cord is long enough—and hook your right foot behind your left ankle. Hold the desk for support, rise on your toes, then slowly lower back down. Repeat with your right leg.

THE VIRTUAL GYM

Most men spend 40 hours a week or more at work. In all that time, you probably never realized that your office is actually a gym in disguise.

"People ask me all the time, 'How do I keep in shape at the office?'" says Joseph Barredo, a personal trainer at the Vertical Club in New York City. "Many people think that they need a gym because they sit behind a desk for 10 to 12 hours a day. But a desk, copy machine, or even your briefcase can be used to get some decent exercise while you're at the office."

To prove his point, Barredo devised a routine of nine exercises that require nothing more than two books or two reams of copy paper, an office chair, a desk, and a briefcase.

"The ideal is to try to do this routine four times a week, but three times weekly should give you visible results over a period of time," Barredo says. He recommends doing 3 sets of 12 repetitions of each exercise, unless otherwise specified.

Biceps
Biceps Curl

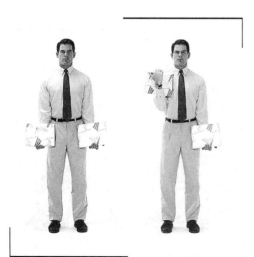

■ Hold a book or a ream of packaged copy paper in each hand. With your feet slightly apart and your knees unlocked, stand straight so that your shoulders are back and your upper torso is upright. Place your hands at your sides with your palms facing out.

■ Bending your elbow, slowly curl your right hand up toward your right biceps, keeping your upper arm straight. Your wrist should be locked, and your palms should continue to face out. Slowly lower to the starting position, then repeat with your left arm.

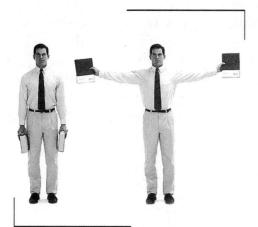

■ Hold a book or a ream of packaged copy paper in each hand. Stand straight with your feet slightly apart and your knees un- locked. Place your hands at your sides with your palms facing in.

■ Slowly raise both arms in unison in a straight line unitl they're at shoulder level, as if you were flapping your arms. Make sure your elbows are slightly bent and your thumbs are higher than your pinkies as you lift. Lower to the starting position. If you can't keep your wrists straight as you lift your arms, you should substitute lighter books or paper that you can lift without bending at your wrists.

Triceps
Seated Overhead Triceps Extension

■ Sit in your office chair with your back straight and your feet flat on the floor. Holding two reams of copy paper between your hands, place both arms straight up over your head.

■ Slowly lower both arms behind your head, bending at the elbows so that the paper touches your shoulders. Your palms should face the sides of your head. Then, raise to the starting position.

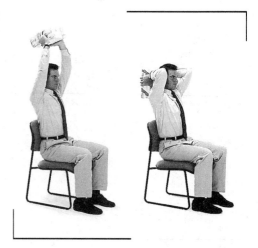

- With your hands shoulder-width apart and your palms facing down, lean forward against the edge of your desk. Your legs and back should form a straight line, and you should be up on the balls of your feet. Your arms should be slightly bent, elbows unlocked.

- Press down against the desk, your elbows bent and facing outward. Then, press back to the starting position.

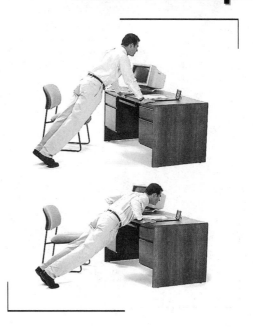

Quadriceps
Leg Extension

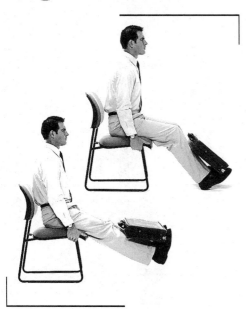

- Sit on the edge of your office chair with your knees slightly bent and your legs together. Place your briefcase or a big book on top of your shins, bending your feet upward so that it doesn't fall off. Stabilize yourself by holding the sides of your chair with your hands.

- Straighten your legs by lifting with your ankles. Don't lock your knees at full extension, but rather keep a slight bend. Your toes should point up and out at about a 45-degree angle. Hold the extension for 2 or 3 seconds, then slowly lower to the starting position.

Adductor Resistance

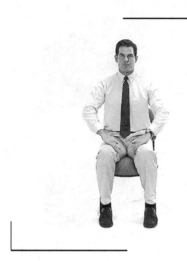

■ Sit comfortably in your office chair with your back straight, your knees bent, and your feet flat on the floor. Place your hands on your inner thighs, just above the knee joints. Pull your hands outward while you move your knees together. Hold for 6 seconds. Repeat five times.

Abductor (Outer Thigh) Muscles
Abductor Resistance

■ Sit comfortably in your office chair with your back straight, your knees bent, and your feet flat on the floor. Place your hands on your outer thighs, just above the knee joints. Press your hands together while you move your knees apart. Hold for 6 seconds. Repeat five times.

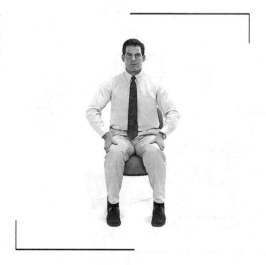

Briefcase Sidebend

- Stand upright with your briefcase in your right hand, your arms resting at your sides with your palms facing in. Your feet should be shoulder-width apart.

- Bend to your right, allowing the briefcase to drop down your right leg until you feel your obliques working. Keep your body facing front in the same plane—don't turn your torso into the sidebend. Once you've gone as low as you can, bring yourself upright to the starting position. Do 20 repetitions. Then, move your brief-case to your left hand and do 20 repetitions on that side.

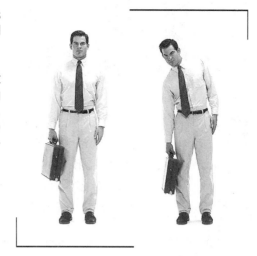

Deltoids and Trapeziuses
Shoulder Press

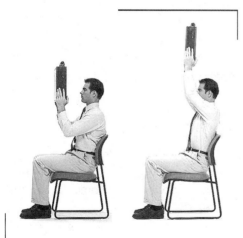

- Sit comfortably in your office chair with your back straight, your knees bent, and your feet flat on the floor. Hold your briefcase by the bottom corners with your palms facing in, and lift it directly in front of your face with your elbows bent and in at your sides.

- Slowly press the briefcase straight up toward the ceiling until your arms are fully extended above your head. Then, lower the briefcase back to the starting position in front of your face.

Doug Colbeth, Spyglass President and CEO

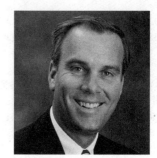

One year, Doug Colbeth didn't know whether he could make his house payments. The next year, he had a net worth in the tens of millions of dollars. The Spyglass president and chief executive officer is one of many small-business men who've cashed in on the current computer craze.

But sudden success has also meant megastress, and Colbeth has found that making time for fitness is essential for keeping his life on track.

Though probably best known for its commercial version of the University of Illinois World Wide Web browser Mosaic, Spyglass provides a suite of embedded networking technologies for the products of more than 100 companies, including Microsoft and IBM.

"We want to get World Wide Web technologies into the hands of all the people in the world who do *not* use computers," Colbeth says.

Spyglass, headquartered in Naperville, Illinois, has offices in four U.S. cities and is expanding into Europe and Asia. Since the company's breakthrough in 1994, the number of employees has been doubling every year, while profits have continued to soar.

All that has meant a worldwide web of responsibility for Colbeth, who works as many as 15 hours a day and spends much of his life in airports and hotel rooms.

"My personal life has suffered some," says Colbeth, now in his forties. "Not with my kids, because I would never sacrifice that. But I have sacrificed what I would call pure fun. My golf is terrible, and I miss it. But I believe that I'm making a temporary trade-off."

A RUNNING START

Colbeth may have lost his grip on his golf clubs, but he firmly grasps the importance of a healthy lifestyle. His average day begins with a 5:30 A.M. jog.

On weekdays, Colbeth puts in 4 to 5

miles on the treadmill or the track. "I plan my workouts a week ahead, based on what my schedule looks like," he says. "I'm looking to get in 20 miles a week over 4 to 5 days. I may miss a day if I'm taking an early-morning flight, but then I always run the next day."

Colbeth says that he feels lethargic on days when he misses his morning run.

"I feel more alert after I jog, and that feeling lasts all day," he says. "Obviously, it's most intense right after a workout, but I feel good even toward the latter part of the day. Everyone has optimistic and pessimistic sides, and my optimistic side comes out much more with regular exercise."

That's why the Colbeths keep a treadmill, a stairclimber, and weights in the room over their garage—in what was once Spyglass headquarters.

"Time is very important. I don't even go to health clubs anymore because of the 15 minutes you spend going each way. But I can always roll out of bed and get on a treadmill."

A former football player, the 6-foot-2, 210-pound executive still lifts weights three times a week to tone his arms, doing high repetitions with relatively light weights. But he considers running to be the mainstay of his fitness routine.

"Jogging works for me because I'm not depending on someone else," he says. "True, a racquetball game would be more fun, and I love to play basketball in the driveway with my son. But that's not something you can do when you travel. Those are just fun weekend things."

Colbeth follows his morning run with a breakfast packed with plenty of fiber and fruit. By 7:30 A.M., he's on his way to the office or the airport. Either way, he can look forward to a day of constant discussion with customers, potential partners, and fellow executives.

"I often have speaking engagements, which are typically around noon," Colbeth says. "I don't like to eat before I speak, and usually, the meal is cold by the time I'm done talking, so I don't end up eating much."

To compensate, he reaches for some fruit between his afternoon meetings, which are scheduled in precise 30-minute blocks. Work tends to extend into the evening, especially during the 2 or 3 days a week that he typically spends on the road.

"Over the years, I've learned that I need a very controlled diet when I travel or else it's much more exhausting," he says. "At first, I ate too much and drank too much. Now, I'm much more careful. I don't drink alcohol on the road, and I don't eat late-night meals. I eat at 6:00 P.M. or 7:00 P.M., then schedule a meeting after dinner. That way, I don't go to bed on a full stomach."

With his stomach settled, Colbeth can turn to settling his mind. He insists on having an hour to himself before getting his 6½ hours of sleep.

"The 2 sane hours of my life are when I'm running in the morning and at 10:00 P.M.," he says. "I'm a sports fanatic, so I catch the nightly wrap-up on ESPN. But I'm always in bed by 11:00 P.M. because if

I try to function on 3 to 4 hours of sleep, I really start dragging at the end of the next day."

WORKING THINGS OUT

Organizing a training schedule is a tiny challenge compared with some that Colbeth has faced. In 1994, Spyglass was on the verge of going broke, and his family didn't know how—or if—they'd be able to pay the three mortgages they had taken out on their house.

"I used to wake up in cold sweats a lot of nights," he says. "There were three things that were really gnawing at me. One was that we'd gone through the savings for our kids' college. Second was that I felt like the employees were going to be let down if the company couldn't continue. Then there was the personal pressure of wanting to be successful."

Unable to find any solutions himself but unwilling to give up, he put his 17 employees in a room and asked them to brainstorm new markets and investors that Spyglass could pursue. From that meeting came the idea that would eventually earn the company millions.

"When you don't have anything, you really learn how to build partnerships,"

Colbeth says. "We had to build, first, with the employees. We had to let them be a part of deciding what to do next. Then, we had to build with the University of Illinois. We told them, 'We have a great idea. You have a great technology with Mosaic. Let us take it over commercially.'"

Colbeth's relationships, at work and at home, remain the key to minimizing the pressure he feels as he tries to direct the company's frenzied growth.

"As my executive staff gets better, that takes stress off me," he says. "Two years ago, I didn't have that infrastructure. Now, I have the support staff that makes my days easier—not easy, but easier."

He's also learned that a social calendar can be as much of a strain as a business calendar. Colbeth and his wife, Margey, have two children—a daughter, Jackie, and son, Brett—who help keep them plenty busy.

But no matter what parts of his personal schedule are shuffled, one thing that Colbeth will never give up is his exercise.

"I want to contribute to this industry when I'm in my fifties and potentially in my sixties," he says. "To do that, I have to stay in shape in my forties. I look at those 45 minutes a day I run as an investment so I'll have a longer career and feel better."

Gary Barnett, University of Colorado Football Coach

Being a miracle worker has a way of keeping a guy on the move. Just look at Gary Barnett, the man who turned the once hopelessly pathetic Northwestern University football team into a Big 10 conference champion.

How did he do it? By working 15 hours a day, 7 days a week; by telling anyone and everyone that his team was going to succeed—no matter how often people laughed in his face; by staking a claim on a program that everyone else had given up on.

"We were in the epitome of a situation where you want to feel like you can't change the system," he says. "But what we did is *prove* that no matter where you are, you are in control. Most of us prefer to point fingers somewhere else and say, 'That's the reason I'm not where I want to be.' But you really do have control. You have to believe that, because if you choose to look at it the other way, you'll be right. You'll never make a difference."

EXERCISING CONTROL

Barnett's no-excuses philosophy extends directly to his personal fitness regimen. While some of his head-coaching counterparts look as though they're living on double cheeseburgers and cigars, Barnett, now in his mid-fifties and the coach of the University of Colorado's Golden Buffaloes, has made his health a high priority.

It all started when he took up running in 1976, and it gained momentum when he drastically reduced his red meat consumption 2 years later.

"During the season, now, I really watch my diet—especially during two-a-days," he says. "In the morning, I have fruit. At noon, I have salad. And in the evening, I make sure that I get my vegetables. I try not to eat anything after dinner."

When it comes to strength training, Barnett prefers to do things the old-fashioned way: alternating each morning between doing 60 pushups or 200 situps. He keeps his aerobic exercise simple, too, especially when he has to make recruiting trips in December and January.

"I don't really like the other exercise machines, but I do try to stay at places that have treadmills," he says. "Otherwise, what I can do depends on where I have to go. If I go south or west, I can usually run outside. But if I'm in the Northeast or the Midwest that time of year, it's very hard."

The weather may not always cooperate with his plans, but at least Barnett's body is holding up. While a lot of men his age are hobbled by old football injuries, Barnett managed to emerge relatively unscathed from his playing days at the University of Missouri in the late 1960s. Though he has had knee surgery and sometimes contends with a troublesome calf muscle, he has no chronic aches or pains that would interfere with his workouts.

That means almost nothing can keep him from a 3½-mile run, 6 days a week.

"It's aerobic obviously, but honestly, I do it for my head," he says. "It gets me a break in the middle of the day. I walk out the door with all my problems, and by the time I'm finished, they're solved. I just try to get into an unconscious state. I usually do not even know where I have run."

RUNNING OUT THE CLOCK

Barnett cherishes the chance to clear his head, because the rest of his day is a study in time micromanagement. From the beginning of August to Thanksgiving, there are no days off—just a never-ending stream of decisions to make and questions to answer.

Practice days begin with a 7:00 A.M.

meeting of the full coaching staff, to coordinate plans and discuss personnel issues. From 8:00 to 11:00 A.M., Barnett sits in on strategy sessions with either the offensive or defensive staffs.

"At these meetings, our goal is to make a plan for each potential game situation—for instance, what we are going to do this week on second and long," he says. "We make these decisions based on the game films and what we see at practice."

Fans who think that this process sounds more like fun than work are mistaken.

"You would be amazed at the amount of time that goes into just planning a practice," Barnett says. "We watch video on each opponent that's broken down by computers to chart their tendencies. And we do the same thing to ourselves, to be aware of what other people are looking at as our own tendencies."

One off-field tendency that Barnett is known for is his prompt, direct dealings with members of the media. He leaves a 2-hour block open for interviews, starting at 11:00 A.M. By 1:00 P.M., he's ready to run.

When he returns from his workout at 2:00 P.M., the coaches meet for a final review of the afternoon's practice schedule, which begins with a brief team meeting at 2:45. From there, players break off into position meetings. Everyone takes the field at 3:40.

"We script every minute of practice," Barnett says. "In every 10-minute interval, we run 15 plays. Every one of those plays has a purpose. It's been thought through carefully. We can't afford to fall behind."

Things are scheduled to wrap up at 6:00

P.M. Barnett often takes questions from reporters and fans who attend practice, then eats dinner with the team. His work isn't done, though.

"At 7:00 P.M., I come back to my office and make recruiting calls or put on the practice film from that afternoon," he says. "I generally finish up after 9:30 P.M. and get home at about 10:00 P.M."

ALL IN THE FAMILY

The in-season schedule obviously doesn't allow for much time at home with his wife, Mary. Off-seasons are somewhat more relaxed, though there are still clinics and camps to run—and award ceremonies to attend. But Barnett says that his children have benefited from his career in football, although he acknowledges that his family life may not be what most people would consider normal.

"I don't know if someone on the outside can understand it, but college football is a way of life for a coach's family," he says. "Everything revolves around football. Instead of taking family vacations, you go to bowl games."

Well, they do now. But during Barnett's first three seasons at Northwestern—in which his teams won a total of eight games—the Wildcats didn't look to be any closer to a bowl bid than they'd been in any other year since their 1949 Rose Bowl victory. That didn't sit well with Barnett, who believed that he was building a better program, not just adding to the school's losing tradition.

"That pressure is very personal," he says. "It's the pride of wanting to do a good job, knowing that every Saturday your work is laid out in front of everybody. People do judge you based on your wins and losses."

For Barnett, coping with success is a lot more fun.

"When you go 24 years without a winning season, *that's* pressure," he says.

Phil Jackson, Los Angeles Lakers Coach

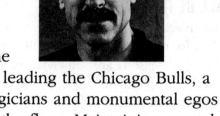

To be a coach in the NBA would be enough stress for most men. But imagine the added pressure Phil Jackson felt while leading the Chicago Bulls, a team blessed with a bunch of physical magicians and monumental egos that is expected to win every time it is on the floor. Maintaining mental and physical alertness isn't a luxury; it's part of his job.

Jackson coached the Chicago Bulls to six NBA titles and was himself a former championship player with the New York Knicks from 1967 to 1978. How does he handle the stress? He achieves a level of equilibrium by breathing deeply at critical moments, by practicing Zen meditation each morning, and by getting exercise when he can.

The son of Pentecostal preachers, Jackson has been meditating regularly for more than 20 years. "I enjoy doing it first thing in the morning instead of jumping fast-forward into life. Meditation allows you to sit and let the mind realize who's in control."

It's difficult to imagine how Jackson maintains his cool in the midst of a fast-paced game, pacing up and down the side-lines with refs making bad calls and plays unraveling before his eyes.

The hard part, Jackson says, is finding the time to meditate in a busy schedule on the road. "Nowadays, I carry a foldable wooden meditation stool and I sit first thing in the morning. That's how I make sure that it's a necessary part of my life."

Because of injuries incurred during his playing career—first a torn shoulder from his high school pitching days and later a debilitating double-herniated disk with the Knicks that sidelined him for two sea-sons—his ability to get regular exercise is severely limited. Jackson's regimen consists largely of walking—when the pain is not too great.

"I lost a nerve in my leg after that in-jury in 1968," he says, "so when I can't walk, I meditate. Basically, because of the limits of time and my own body, I can only do one."

There's another stressor that basketball professionals face. Being on the road 100 days a year takes a toll on family life. "The biggest stress is balancing family and work," Jackson says. "It's not just being away that causes stress. It's the little work stresses that keep me from being attentive to my kids. Trading deadlines, watching game tapes at home, all those niggling things that come along and create a little more job pressure, which forces you to put in a few extra hours. Then suddenly, you don't know your kids' teachers, you're unfamiliar with their classes, and you don't know their friends' names. You realize that you're not participating in their lives."

Ultimately, whether in family or basketball, for Phil Jackson, dealing with stress comes down to awareness and selfless compassion. As he puts it in his book, *Sacred Hoops*, "The power of We is stronger than the power of Me."

Part 13

EATING FOR PEAK PERFORMANCE

The Killer Fats

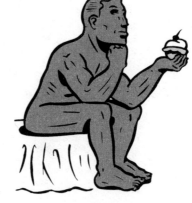

It has been reported that when a murderer named Donald Snyder entered Sing Sing, he weighed 150 pounds. He doubled his weight with heaping meals, and even on his last day, he demanded mounds of pork chops and eggs. Snyder's plan: to grow too large for his final seating.

Nevertheless, on July 16, 1953, the electric chair still fit him like a warm glove.

A high-fat diet isn't likely to extend *your* life either. What it will do is expand your belly. No matter how much you exercise, and no matter how many other things you do to keep your weight under control, nothing—*nothing*—will have more impact on your gut than the foods you eat. And nothing affects diet more than the fats that it includes.

But weight loss is just part of the equation. You aren't going to be fit if you're sick, and too much fat in your diet can make you very sick indeed. So before we discuss the ways in which you can use diet to trim your waist, we'll talk about ways that it keeps you alive.

Back to fat. Sure, you need some of it. Besides serving as an energy source, it gives structure to every cell in your body. It helps to regulate bodily functions, it insulates you against heat loss, and it cushions your vital organs.

But men take in about 34 percent of their calories from fat. You don't need nearly that much, and this overconsumption of fat can lead to killer conditions such as heart disease and cancer.

"The national recommendation is to consume no more than 30 percent of your daily calories as fat, but that is sort of a compromise by committee," explains Benjamin Caballero, M.D., Ph.D., director of the Center for Human Nutrition at Johns Hopkins University in Baltimore. "There is nothing magic about 30 percent. I think that 20 to 25 percent is reachable without being a Tibetan monk.

"A few fats are essential for us, but you can fulfill all those needs with a little over 5 percent fat in your diet. A diet completely free of fat is not healthy, but you have a very wide margin between 5 and 30 percent."

THE MAMMOTH APPETITE

Thog, your Cro-Magnon grandpa 35,000 years removed, feasted on bison, reindeer, horse, and mammoth. When he gobbled down meat, his body wisely stored any excess fat to get him through lean times.

"Evolutionarily, we were prepared to have these periods of starvation. That's why we accumulate fat so easily," says Michael J. González, D.Sc., Ph.D., assistant professor of nutritional biochemistry and advanced nutrition at the University of Puerto Rico Medical Sciences Campus School of Public Health in San Juan. "As my nutritionist friends say, the problem today is the refrigerator. We used to go search and hunt for food, and now we just open the refrigerator. Calories are very accessible."

For Thog, fat was a conveniently dense energy source—9 calories per gram. Carbohydrates and protein each provide only 4 calories per gram. Unfortunately, Thog's modern descendants have inherited bodies that are programmed to railroad excess fat right to their waistlines. Chemically, the fat you eat is pretty much ready-to-store, and it takes minimal effort for your body to sock it away. Your body is able to convert excess protein and carbohydrates into storable fat, but that process requires extra energy.

A CHOKE HOLD ON YOUR HEART

Excess fat in your diet may throw your body out of whack in several serious ways, contributing to heart disease, high cholesterol, obesity, diabetes, and some cancers. Saturated fat (the stuff found in meat, poultry, and dairy foods) and trans fats (found in margarine and shortening) seem to be the most dangerous kinds.

Coronary heart disease is the leading cause of death in the United States and other affluent countries. Much of it is traceable to saturated fat. This fat raises the level of LDL (low-density lipoprotein, or "bad," cholesterol) in your blood. LDL leaves fatty deposits in your coronary blood vessels. Narrowed blood vessels leading to your heart can cause a heart attack. Strokes can be caused by narrowed blood vessels leading to your brain.

In a program called the Seven Countries Study, scientists tracked 12,763 middle-age men for 25 years. The more saturated fat and trans fats the men consumed, the more likely they were to die of coronary heart disease. For instance, the men in Tanushimaru, Japan, received just 3.8 percent of their energy from saturated fat and had a 4.5 percent death rate from heart disease. At the other extreme, men in east Finland received 22.7 percent of their energy from saturated fat and had more than six times the Japanese death rate from heart disease.

Scientists generally agree that monounsaturated fat (such as olive oil) and polyunsaturated fat (such as corn oil) are much more heart-friendly than saturated fat. Those fats either have no effect on or actually *lower* your blood cholesterol. But which kind of fat is more beneficial? Christopher Gardner, Ph.D., who studies disease prevention at Stanford University, combined the results of 14 cholesterol studies. The resulting overview surprised him: It's a tie—they're equally beneficial to your cholesterol levels.

"We were stunned because we expected it to be one way or the other," says Dr. Gardner. "They were really virtually equivalent." This doesn't mean that the two oils are equal in all respects, he notes. Polyunsaturated fatty acids, such as in sunflower or safflower oil, might encourage tumor growth.

CORRALLING CHOLESTEROL

Good cholesterol, bad cholesterol. Sounds like a B western being played out in your bloodstream. Fine—go buy a white hat. You have the lead role.

Your body actually needs some cholesterol, but it makes a sufficient amount all on its own. The extra cholesterol you get from food is just icing on your arteries. When doctors test your blood, they measure the cholesterol in terms of milligrams per deciliter. This is the famous "count" for total cholesterol, which is best kept under 200. Almost half of all Americans fall on the dangerous side of that figure.

To get a really meaningful measure of your health status, make sure that your cholesterol test gives a breakdown for both LDL and HDL (high-density lipoprotein). Your count for the harmful LDL should be below 130. For the protective HDL, you want a count above 35. An HDL count below 35 could mean danger even if your *total* cholesterol is at or below the 200 mark.

Cholesterol is found only in animal food: meat, fish, eggs, and dairy. In food, there's no good or bad cholesterol. That issue applies only to how your body transports cholesterol once it's in your body. HDL ushers cholesterol out of your body; LDL paints it onto the walls of your blood vessels.

Identifying the cholesterol in your food is not hard. In general, the same foods that are high in saturated fat are also high in cholesterol—beef, ice cream, and béarnaise sauce, for instance. So a low-fat approach to eating will also cut your cholesterol consumption. Eggs and seafood are exceptions: Although they are low in fat, they have more cholesterol, ounce for ounce, than any other food.

So aside from eating low-fat, what can you do to lower cholesterol? Scientists offer these suggestions.

Eat more fiber. Studies show that eating foods that are high in soluble fiber helps to lower cholesterol, even for people who are already on a low-fat diet. Doctors say that adding 3 grams per day of oat fiber, for example, can lower your total cholesterol level by 5 to 6 points. So order up the beans, whole-wheat pasta, oat and wheat bran cereals, fruits like apples and oranges (eat the white stuff under the peel, too), and just about any vegetables.

Grab a grapefruit. Antioxidant vitamins are on your side in preventing heart disease. Government researchers say that men who get lots of vitamin C, for instance, have elevated HDL levels. (Go for the citrus fruits and juices.) In Finland, researchers found that arteries clogged more slowly in men with high LDL levels when they got lots of beta-carotene (carrots and sweet potatoes) and vitamin E (wheat germ and mangoes).

Hit the bricks. If you're overweight, dropping excess poundage is essential to controlling your cholesterol, doctors say. A one-two punch of weight loss and exercise will lower total cholesterol, reduce the level of triglycerides in your blood, raise your

FAT IN YOUR FOOD

Here is the fat content of some common foods.

Food	Total Fat (g)
Apple pie (⅛ of a 9" pie)	13.8
Bagel, plain, 1	1.1
Beef frankfurter, 1	12.8
Cheese, Monterey Jack, 1 oz	8.5
Chocolate chip cookie, store-bought, 1 small	2.3
Cornflakes cereal, 1 cup	0
Cottage cheese, 1%, ¼ cup	0.6
Croissant, butter, 1 medium	12.0
Doughnut, plain, 1 medium	10.8
Egg, scrambled	7.3
Ice cream, regular vanilla, ½ cup	7.2
Milk, 1%, 1 cup	2.6
Milk chocolate, 1.55-oz bar	13.5
Peanut butter, 2 Tbsp	16.0
Pork sausage, smoked, grilled, 1 link	21.6
Sandwich, ham and cheese	15.5
Sandwich, roast beef	13.8
Spaghetti, cooked, 1 cup	0.9

HDL level, reduce blood pressure, and reduce the risk of diabetes. And when you weigh less, reducing saturated fat and dietary cholesterol does a better job of lowering your LDL. To lose weight, try aerobic exercise, such as jogging or cycling, for 30 minutes, 4 or more days a week.

THE FAT-CANCER LINK

Dietary fat has been linked to colorectal cancer, prostate cancer, pancreatic cancer, and breast cancer, among others—even to lung cancer in nonsmokers. Scientists aren't sure whether a high-fat diet directly creates cancer tumors, but there's strong evidence that a steady diet of some fats will grease the skids for tumors that do appear.

Dr. González says that animal studies show that omega-6 fatty acids, found in corn oil, promote tumor growth, while omega-3 fatty acids, found in fish and fish oil capsules, slow tumor growth. "Let's say we had a 20 percent corn oil diet. You would have tumor growth that was very high. If you had 15 percent corn oil and 5 percent fish oil, the tumors would grow, but they would grow less. And as you increase the fish oil, they would keep decreasing in size."

It's tough to say how much of that applies to people, Dr. González says. You can't do such experiments on humans, and our complex metabolisms and varied diets cloud the issue still further.

But cutting back on fat overall is a good cancer-fighting move, he says. "There's no good fat, just as there's no sweet lemon, like my grandmother used to say. If I had to use one, I'd rather use olive oil. About half the studies show that it doesn't enhance tumor growth. In other studies, it enhances, but it never enhances as much as corn oil."

Let's cut to the chase and trim the fat.

Treat your meat. When you buy beef, go for the lean stuff: USDA choice or select. Prime meats have more marbling and, therefore, more fat. Lean meat doesn't have to be tough. When you soak beef in a marinade, the acids tenderize the meat and add taste. Try citrus juice and herbs, low-sodium soy sauce, vinegar, or yogurt. And

THE FAT BUDGET MADE EASY

If you want to be totally fastidious about tracking your fat intake, you'd better hire an accountant and a nutritionist to follow you around with one of those little food scales. But here's an easy way of tallying it all in your head—without the entourage.

In the table shown here, find the fat limit that's appropriate for your weight. This figure represents 20 percent of the calories that a guy your size would typically consume in a day, says Robert Kushner, M.D., director of the nutrition and weight-control clinic at the University of Chicago. Eat more, and you're destined to gain body fat. Eat less, and you'll lose.

Anytime you fix something to eat, check the nutrition label. Look at the serving size and look at the amount of fat in each serving. If you're eating, say, twice the serving size listed, you'll have to double the amount of fat listed. In your head, keep a running total of the fat you consume. When you're finished putting things in your stomach for the day, check your actual total against your limit.

That was easy, huh? Now send your accountant home. Tell him you might have a job for him next April.

Your Weight (lb)	Fat Limit (g)
130	40
140	44
150	46
160	49
170	53
180	55
190	60
200	62

here's a no-brainer: Organ and lunchmeats are high in fat, so avoid brains, hearts, kidneys, livers, sweetbreads (that's the thymus gland of an animal), bologna, hot dogs, and sausages.

Read the package. Check the nutrition and ingredients labels on food packages before you buy. In a split second, you can find out the total fat and saturated fat content.

Eat early. Consume at least 60 percent of your calories in the morning. Even if you made no changes in your diet and exercise, this move would trim fat from your frame,

according to A. Scott Connelly, M.D., a California researcher specializing in nutrition and metabolism. In the evening, the excess blood sugar in your system is more likely to be converted into body fat.

Bake to shake fat. If you gravitate toward fruits, vegetables, and grain foods, you'll automatically sidestep a good amount of fat lurking out there. But keep an eye on the chef. A baked spud, for example, is virtually fat-free (unless you smear it with butter), but you'll get 11 grams of fat in just 14 french fries.

Nutrition Made Easy

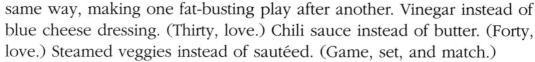

You win your tennis matches one stroke at a time—whop, crosscourt with topspin. You win the showdown with fat the same way, making one fat-busting play after another. Vinegar instead of blue cheese dressing. (Thirty, love.) Chili sauce instead of butter. (Forty, love.) Steamed veggies instead of sautéed. (Game, set, and match.)

The overall strategy in the fat-fighting game is to forgo fat calories and replace them (because your body won't run on thin air) with carbohydrate calories.

When you consume fat, your metabolic processes burn off only about 3 percent of those calories before they start adding an extra layer of tread to the spare tire around your waist. But when you consume carbohydrates—from grains, fruits, and vegetables—your metabolism flames 23 percent of the calories before they're available for conversion to fat. With luck, any excess calories you consume will be burned up by your daily activities before they become long-term blubber.

MAKING SENSE OUT OF MEALS

It's a familiar pattern. There was no time to prepare oatmeal and orange juice for breakfast, so you grabbed a Danish at the office. You had a craving for grilled chicken breast at lunch, but time ran out, so you had a Twinkie at your desk. After going hungry all day, you had the appetite of a crocodile when you got home. So you raided the refrigerator and half the pantry, plus the carton of ice cream in the freezer.

That's a meal pattern out of control. "The object is to curb your appetite before it gets to be too much, overwhelming, that famished feeling," says Pat Harper, R.D., a Pittsburgh nutritionist and spokesperson for the American Dietetic Association. "Then, you lose control and you eat too much. So plan ahead—that's the big message. Be prepared."

Eat a solid breakfast. A morning meal as simple as juice and a high-fiber cereal with 1% or fat-free milk will help protect you from fat as the day wears on. It's filling, so you'll be less tempted to graze on vending machine junk or overeat at lunch. It can also cause you to burn calories faster. Researchers at George Washington University in Washington, D.C., found that people who skipped breakfast burned 5 percent fewer calories than folks who ate three or more meals a day.

Munch often. "The guideline—the ideal—is not to go more than 4 or 5 hours without either a meal or a snack," Harper says. This will prevent you from becoming famished and gobbling down an entire sausage pizza as a midafternoon snack.

Load up early. Rather than having your big meal at night, try having it at noon instead. "Sometimes, all men need to do is eat more in the first half of the day and less in the second half," says Harper. "In the first half of the day, they're up and about and burning up those calories. In the evening, they're sitting and watching television, and they're not burning so many calories."

Practice portion control. To keep serving sizes down, make like a farmer: Devote most of the real estate on your dinner plate to plants and reserve just a little for livestock. "The way to deal with portions is to fill up your plate with vegetables and starches and go easy on the meat," says Harper.

HAVE IT FAST AND LEAN

When you're starved for time—as well as just starved—snack cakes, burgers, and candy bars are so available that they seem to leap into your hands. But fast food doesn't have to be junk food. Here are a few healthy ideas for when you're on the run.

Make it mobile. Dried fruits such as raisins, dates, and apricots are perfect for the man on the move. "They're concentrated in calories, and they're loaded with vitamins and minerals," says Chris Rosenbloom, R.D., Ph.D., associate professor in the department of nutrition and dietetics at Georgia State University and nutrition consultant for the Georgia Tech Athletic Association, both in Atlanta. "I always encourage people to keep some in their desk drawers or, for students, in their backpacks."

Grab a bagel to go. If there's no time for breakfast, grab a bagel as you head for the door. It's compact and neat and doesn't require toasting. Bagels also come in a variety of flavors, so you'll never get bored. "Bagels are virtually fat-free," Harper adds. "They give you nutritional value, plus they fill you up and stay with you."

Slow-cook your supper. Slow-cooking Crock-Pots, stoked in the morning with things such as chicken, potatoes, and onions, can have dinner ready for you the minute you walk in the door. In addition, they can keep food moist with virtually no added oil. Current models will not get you a beer or clear the table, however.

Grab a salad on the fly. Many fast-food restaurants and groceries now offer salad bars, so it's easy to make a salad raid part of your routine. Load up on the vegetables and darker salad greens, which have more nutrients. Add the low-fat dressing. Skip the croutons. In the fat-fighting game, you'll be miles ahead of the guys who snapped up double cheeseburgers.

SWITCHIN' IN THE KITCHEN

A lean lifestyle depends heavily on swapping one food for a substitute that's lower in fat. Sometimes, the choices are clear, as when you swap the bacon and eggs for a bagel with jelly. More often, however, what's involved is an incremental rollback of the fat content—small changes that add up, like drinking 1% or 2% milk instead of whole milk.

"In the past few years, the food industry has really tried to change its products to accommodate the low-fat recommendations," says Lisa Litin, R.D., a research dietitian at Harvard School of Public Health. "Many of these products actually do provide a lower-fat alternative—not necessarily low-fat, but definitely lower-fat."

A good general rule is always to reach for "natural" foods as opposed to their highly processed counterparts.

You'll also want to rethink the preparation and presentation of food. What's the point in giving vegetables a lean steaming, for instance, if you're just going to smother them in butter once they get to the table? "You need to watch the total fat that's added to the food, either before it gets to the table or at the table," says Litin.

To get into the swing of swapping away fat, try these tips from the food pros.

Know beans. Rather than stuffing yourself with red meat 5 days a week, make a move toward a healthier source of protein. Three-quarters of a cup of lima beans, for example, has 7 grams of protein. The same amount of peas has more protein than an egg—with virtually no fat.

Though you can use beans as a standalone dish, they can also be combined with traditional favorites. Instead of using ground beef in lasagna, for example, try substituting cooked and mashed chickpeas or pintos, suggests Michele Tuttle, R.D., director of consumer affairs for the Food Marketing Institute in Washington, D.C.

Swear off the oils. Although cake and pancake recipes typically call for lots of butter or oil, you can usually substitute fat-free sour cream in equal portions without substantially altering the flavor or texture of the food.

Hit the sauce. Who says that white sauces have to clog your arteries? In lieu of a cream-based sauce, toss some low-fat or fat-free cottage cheese into the food processor and thin it with fat-free milk. Then, stir in sautéed onions, garlic, and basil.

Dress with less. When you're making salad dressing, toss out one-third of the oil and substitute water. The taste and texture will barely change, and you'll be saving yourself 33 percent pure fat.

Try it on the side. Making a switch in presentation styles can shave off fat. Instead of sopping down salads with fatty dressing, serve the dressing in a small container at the side of the plate. "You dip the fork into the dressing and then pick up a forkful of salad," says Dr. Rosenbloom. "You use so little dressing that way, but you get a little flavor with each bite."

Use your noodle. Egg noodles are delicious. They're also loaded with fat. So switch to spaghetti instead. You probably won't notice the difference—it's under a sauce, right?—and you'll save 1 gram of fat and 16 calories per cup.

Catch a lean tuna. Fish belong in water, so why would you buy tuna that's packed in oil? Using the kind packed in H_2O will save you 6 grams of fat and 70 calories per 3-ounce can.

Spice your java. Although those elegant little tins of instant gourmet coffee are convenient and delicious, they are decidedly high in fat. To get the flavor without the fat, try spicing up your regular brew with a pinch of cinnamon or nutmeg. "I put cinnamon in the grounds, and that gives it a nice flavor and aroma, and it doesn't add any calories," says Dr. Rosenbloom.

Do some reading. The food industry knows that you're cruising for ideas, and many companies print recipes—both traditional and low-fat versions—on the backs of their packages. A pancake mix, for example, might recommend substituting 2 egg whites for each whole egg and using fat-free milk instead of whole.

OLIVE OIL: KING OF HEARTS

Who'da thunk a lunk like Popeye would be such a visionary? Not only did he gobble nutrient-rich spinach, he also was fond of Olive Oyl.

These days, olive oil—the foodstuff, not the cartoon character—is a dietary darling. While it's still pure fat and loaded with calories, studies show that it may help lower levels of harmful low-density lipoprotein (LDL) cholesterol while leaving the "good"

high-density lipoprotein (HDL) cholesterol unchanged.

In one study, researchers tested lipid levels of 12 people who consumed 30 percent of total calories from fat. Some got their fat from milk fats, while others got it in the form of sunflower, rapeseed, or olive oils. With the olive oil diet, researchers not only saw the greatest drop in LDL levels but they also saw HDL become smaller and more fluid, which may help it remove cholesterol from cells more effectively.

"This finding helps explain how higher HDL levels may protect against heart disease and how monounsaturated fat might play a helpful role; however, more research is needed," says lipid expert Margo Denke, M.D., assistant professor of medicine at the University of Texas Health Science Center at Dallas Southwestern Medical School Center for Human Nutrition.

You can use olive oil as a substitute for every oil in the kitchen—not only for frying and sautéing but for baking as well.

Incidentally, of the three grades of olive oil commonly available—virgin, extra-virgin, and pure—only the pure oil should be used for frying. The virgin and extra-virgin are higher-grade oils. Their delicate nature—and considerably higher price—means that they're best used for light sautés or just for drizzling on pasta, vegetables, or bread.

How to Make Fast Food Good for You

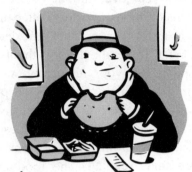

For men who are fighting fat, a shopping-mall food court is the demilitarized zone. Only the danger isn't friendly fire. It's friendly fries. When you find yourself hungry, short on time, and surrounded by fast-food joints, the temptation to wave the white flag and chow down is nearly irresistible.

Before you wolf down the super-deluxe-mega-triple-cheeseburger-with-bacon, ask yourself, How will I feel afterward, mentally and physically?

"It changes your food choices," says Phillip M. Sinaikin, M.D., a Longwood, Florida, psychiatrist who specializes in the treatment of obesity, and the author of *Fat Madness: How to Stop the Diet Cycle and Achieve Permanent Well-Being.* "If it's going to sit like a lump in your stomach and not give you the pleasant sense of energy that carbohydrates do, then that probably makes it a bad choice."

PENNY-WISE, POUND-FOOLISH

One national survey found that 58 percent of men eat in fast-food restaurants at least once a week.

Sure, you can go low-fat and buy a regular hamburger, salad, and diet soda at most places. But it will probably cost you more than if you bought a combination meal with a huge burger, large fries, and big drink. Yes, you can buy a small order of fries—but the large order often doesn't cost much more.

"It's ridiculous. They convince you that you've got to be out of your mind to get small fries," says Bonnie Liebman, a licensed nutritionist and director of nutrition for the Center for Science in the Public Interest in Washington, D.C.

What you're gaining in quantity, however, you're paying for in fat. "We can't make the world stop advertising fast food," Dr. Sinaikin notes. "But we can step back from the world and look at it a bit and say, 'Hey, what about the quality of my life—my single individual

FAST FOOD: THE NEXT GENERATION

Daily's Fit & Fresh, a health-conscious restaurant chain based in San Diego, hopes to follow the trail blazed by McDonald's 40 years ago.

Daily's, which opened its doors in 1992, offers speed and convenience but goes a step further: Nothing on the menu contains more than 10 grams of fat or 20 percent of calories from fat.

Daily's is the dream-come-true of cardiac surgeon Pat Daily, M.D. "The vision for this concept is the wave of the future," says dietitian Patti Tveit Milligan, R.D., director of nutrition for Daily's. "We do hope it can be a national chain."

Pasta, potatoes, and rice receive star billing among entrées, along with poultry and fish. Selections include grilled chicken breast in a pita pocket with salad greens and ginger-and-sesame dressing, and a chili-stuffed baked potato. But don't order a burger. Milligan says that Daily's decided not to mimic high-fat offerings from other fast-food restaurants. Instead, Daily's offers a veggie burger with brown rice and vegetables served on a whole-wheat bun.

Milligan admits that she was skeptical when Dr. Daily first approached her in 1989 with the idea of starting a healthy fast-food restaurant. "People talk about how they want to eat healthy, but do they put their money where their mouth is?" She now believes that if you offer people tasty, low-fat food at a reasonable price with fast service, they will buy it—again and again.

---

life? What can I do to enhance the quality of my life?'"

FAST AND GOOD

The world isn't going to slow down anytime soon, and until it does, we're always going to appreciate fast food. But it's still possible to get good food fast. Here's what you can do.

Start the day right. Most fast-food restaurants offer healthy breakfasts. Pancakes are almost always a good choice, assuming you hold the butter or margarine and go easy on the syrup. English muffins, toast, bagels, or cereal with 1% or fat-free milk can also get your engine humming in the morning. But avoid croissants, pastries, and Danish. The high levels of sugar and fat

can turn your idle way down—and push your waist out, says Megan Cordova, R.D., an outpatient dietitian at Johnston-Willis Hospital in Richmond, Virginia.

Don't be biased against burgers. You want one, get one—but use common sense. A single-patty burger at most fast-food restaurants has more than 10 grams of fat. That's no problem, says Dale L. Anderson, M.D., head of the complementary medicine department at Park Nicollet Medical Center in Minneapolis. But what happens when you pile burger on top of burger and cover both with cheese, mayonnaise, or "special sauces"?

Dr. Anderson has a term for this: Rather than calling them double or triple burgers, he jokes, we should call them double or triple bypasses.

Consider that a Double Whopper with Cheese at Burger King packs 63 grams of fat. For a lot of guys, that's more than a day's worth in one sitting.

Lean toward roast beef. Beef doesn't have to mean hamburger. A Roy Rogers roast beef sandwich has 4 grams of fat, while a hamburger carries 9 grams. So if you like beef, make the leaner choice and go with the roasted kind, says Liebman.

Go ahead, chicken. Grilled, baked, or broiled chicken sandwiches are a good bet most of the time. Again, watch the toppings and be sure to order them without mayonaisse.

Flee fries. A burger and fries go together like Abbott and Costello. But for your health's sake, it would be better if they were more like Dean Martin and Jerry Lewis—ex-partners.

"A large order of fries is almost like having two sandwiches," Liebman says. "We think of it as a side dish, but it's really as fatty and caloric as a main dish. Large fries have 450 calories, compared with 420 in a Quarter Pounder at McDonald's. And the fries have 22 grams of fat, compared with 20 in the Quarter Pounder."

Pizza delivers. Great news, guys. Pizza can actually be part of a healthy, balanced meal.

Order the thin crust; it has less fat. And go for the vegetable toppings like green pepper and onion, not the pepperoni and sausage.

Go convenient. It used to be that hitting the 7-Eleven or other convenience stores meant having a hot dog or—shudder—a microwave burrito. These days, a number of quick-stop stores carry items such as low-fat yogurt, turkey sandwiches, fresh fruits, and salad fixings. Pick the one nearest you and shop around. You may be pleasantly surprised.

Frozen Convenience

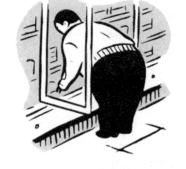

They used to be called TV dinners, and they were manly meals. Meat loaf, mashed potatoes, gravy, peas, and—if you were lucky—even some applesauce for dessert. All in one convenient container. In the 1950s and 1960s, they were what men cooked—or burned—when their wives weren't home for dinner.

Those were simpler times, and your choices in the freezer section of the local grocery store were uncomplicated by matters such as calories or fat content. TV dinners were quick, easy, and filling, and that was sufficient.

No more. In the health-conscious 1990s, we demand more from frozen foods. And mainly, we do it by demanding less—less fat, less sodium, and fewer calories.

For harried men who want to fight fat, learning to choose the right frozen dinners can make a big difference because we tend to eat higher-fat foods when we're short for time. Nearly one-half of the shoppers who eat high-fat foods do so when they're in a hurry, according to a survey.

TV dinners now go by the more upscale moniker of *frozen entrées*, and manufacturers have responded with an array of offerings that are labeled "healthy" or "low-fat."

But beware: You can't always judge a frozen entrée by its cover. At least not solely from the sumptuous photograph and catchy name.

"The definition of low-fat for dinners and entrées is more liberal than it is for individual foods," says Bonnie Liebman, a licensed nutritionist and director of nutrition for the Center for Science in the Public Interest in Washington, D.C. "So you can often get up to 9 or 10 grams of fat in a dinner that's labeled 'low-fat.' Don't look at just the word 'low-fat' and assume that it's the lowest possible you can get."

THE LOWDOWN ON CALORIES

With frozen foods, it pays to read the labels. First, check total calories. Today, you may have more of a problem with low-fat entrées having too few calories than too many.

Portion sizes probably are smaller than you're accustomed to. This is one of the ways that packagers keep fat levels down. Most low-fat frozen dinners come with some type of sauce, which actually makes them more filling than they look, but side dishes such as a salad and a piece of fruit are needed to satisfy a realistic appetite.

Concentrate on percentage of calories from fat, not on the number of calories. Often, fewer calories means less food, not necessarily less fat.

"Interestingly, for men, who tend to want more calories, we don't tell people to just get the fewest calories possible, because frankly, that isn't much of a dinner," Liebman says.

A frozen dinner with only 250 calories is about the same as what you'd get in a plain bagel or a cup of fruit yogurt. Now be honest: Would you ever consider a bagel or a cup of yogurt to be a complete dinner?

"We actually recommend that people look for dinners that supply a larger amount of food but are still low in fat," Liebman explains.

Once again, percentage of calories from fat is what really counts. As a quick rule of thumb, look for frozen dinners that have 7 grams of fat or less. And in the key category of saturated fat—what Liebman calls "the kind that clogs the arteries"—dinners should generally check in at about 3 to 4 grams or even less.

AVOID FREEZER BURN

To keep from getting burned by frozen foods, here are some important things to keep in mind.

Investigate ingredients. Not all meat is really all-meat—some is mixed with soy or wheat products to make it lower in fat. This doesn't always make a big difference in taste, however, and in some cases it allows for heartier portions.

Check the order of ingredients on the package. If it's supposed to be a cheese dish and you see cheese way down on the list, after things like xanthan gum, you know that somebody is skimping. It's a good idea to look for products with generous amounts of low-fat cheese.

Stay off the sauce. Pass on the frozen vegetables with butter or cream sauces. "That's where the fat content really goes up," says Chris Rosenbloom, R.D., Ph.D., associate professor in the department of nutrition and dietetics at Georgia State University and nutrition consultant for the Georgia Tech Athletic Association, both in Atlanta.

Keep it simple. Frozen chicken potpies, for example, are almost always higher in everything you don't want than are one-ingredient meals, such as roasted chicken entrées.

Be wary of the all-in-one meals. The four-course dinner may look appetizing, but looks can be deceiving. Better to get just a nice pasta or rice dish. You can throw together a quick salad on the side.

Prepare extra vegetables. An analysis by the Center for Science in the Public Interest found that most frozen dinners shortchange you on vegetables.

"While the industry has made great strides in cutting fat and sodium, one thing it hasn't done is provide a decent amount of vegetables, which is not inconsequential considering that the National Cancer Institute recommends five to nine servings of fruits and vegetables a day," Liebman says.

"Most people figure that if you're eating a frozen dinner, it should at least have a serving or two. Many have less than a single ½-cup serving, and very few of them have two servings, which is only a cup of vegetables."

Your best bet: Supplement your frozen dinner with either frozen or steamed vegetables, which are quick and convenient.

Chill out with desserts. Among the frozen desserts, grab up the fat-free yogurt, fruit bars, sorbets, and pops. Don't forget that they are still sweetened with sugar and can be high in calories.

Consider the serving size. When you're checking a frozen food item's label for fat content, don't forget to factor in the serving size that's being used. For instance, your favorite frozen yogurt may boast only 3 grams of fat per serving. The serving size listed is ½ cup, however, and you usually spoon down 1½ cups of frozen yogurt in one sitting. That adds up to 9 grams of fat per actual serving. Frozen pizzas often list the serving size as two slices. Be honest: When was the last time you ate two slices of a frozen pizza and put the rest in the fridge for another day?

Dish it out. Unless you have to eat it right from the tray (some are pretty much wedged into plastic cartons), have a separate dish handy to spoon the ingredients into. A nice presentation will make a big difference in how you perceive your meal.

Make your own. Great frozen meals aren't found only in the freezer section of the grocery store; you can make your own at home. During the weekend, whip up a good-size batch of some stew or soup and stick it in the freezer. Then, on a night when you get home from work too late—and too tired—to cook, pop some in the oven or microwave, says Paul R. Thomas, R.D., Ed.D., a staff scientist with the Food and Nutrition Board of the National Academy of Sciences in Washington, D.C. Add some good bread, some fat-free or 1% milk, and a salad. You have an instant, healthy meal.

Health in a Can

Back in World War II, in the First Infantry Division somewhere in North Africa, Fred Seward ate cold Spam for dinner—in the dark, with a sharpened spoon. The next night, he would eat Spam again. It was the same thing the next night. And again the next.

It was the going Army joke during those hellish days whenever C rations were handed out: "Spam again?" But Seward knew that the canned pork concoction was better than nothing. So he ate it.

Once he returned to the United States, he didn't touch Spam until nearly 50 years later. It was the same story with corned beef hash and orange marmalade. "Any canned food, if you have it day after day after day, becomes boring and monotonous and you will not touch it," says Seward, who now lives in Geneva, New York.

As for other foods that come canned—especially corn and peaches—Seward eats them heartily. They're convenient.

And convenience is canned food's main selling point. All the chopping, peeling, and cooking have been done for you. If you come home feeling like a hungry piece of pulp—too hungry to sleep and too tired to eat—there's always that can of ravioli. Rip off the top, find a fork, and you have dinner.

The great thing about canned foods is that they make it possible to have things that you'd never eat otherwise. Take beans. Dried beans take almost forever to cook. They're healthy, but who could be bothered?

"People who would not spend the time it takes to cook dried beans will use the cans. It's so convenient," says Mona R. Sutnick, R.D., Ed.D., a nutrition consultant and spokesperson for the American Dietetic Association. "Beans are such good, nutritious food. They have a lot of the same nutrients as meat, without the fat and cholesterol. And they're versatile. You can really do a lot with them, whether it's soups or stews or chilies or salads."

Canned food's other claim to fame harks back to your Boy Scout days (which, if you're lucky, is the last time you had to eat a lot of food from a can): Be prepared. Just in case Hurricane Elmer wipes out the utility poles in the entire county. Just in case a blizzard dumps enough snow to block access to a grocery store for a month. Just in case an earthquake swallows your refrigerator. According to the Canned Food Information Council in Chicago, this is what you should always have on hand—just in case.

- Canned fruit (pears, mixed assortments, peaches) packed in its own juice
- Canned meats and seafood (tuna, chicken, crabmeat, salmon) packed in water or broth
- Canned vegetables (corn, carrots, tomatoes, potatoes)
- Canned specialty food (chili, chow mein, Mexican dishes)
- Soups (vegetable, chicken noodle, stew), including the low-fat and reduced-sodium varieties
- Beverages (condensed fat-free milk, fruit and vegetable juices)

YOU CAN DO IT

About 1,500 different foods come in cans, including 75 types of juices, 130 vegetable products, and 100 soups and stews. That's a lot to choose from. Here's how to pick out the right stuff and cook it the right way so you can have a nutritious meal. Proviso: Buy fruit packed in juice, not in "syrup."

Drink the juice. When you buy a peach, the vitamins are in the peach. But when you buy a canned peach, only some of the vitamins are in the peach. The rest are in the liquid that the peach is floating in. That's because many nutrients dissolve in water, says Dr. Sutnick.

You can get the most nutrients for your money by using the liquid from canned fruits and vegetables. And you don't have to drink it straight from the can. Here are some more palatable suggestions from Dr. Sutnick.

- Cook vegetables in the juice they come in.
- Use vegetable juice to make soup or stew.
- Put leftover fruit juice in ice-cube trays and freeze it. You can eat it plain or put the cubes into drinks for extra flavor.

Buy water-packed. You don't want to buy tuna that's packed in oil, because it has more fat and more calories than tuna packed in water. Even after you drain the oil, you're looking at three times as much fat and 50 percent more calories, according to researchers at the University of California, Berkeley. And you're getting less of the fish's healthy benefits. The healthy omega-3 fatty acids are oil-soluble. When you drain the oil, you lose 15 to 25 percent of the omega-3's. You don't have the same problem with water-packed tuna.

Bone up on your calcium. If you want to boost your calcium intake, eat the bones from canned sardines and canned salmon. The bones will be soft from the processing. A 3-ounce serving supplies as much calcium as a glass of milk.

Get additional omega-3's with different fish. When we think canned fish, we usually think tuna. On average, each of us eats about 3 pounds of it a year. You may, however, want to consider expanding your tastes. Canned salmon, sardines, and herring have more omega-3's than tuna.

Sardines and herring can vary tremendously in their fat and caloric contents because different packing companies use varying species and sizes of fish from different locations (those from colder waters have more fat). They can have anywhere from 2 to 20 grams of fat in 3 ounces. You need to read the labels.

Watch the syrup. If you're going to buy fruit packed in syrup, make sure it's light, not heavy. Heavy syrup packs more empty sugar calories than you need. The light syrup can be used on pancakes and waffles instead of maple syrup.

Watch the sodium. The National Academy of Sciences recommends that we eat no more than 2,400 milligrams of sodium a day, the amount in 1 teaspoon of salt. The average American takes in close to 4,000 milligrams a day. And 75 percent of it comes from processed food.

Some soups have as much as 1,000 milligrams of salt per cup, so you need to read the labels. Canned-food manufacturers are putting out many reduced-salt products. Some include green beans, sliced beets, diced carrots, whole-kernel corn, sweet peas, mixed vegetables, chickpeas, tuna, salmon, and soups. Here's how to understand the terms.

- *Sodium-free:* Fewer than 5 milligrams of sodium per serving
- *Very low sodium:* Fewer than 35 milligrams per serving
- *Low sodium:* 140 milligrams or fewer per serving

Don't rinse it. Rinsing canned food will reduce the salt content but will also reduce the food's nutrient content. Unfortunately, the most heavily salted canned foods are soups, sauces, gravies, and prepared foods, such as pasta meals, which you couldn't or wouldn't rinse anyway. Dr. Sutnick suggests that you look for low-salt or low-sodium versions of those products.

JUST ADD TASTE

Some canned foods are overcooked and mushy. Some can be downright bland and boring. So what's a guy to do?

You need to get creative.

"Don't ask the food manufacturers to make it taste good. You're in charge of taste," says Diane Wilke, R.D., a nutrition consultant in Columbus, Ohio. "All you want is something that's basically healthy that is safe to eat. If it doesn't taste the way you like it, then you modify it to make it taste better."

So add some zest to canned foods by adding salsa, ketchup, garlic, onions, or fat-free Italian dressing.

And don't overcook the peas—or any other canned foods. Remember, they're already cooked. You only need to warm them up. It only takes a couple of minutes in a saucepan or microwave to get them ready to eat. Technically, you can eat them straight from the can.

We're not saying that you should plop cans of corn, beans, and peas with the lids ripped off on your kitchen table for dinner. We're saying that if you want to save time, you can find ways to use them without even heating them. Make a cold salad out of them. Throw some canned carrots, kidney beans, and lima beans together with a marinade. Or mix canned collard greens with some onion and vinegar.

Here are some other ways to throw together a quick canned-food meal, according to the Canned Food Information Council. Dr. Sutnick recommends that you always look for the light, low-sodium, low-fat versions of the canned foods you choose.

Mix things up. Mix canned fruit with plain fat-free yogurt.

Add them to other cooked foods. Canned vegetables are perfect additions to a variety of soups and stews.

Top it off. Use canned peaches or blueberries on top of low-fat pound cake.

Garnish it. Place canned pineapple rings around various meats and poultry.

Toss it. Toss cooked and cooled rotini or pasta shells with drained canned tomatoes, canned carrots, canned mushrooms, and a vinaigrette dressing.

SHOP SMART

Canned food is inexpensive, but there are some things that you don't need to go wasting your money on. One of them is elegance. Two canned items come to mind: fruit and tuna. Simplest is best—who needs elegance?

First, fruit. You could pay a lot more money for pretty, uniform pear halves. And there are times when you should. If you're cooking up a special dinner, you may want to open up a can of pretty pear halves and arrange them in a pretty bowl.

But if you're just going to rip off the top of the can and jam your fork into the first pear with which it comes in contact, there's no need to pay for elegance. Get the cheaper kind.

Do the same with tuna. There's only one thing to look for in tuna. We already told you about it. You don't want it packed in oil. Other than that, it doesn't matter what you buy. Light meat, dark meat. That's a personal preference, but it won't affect your health, says Dr. Sutnick.

This also goes for the size of the chunks. If you're going to mash it up, don't go wasting your cash on solid tuna, which costs more. Get the flaked kind. Hey, they've done half the work for you already.

The rule applies to any canned item. "Don't buy fancier than you're going to use," says Dr. Sutnick.

ON THE SHELF

As long as it stays in the can and the can is undamaged, the stuff could probably last forever. But you don't want to take chances. The Canned Food Information Council recommends that you use canned foods within a year.

Don't store cans above 80°F. Also, beware of cans that look damaged. If the vacuum seal has been ruptured, the food has not been preserved. And it can make you really sick, so watch out for swelling or leaks.

Some hissing when the can is opened is normal because it's vacuum-packed. But if the can hisses loudly or spurts, the food might be spoiled, according to the council.

What's on the Label?

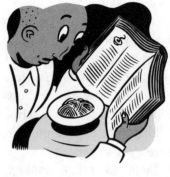

Glance at the Food Guide Pyramid on the opposite page. Does your vision go blurry? Does your mind drift, sleepily reminded of fourth-grade textbook illustrations? Well, smack yourself sharply across the jaw and give it another look.

You've probably been ignoring a tool that's as simple as a paper clip, as versatile as a Swiss Army knife, and as intuitively accessible as a Macintosh computer.

While we're at it, have you ever looked at the Nutrition Facts panel that appears on almost every food item you buy? No? That's worth two smacks because you've really been asleep.

The point is that a lot of the information you need to make wise food choices is right under your nose. It's clear and it's reliable. Even those brightly lettered health claims on food packages have to follow U.S. government guidelines. What you may have been dismissing as hype or inconsequential fine print can help you stay healthy, gain energy, and manage your weight. All you need to do is engage your brain.

"Nutrition labels list nutrients that play a role in chronic disease. The levels of these nutrients have public health significance," says Carole Adler, R.D., a dietitian in the FDA's Office of Food Labeling. "I think that

if men understood that, they would feel more inclined to read them."

Here's how to navigate the Food Guide Pyramid and food labels, including the Nutrition Facts panel. If you master both of these, we'll stop making you slap yourself. People are starting to stare, you know.

HOW THE PYRAMID STACKS UP

The Food Guide Pyramid is a dietary cheat sheet, a visual guide reminding you of several concepts in one glance.

Variety: Eat lots of different stuff, hitting all the food groups.

Moderation: Watch your serving sizes, and go easy on the fats, oils, and sweets.

Proportion: Notice how big a block the grain and pasta group gets on the pyramid? Load up on those foods. See how much smaller the dairy-group block is? A little dab'll do ya.

The pyramid's sections incorporate the five major food groups as defined by the USDA. Sorry, the tip of the pyramid—reserved for soft drinks, candy, butter, oil, and the like—doesn't rate major food group status. The second tier from the top comes mostly from animals. These foods—such as milk, meat, fish, and eggs—are big sources of protein, calcium, iron, and zinc. The third tier is plant food, fruits, and vegetables, which are high in vitamins, minerals, and fiber. Grain foods make up the foundation of the pyramid, providing complex carbohydrates, vitamins, minerals, and fiber.

"The idea is to guide people in balancing amounts of certain products versus others," says Michael J. González, D.Sc., Ph.D., assistant professor of nutritional biochemistry and advanced nutrition at the University of Puerto Rico Medical Sciences Campus School of Public Health in San Juan.

Check out the number of servings a day listed for each food group. Men are supposed to gravitate toward the high end of the range, particularly if they're active. Does 11 servings of grain sound like a belly buster of an eating plan? Maybe not, if you consider what counts for a serving: one slice of bread, 1 ounce of cold cereal, or ½ cup of cooked cereal, rice, or pasta. The servings add up quickly: If you eat cereal and a slice of toast at breakfast, a sandwich at lunch, 1 cup of pasta at dinner, and three or four small, plain crackers for a snack, you're at 7 servings already.

Here's what counts for a serving in the other food groups.

Vegetables: 1 cup of raw, leafy veggies; ½ cup of other vegetables, cooked or chopped raw; or ¾ cup of vegetable juice

Fruits: a medium apple, banana, or orange; ½ cup of chopped, cooked, or canned fruit; or ¾ cup of fruit juice

Dairy foods: 1 cup of milk or yogurt; 1½ ounces of natural cheese; or 2 ounces of processed cheese

Meats: 2 to 3 ounces of cooked lean meat, poultry, or fish; ½ cup of cooked dry beans; one egg; or 2 tablespoons of peanut butter

The food guide's illustrations are a helpful touch, Dr. González says. It's no coincidence that broccoli appears, for example. High in vitamins and fiber, "it's almost the perfect food," he says.

Speaking of illustrations, most folks don't notice those tiny circles and triangles sprinkled over the pyramid. They represent the fat (circles) and added sugar (triangles) that appear in various foods. The more fat and sugar a food group is likely to have, the

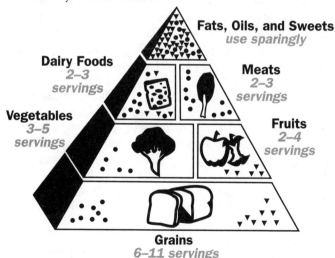

Fats, Oils, and Sweets
use sparingly

Dairy Foods
2–3 servings

Meats
2–3 servings

Vegetables
3–5 servings

Fruits
2–4 servings

Grains
6–11 servings

more little circles and triangles you'll see in that section of the pyramid.

WHAT'S IN THIS STUFF, ANYWAY?

If the Food Guide Pyramid is your overall battle plan, then the Nutrition Facts panel is your ammunition in the trenches. Okay, the trenches look an awful lot like grocery aisles, and you're lugging granola bars instead of grenades. But this is where the nu-tritional battle is won or lost—the moment when you decide whether to toss an item into your cart or to leave it on the shelf.

When you're considering buying a packaged food, turn the item around until you find that little box with the words *Nutrition Facts* at the top. For most foods, the FDA requires manufacturers to list the amounts of 13 nutrients and the number of calories from fat, and it allows the voluntary

WHY A PYRAMID?

Remember *The $100,000 Pyramid* game show? Not to be outdone, the federal government spent nearly $1 million test-marketing the Food Guide Pyramid before introducing it in 1992. Among the other hot contenders were a jigsaw design (which test subjects found puzzling), a circular pie chart (which reminded kids of pizza), and a grocery cart filled with paper sacks of varying size (they bagged it—too ambiguous).

"A couple of things make the pyramid work. For one thing, it's very simple. Also, it's not a new shape," says Dan D. Snyder, of the communications company Porter/Novelli. Snyder was the designer on the case when the USDA commissioned a new food guide in the late 1980s. "Everybody knows what a triangle looks like, so it's not trying to teach a consumer a new shape, like a shopping basket or a fruit bowl."

The Food Guide Pyramid first took shape on Snyder's sketch pad as he watched a focus group from behind a two-way mirror. He and a government staffer were toying with block shapes that represented different food groups when they decided to stack the blocks to form a triangle.

That pyramid is now a cultural icon. Sixty-three percent of Americans are familiar with it, according to a *Parade* magazine survey, and 57 percent of those people say that they obey its recommendations an average of four times a week.

If you're among its followers, remember this about the pyramid's design: Higher is not better. "The things that you should eat the most are at the lower part," notes Michael J. González, D.Sc., Ph.D., assistant professor of nutritional biochemistry and advanced nutrition at the University of Puerto Rico Medical Sciences Campus School of Public Health in San Juan. "Sometimes, people will say, 'Hey, why are grains down low when we should be eating more? They should be up there.'"

Snyder says that an upside-down pyramid was actually tested, but "people thought it was not stable. It looked like it was going to fall over." Besides, the name "Food Guide Yield-Sign-Shape" doesn't have the same ring to it.

listing of 10 additional dietary components. If you want to ponder as many as 23 nutrients for every food item you buy, be our guest. Just don't forget to take your laptop computer, and turn off the lights when you leave the supermarket. In the real world, you're more likely to zero in on the handful of items on the nutrition label that most concern you.

"It really depends on what your goals are," Adler says. "Let's say that you're a man trying to focus on weight management and a low-fat diet. Then you may want to look at the information on calories, calories from fat, total fat, saturated fat, and cholesterol. Of course, if your doctor says that you're sodium-sensitive and you're trying to lower your blood pressure, then you would also focus on the amount of sodium in the product."

Suppose you're looking for a snack cracker and you pull a box of chili-and-cheese-flavored Munch 'Ems off the shelf. You see at the top of the chart that a single serving is 28 crackers. (This serving size is not a recommendation—it's just what the FDA says is an amount customarily consumed in one sitting.) If you eat twice that many when you snack on crackers, then you need to double all of the nutrient amounts you find on the chart.

But let's assume you're a 28-cracker snacker. If you're concerned about calories and fat, you check out these figures next: 140 calories, 35 of them from fat. A quick calculation tells you that this food gets 25 percent of its calories from fat. You're trying to keep your fat consumption to less than 30 percent of calories, so these Munch 'Ems won't throw you seriously off track, if you've kept your fat intake in check during the rest of the day.

You also see that there is a total of 4 grams of fat in a serving, and beside that figure is the notation 6%. That is the percentage of what's called a Daily Value, which gives you an idea of how this snack fits into your overall eating plan. A serving of these crackers will give you 6 percent of the maximum amount of fat you should be eating in a day for a 2,000-calorie diet. So you make the call: How does that jibe with whatever else you want to eat? How do these crackers stand up nutritionally against other snacks?

Two important points about those Daily Values. First, they're based on the assumption that you consume 2,000 calories a day, which is low for lots of men. Generally speaking, a guy who's 5 feet 11 inches tall, medium-framed, and moderately active needs about 2,750 calories a day. Second, for troublesome nutrients, such as fat, cholesterol, and sodium, consider 100 percent of the Daily Value to be a maximum, a mark you want to come under. For user-friendly stuff, such as carbohydrates and dietary fiber, think of the Daily Value as a minimum, a target you want to hit or surpass.

JUDGING A FOOD BY ITS COVER

One reason you pulled that box of crackers off the shelf was the inviting phrase ". . . but with 33% less fat than regular tortilla chips." Hmmm, sounds good. But years of dubious nutrition advertising claims have left you with a powerful knee-jerk cynicism. The fact is that health and nutrient claims on food packages are now closely regulated. Knowing the rules that manufacturers have to play by will make you a more confident shopper.

"There used to be consumer confusion," says Adler. "A firm would state on the label that a food product was low-fat, and the firm itself would make that determination with its own definition. Now, those definitions are provided by the FDA, so they have to be accurate."

Here's how the FDA defines some of the most common terms found on food packages.

- *Free:* Contains none, or only a trivial amount, of the nutrient named. *Fat-free,* for example, means that there's less than ½ gram of fat per serving.
- *Low:* You can eat this food frequently without blowing your limit for the nutrient named. *Low-fat* means 3 grams of fat or less per serving, for example.
- *Lean* and *extra lean:* These terms describe the fat content of meat. Generally speaking, *lean* means fewer than 10 grams of fat per serving (and per 100 grams). *Extra lean* means fewer than 5 grams of fat per serving (and per 100 grams).
- *High:* Contains 20 percent or more of the Daily Value for the nutrient named.
- *Good source:* A notch below "high." Contains 10 to 19 percent of the Daily Value.

- *Reduced:* Somebody has monkeyed with this food to get at least 25 percent less of a nutrient or calories than the regular product.
- *Less:* Contains 25 percent less of a nutrient or calories than some similar food we'd like to point an accusing finger at. (See the tortilla chip claim mentioned previously.)
- *Light:* One-third of the calories or half the fat has been booted out of this food. Or, for a food that's already low-calorie and low-fat, half the sodium has been removed. Careful: Packages may still use the word *light* when speaking of color, as in *light brown sugar.*
- *More:* Contains at least 10 percent of the Daily Value of a nutrient above what's in the regular version of the food. For example, if a regular juice contains 34 percent of the Daily Value of vitamin C, then the high-test version claiming *more* vitamin C must have at least 44 percent.

Food packages also are allowed to carry statements associating nutrition and prevention of specific diseases. Examples are calcium and osteoporosis, and fiber and cancer. Such a statement might read, "While many factors affect heart disease, diets low in saturated fat and cholesterol may reduce the risk of this disease." Foods carrying these reminders generally have to contain significant amounts of the nutrient being touted.

Jacques Pépin, World-Class Chef

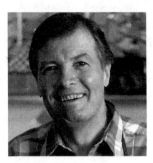

Jacques Pépin does a lot of talking about food. He roams the United States for at least 30 weeks out of the year teaching and making appearances. He banters with David Letterman now and then on the *Late Show*.

He shares secrets with PBS viewers during his *Jacques Pépin's Kitchen: Encore with Claudine* series and speaks to readers from the pages of *Food & Wine* magazine and more than a dozen books.

So when he's between classes, the TV shows are in the can, all the recipes are written, and he's home in Connecticut, what does he do? He talks to himself—about food.

"I would say that it is very important to listen to your body, to what it tells you as you get older," says Pépin, who's in his sixties. "I'm not a macrobiotic guru trying to tell people to get into some type of inner experience. It's really not that complicated."

A LIFELONG LOVE AFFAIR WITH FOOD

Pépin grew up in the kitchen. His mother was the chef in the family restaurant near Lyons, France, and as a child, young Jacques was her helper. At age 13, Pépin began his formal apprenticeship as a chef at the Grand Hotel de L'Europe in his hometown.

Eventually, he made his way to the bright lights of Paris, where he continued his training at two of the city's finest restaurants. In the mid-1950s, Pépin served as personal chef to three French heads of state, including the legendary Charles de Gaulle.

In 1959, Pépin decided to seek his fame and fortune across the Atlantic Ocean. Starting in the kitchen of New York's historic Le Pavillon, he moved on to the Howard Johnson Company, where he served as director of research and new development for 10 years. While establishing his reputation as one of the world's most creative and colorful chefs, Pépin earned his master's degree in eighteenth-century French literature from Columbia University in New York City.

CHANGING WITH THE TIMES

Pépin's philosophy on cooking is still very much rooted in his mother's kitchen and his childhood.

"I try to eat not much differently than when I was much younger," Pépin says.

"When I was a kid living in France, we didn't really eat meat more than once or twice a week. Not because it was a fad or for health purposes—we didn't know anything about that—but probably more because of economic conditions. I was never the type of person who ate a lot of meat every day, because I just didn't feel like it."

Over the years, though, Pépin has gradually moved away from using ingredients high in saturated fat and cholesterol, such as butter. He has also cut back considerably on the use of desserts. Part of it has been the growing awareness about what constitutes healthy eating. And part of it has been Pépin's personal journey.

"There has been a great deal of change in the last 20 years or so in the eating habits of people," Pépin notes. "And I feel that I have been part of it, as I have been here doing recipes for many, many years. I would also say that I am 20 years older, and you kind of follow your body, you know?

"I am sure that I am eating things now that I would not have been that crazy about 20 or 30 years ago. It's just that I'm older and I don't feel like eating the same way. I'm eating more soup, more vegetables, things like this, because that's what I feel like eating."

A MATTER OF TASTE

Don't think for a moment, however, that Pépin would sacrifice taste on the altar of low-fat living. He is, first and foremost, a chef. Pépin has not eliminated any ingredients—including butter, beef, or sugar—from his kitchen. He has merely scaled them back and found innovative ways to trim the fat while maintaining the flavor.

Pépin believes that chefs should never say never. Take cream sauces, for example. "I haven't seen cream sauce in a restaurant in at least 2 or 3 years," Pépin says. "But very often, I have made it on my show to purposely show that it can be done with much fewer calories."

So Pépin will take scrod and mix together a sauce with white wine, horseradish, black olives, and—gasp!—some sour cream.

"Now, it comes out to about 1 tablespoon of sour cream per person, and that's 20 calories. So it's really nothing much at all, much less than if you had grilled it with olive oil. But the point is that people look at that dish, with the white sauce oozing out of it, and say, 'That's it. I'm dead.' They won't touch it, you know?"

When it comes to eating, Pépin suffers from the same temptations as the rest of us. "I am the type of person who can probably do without a meal, but if it's in front of my nose, I am going to eat it, which is not necessarily good," he confesses.

The key to healthy eating, Pépin says, is smart shopping.

"I love to go to the market. Unless I have to write a recipe and I go specifically for one thing that I need, I like to see what's good, what's interesting there. I'm talking mostly about vegetables and fruits. I start buying this way, listening to what I feel like eating these days. It's a natural way of doing it. It works for me."

Pépin is a big fan of salads, and they're tossed together in a similarly intuitive fashion. And the simple fact that fresh salad ingredients are always easily at hand in his refrigerator makes it more likely that he will make wise eating decisions.

"We had a big salad last night," he says. "I think it was romaine. I opened the refrigerator and I had a piece of cucumber, half a lettuce and half a tomato or whatever, and we used that."

As a rule, Pépin doesn't eat between meals. "That would be very rare. Unless I'm cooking," he says. "But usually, if I have lunch, I do not have anything before dinner. It's not part of the way I live, so I don't try to get bad habits if I don't have them."

And he doesn't care much for dessert either—at least nothing from the oozing-with-chocolate food group. "Last night, I had a very nice, ripe peach, so I peeled some and that's what we had for dessert. I mean, most of the time, except for fruit or maybe a piece of cheese, we really don't have dessert."

That's normally something he saves for special occasions. "Very often in our house, that's what makes the difference between an everyday meal and a guest meal," Pépin says. "Because if people come over on the weekend, or we have guests unexpectedly, I may serve the same meal that I was going to serve, but then add a dessert."

Kareem Abdul-Jabbar, Hall of Fame Basketball Player

To see him play, Kareem Abdul-Jabbar's millions of fans would never have guessed that the basketball legend could ever have to worry about his weight. "I think most people saw just the opposite—a tall, skinny guy who looked like he could use a good meal," Abdul-Jabbar says.

And while that was true for most of his career, in his final basketball season before retirement in 1989 at the age of 42, the former center for the Los Angeles Lakers found himself trying to shed a nagging 8 pounds that refused to leave his 7-foot-2 frame.

"A lot of that was just needing to get back into shape for the season after laying off for a few months. But I won't deny that the extra pounds had to get on there some way, and how much I ate was playing a role," he says.

When he was playing basketball, the solution was to double up his training and burn off the extra pounds. But now, as an entrepreneur—the Hall of Famer heads his own company, Kareem Enterprises, in Los Angeles—Abdul-Jabbar says that he shares the same fitness concerns as many suc-

cessful businessmen, namely finding the right time and place to get all the right foods.

"Now, I'm traveling all over the world on business," he says. "It does take a bite out of my time for exercise and good eating."

A SEA OF SMART CHOICES

During his playing days, Abdul-Jabbar burned calories as routinely as he torched opposing centers. He retired with the all-time NBA record for most points scored—a staggering 38,387, nearly 7,000 more than Wilt Chamberlain. He also held the all-time career marks for games played and blocked shots and was third on the all-time rebounding list, behind only Chamberlain and Bill Russell.

Once he stopped running the hardwood floors of basketball arenas night after grueling night, though, Abdul-Jabbar realized that he had to change his eating habits.

"Initially, it was hard to make the transition from sports to business, at least in terms of my diet," says Abdul-Jabbar. "When I stopped playing, I started to gain all this weight—all of a sudden I noticed this gut growing on this long frame, and I was just appalled. I was still working out, but I wasn't burning the calories the way I had on the court. I realized then that I had to make modifications."

Abdul-Jabbar started by modifying the portions he was eating—"I just didn't need all that fuel anymore"—and then he focused on sticking to a diet that emphasized lean meats, grains, and plenty of fruits and vegetables. "Once you learn what to eat, having a healthy diet—even when you're on the road—is not that tough. Although I'm on the road for many months of the year, I still eat a balanced diet," he says.

A large part of that diet is fresh seafood. "Wherever I am, I try to seek out the local seafood, whatever it is, be it soft-shell crab or salmon. Especially salmon. I love it. I'll even have it for breakfast from time to time," he says.

ENTER THE DRAGON

Abdul-Jabbar isn't content to let 20 years of NBA muscle degenerate into postgame flab. Like most professional athletes, Abdul-Jabbar knows that the secret to being fit—and having fewer restrictions on his diet—is to build and keep calorie-burning muscle. "I didn't always feel this way. When I was

playing, for a long time it was considered taboo to build up any muscle. Players thought it would make them slow," he recalls.

Indeed, Abdul-Jabbar was first pushed to do weight training by a nonbasketball superstar—karate legend Bruce Lee, whom Abdul-Jabbar met during his college days. "He was always pushing me to build muscle, but I resisted him. Eventually, I tried it and noticed a tremendous difference in my game and in my general fitness. If you look at professional athletes today, you know that most of them see the value of it, too. And it helps you off the field as well," he says.

STAYING FLEXIBLE

Today, Abdul-Jabbar's workout consists of a 6-day-a-week cross-training schedule. "It varies day to day, depending on my schedule and how I feel, but I try to do some lifting and some running." Finally, Abdul-Jabbar rounds out his workouts with a yoga routine. "I've been doing stretches since my days with coach John Wooden when I was at UCLA. Absolutely, that's what allowed me to stay in the game longer than anyone. But even if you've never played professional sports, stretching is a vital part of your total fitness. The more flexible I am, the more I can use my body to do whatever I want."

And it's not like Abdul-Jabbar has retired to a life of leisure. He can still play a little ball. Just ask the Harlem Globetrotters. In September 1995, Abdul-Jabbar led a team of former pro players against the legendary clown princes of basketball. Showing his old touch, he poured in 34 points on 15-of-16 shooting to lead the Kareem Abdul-Jabbar All-Stars to a 91-85 victory—ending the Trotters's amazing 8,829-game winning streak that dated back to 1971.

The six-time NBA champion realizes that by staying in shape, he can continue to burn calories, even from the foods he knows he shouldn't eat. Even legendary sports figures have foods that they know they should avoid. As a Muslim, Abdul-Jabbar has two important dietary restrictions: no pork and no alcohol. And while that means that he never has to worry about getting a beer gut, Abdul-Jabbar does have his weaknesses.

"I love ice cream, oh yes," he confides. "I'll seek it out wherever I am. Overseas, when I was in Italy, I loved the kind they call gelati—I can get into that pretty good if I'm not careful. It's my one guilty pleasure. But you know, after a long day of work you have to give yourself something to shoot for."

As the man who took—and made—more shots than anyone else in NBA history, Abdul-Jabbar ought to know.

Part 14
MASTER OF THE KITCHEN

The Leanest Techniques

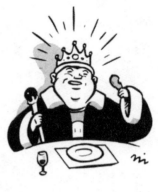

Maybe you've dreamed of being a sculptor, a wilderness guide, or coach of the Dallas Cowboys. If being creative and in control appeals to you, then you should also explore the kitchen. Cooking is fun. You'll impress friends and turn out some delectable chow. And for fighting the fat around your waist, the kitchen is the best place to take a stand.

In a country awash in convenient but larded foods, taking spatula in hand can be your best defense.

Cooking is a guy thing, you know. An American Dietetic Association survey found that 49.8 percent of men say that they do at least half the cooking at home. In addition, the U.S. Department of Labor says that 54 percent of professional cooks in the United States are men.

One of these chefs is Tuan Lam, owner and head chef of Thuy Hoa restaurant in Denver.

"We don't use many things like cheese or butter," Lam says. "We have lots of customers now who don't want lots of oil. So we're using lots of vegetables and we're using lots of broth, adding them together."

The fat-busting techniques used by Lam and other cooks nationwide are easily adapted to your kitchen. The principles are basic: Invest in good hardware; keep lots of versatile, low-fat ingredients in the kitchen;

and most important, be inventive—and have fun.

GEARING UP

You have to have the right tool for the right job. That was true in shop class, and it applies in the kitchen, too. To help yourself work efficiently in the kitchen and, while you're at it, whittle fat from your food, here's what food experts recommend.

Put a blender in the mix. Yes, a blender is good for more than making margaritas. You can use it to whip up low-fat sauces as well. For example, Susan Harville, a member of the collective that owns Moosewood Restaurant in Ithaca, New York, recommends using a blender to make this tasty, no-oil pesto.

Combine 1 cup of basil leaves (packed), 1 teaspoon of salt, 1 tablespoon of toasted pine nuts, a whole fresh tomato, and a clove or two of fresh garlic. Blend until smooth, then serve over pasta, steamed fish, or vegetables. You can also use it as a sandwich spread or put it on a baked potato.

Rack up fat savings. Oven roasting makes meat crisp and brown on the outside and tender and juicy inside. Cooking a roast or chicken without a rack means that the meat lolls around in its own fat, picking up surplus calories along the way. Putting a rack underneath allows the fat to drain away, giving meat a crisper skin in the process.

Skim the risks. When making soup or stew, you'll see globules of fat rising to the surface. Fat is easy to remove using a specially designed slotted spoon or ladle. Or if you're working ahead of time, cool your masterpiece in the fridge overnight. The fat will rise and congeal into a waxy film on the surface. Gently spoon it off. Nobody will miss it.

Make waves. Microwaves are not only fast, they can also cook food with little or no added fat. At the same time, they help preserve many of the nutrients that are lost when you boil.

"You can cook vegetables in a microwave quite easily," says Dan Remark, executive chef of Mustard Seed Market and Cafe in Akron, Ohio. "Place the vegetables on a plate, add a slight amount of water to create steam, put plastic wrap over the top, and then microwave to the desired consistency. Great method."

Get past the sticking point. No-stick cookware is a blessing for the working chef. Not only does it help reduce cleanup time, it also allows you to sauté or bake without adding oil. Kitchen stores stock a large variety of no-stick pots and pans. The more expensive kinds are more likely to hold up to the rigors of hard kitchen use. But regardless of the kind you buy, treat the slick surface gingerly: Use wood and plastic utensils only.

Cook under pressure. Because pressure cookers can substantially shave the preparation time needed for slow-cooking foods such as dried beans, brown rice, potatoes, and stews, they're a must for any chef living in the fast lane.

"Chickpeas would take 2 to 4 hours to cook just boiling them, but a pressure cooker will cut the time down to an hour and a half," says Tom Flener, a cook at the Sunlight Cafe in Seattle. "They're pretty convenient for things that take a long time to cook."

Try steam power. Like the microwave, steam can cook food fast with no oil added. At the same time, it helps preserve the color, flavor, and nutrients that can be lost to boiling.

To steam vegetables, first allow the water to boil. Then, throw the vegetables into the steamer and put the lid on. Make sure that the water isn't so high that it touches the vegetables—contact with the boiling water will sap away nutrients.

"We combine carrots, broccoli, cauliflower, and green peppers," says Roger Brown, co-owner and cook at Valley Restaurant in Corvallis, Oregon. "Then, we steam them until they are cooked but still have a slight crunch. We add onions right toward the end of the cooking. Mushrooms

TAKING STOCK

To truly master low-fat cuisine at home, you have to plan ahead and lay in supplies.

"I like to look at it from a standpoint of 'What do I have in my pantry or my refrigerator that, when I get home and it's late and I'm hungry, I can throw together in 10 minutes and still eat healthy?'" says Chris Rosenbloom, R.D., Ph.D., associate professor in the department of nutrition and dietetics at Georgia State University and nutrition consultant for the Georgia Tech Athletic Association, both in Atlanta.

Here are 20 ingredients that no man's kitchen should be without.

In the Pantry
Dried and canned beans
Canned tomatoes, tomato puree, and
  tomato paste
Canned corn
Canned peas
Canned chicken broth
White and brown rice
Quick-cooking grains, such as bulgur
  and millet
Onions
Garlic
Fresh ginger
Olive oil
Pasta

In the Refrigerator
A variety of fruits and vegetables
Dijon mustard
Fat-free yogurt
Fat-free buttermilk
Tortillas

In the Freezer
Boneless chicken breast
Turkey cutlets
Frozen vegetables

take the least amount of time, so they go in last."

Don't neglect man's best disposal. Canine disposal units come in a variety of sizes and colors and are a handy way of getting rid of trimmed fat, unwanted egg yolks, and other scraps. "I give all that to my dog, and he loves it," says Chris Rosenbloom, R.D., Ph.D., associate professor in the department of nutrition and dietetics at Georgia State University and nutrition consultant for the Georgia Tech Athletic Association, both in Atlanta. "Dogs don't get atherosclerosis. So my dog's happy."

INGREDIENTS FOR SUCCESS

The foods you stock in the refrigerator and pantry are the building blocks of your diet—and of any recipes you dream up. On the most basic level, taking low-fat ingredients and cooking them with low-fat techniques guarantees that you're going to have healthy chow to take to the table. But there are other things to consider before laying in inventory.

- Are the ingredients easy to use? If preparing a certain food is as complex as the Manhattan Project, it's going to bomb as a menu item.
- Is it versatile? You don't want to waste shelf space on something you'll use only when you make rattlesnake fritters.
- Is it quick? Can you open a container and dump it in a pan, or do you have to whittle, soak, pound, or otherwise negotiate with it?

The bottom line is that low-fat ingredients that slide easily into active duty are much more likely to wind up in your belly than the exotics you bought on a whim—those dried mushrooms, for example, that you shoved behind the canned brussels sprouts 5 years ago and that by now are harder than the concrete in Hoover Dam.

Use the ol' bean. Canned beans, be they pintos, black beans, kidney beans, split peas, or any other kind, are great staples to have on the shelf. Not only are they used in a vast array of recipes but they also cook a heck of lot faster than the dried kind.

Explore combinations. Loosen up, man. There's no kitchen cop telling you not to dump a can of corn into a stir-fry or add anchovies to a tomato paste. So the next time you're shopping or perusing the pantry, make some educated guesses about what combinations will taste good together. Then, toss them together.

"I've been buying a lot of reduced-fat cream soups—the low-fat mushroom soups and potato soups," says Dr. Rosenbloom. "Those are a quick, good basis for a casserole. You can take a chicken breast and a can of vegetables and one of those soups, mix them together, heat, and serve the casserole with bread—it's real fast and it tastes pretty good."

Grab a cold one. Bags of frozen vegetables deserve top marks both for saving time and for cooking versatility. The vegetables taste almost as good as fresh and are ready to toss right in the pot with no cleaning or chopping necessary. "You can take out a single serving size and put the rest back in the freezer," says Dr. Rosenbloom. "But don't get the ones with the butter sauces or cream sauces. That's where the fat content really goes up."

Put on the spritz. It's a good idea to keep a can of no-stick spray handy. Shooshing your frying pan with this stuff will add just 2 calories and a trace of fat to your meal, as opposed to the 102 calories and 11 grams of fat that come with a tablespoon of butter.

Spice up your life. The addition of spices to food is a wonderful and tasty way to fill the void left when fat and salt are reduced or eliminated. You probably already have the basics: black pepper, cinnamon, basil, dill, paprika, and oregano. For more exotic offerings, check out the spice chart included in many cookbooks.

"If you're not familiar with the flavor of a spice, we suggest that you try it in something bland like rice or scrambled eggs," says Camille Appel, manager of consumer communications at McCormick and Company in Hunt Valley, Maryland, the world's largest spice company.

Grow your own. Many herbs lose flavor in the drying process, so nothing will add kick to your low-fat cooking like using the fresh stuff. The problem with fresh herbs is that they're usually sold only in huge bunches, most of which will turn into a science experiment at the bottom of the vegetable bin before you get around to using them.

An alternative is to grow your own, says Dr. Rosenbloom. "Keep them on the windowsill, and you can just snip off what you might want for cooking." Since fresh herbs begin losing flavor and color with long cooking, it's best to stir them in just before serving.

COOKING OVER THE COALS

That grill in the backyard means a hump of fatty pork ribs slathered in barbecue sauce, right? Well, the ol' Weber grill can turn out lean chow as well, adding a distinctive smoky flavor to boot.

"We have the perception that healthy food is boring. But we're able to throw a piece of fish on the grill, or even a vegetable, and have it take on a lot of flavors," says Chris Schlesinger, chef and co-owner of the restaurants East Coast Grill, Blue Room, and Jake and Earl's Dixie BBQ, all in Cambridge, Massachusetts.

To make your grill a lean machine, here's what chefs recommend.

- Rather than slathering oil onto your ingredients, brush the oil directly onto the hot bars of the grill. Then, wipe it off with a rag or paper towel before cooking.
- When grilling chicken, remove the skin and rub the meat with a garlic-herb paste made by mixing ½ cup of chopped fresh basil, 2 tablespoons of minced garlic, and a little salt and cracked black pepper.
- Eggplant, onions, summer squash, and peppers all make good grilling candidates. Char, let them cool, then peel the black stuff off. Eat with minced garlic, olive oil, and crusty bread.
- Corn on the cob needs gentle handling. Shuck the ears and soak them in water for 20 minutes, then cook them over low coals.
- Roasting eggplant gives it a delectably smoky flavor. Wrap it in foil and put it on the grill for 12 to 15 minutes. Then, let it cool, peel away the skin, and spread the innards on bread, crackers, sandwiches, or a baked potato.
- Tuna, salmon, swordfish, shark, and halibut steaks all grill well because they're compact and of one thickness and because they don't fall apart on the grill as fillets do. If they're the usual 1-inch-thick steaks, grill for 4 to 5 minutes on each side.
- The most flavorful beefsteaks also tend to be the fattiest. Rather than sacrificing flavor by using leaner cuts, Schlesinger prefers to reduce the portion size. He recommends grilling a 6-ounce steak, then slicing it over salad greens and tomatoes to make a steak salad.

Put ginger on ice. When added to sauces, stir-fries, and marinades, fresh ginger packs a punch that you just don't get from the powdered stuff. Problem is, this ugly root is perishable, and after a few weeks in the refrigerator, it generally resembles a Henry Moore sculpture made from blue cheese.

To keep fresh ginger handy, try grating the entire root, then freezing it in a plastic bag or small container. The shavings will stay loose and separate, so it's easy to scoop out small amounts as needed. Or freeze it whole, then grate it only as needed.

Freeze a block o' stock. Although bouillon cubes are a passable substitute, nothing can match the rich flavors and cooking versatility of a homemade vegetable stock. It makes a fantastic soup, stew, or gravy and contains virtually no fat.

Basically, all you need to do is throw leftover vegetables—including peelings and onion skins—into a large pot of water. Fruits are good to use, too, especially apples and pears. "Put them on to cook for an hour while you're doing other things," says Harville. "Then, strain out the vegetables and freeze the liquid. That way, you're ahead."

Ready the radicchio. Experts agree that greens such as spinach and other dark green leafy vegetables should be a mainstay of your refrigerator. They're packed with vitamins and have zero fat. They also tend to turn to mush before you get around to eating them.

To keep greens fresh, wash them as soon as you get home. Then, shake off the excess water, roll them in paper towels or kitchen towels, place them in a plastic bag, and pop them in the fridge. That way, they'll stay fresh for at least 3 to 4 days, and often longer.

MASTERING MEAT

What man is not familiar with temptations of the flesh? We mean, of course, a sizzling slab of beef on the backyard grill, a thick puck of hamburger oozing juice into a seeded bun, or those crisp brown strips that transform a mere plate of eggs into a bona fide breakfast.

While we're indulging, however, there's a relentless accountant tallying up the fat: 60 grams in the 12-ounce sirloin, 48 grams in the ½-pound burger, and 9 grams for three slices of bacon. With those kinds of numbers, it's not surprising that health experts typically view cows or pigs as obesity on the hoof.

But with a little moderation and advance planning, it is still possible to make peace with pork and say "Wow!" to cow chow. Here's what experts recommend.

Give it a trim. The next time you have a craving for a thick pork chop or juicy New York strip, trim away the outer rim of fat before slapping it on the grill. It's easier to trim the fat if you first pop the meat in the freezer for 20 minutes. Chilling also causes hidden fat to turn white, making it easier to spot and lop off.

Let the fat flow. Trimming away visible fat is just one way to keep your meat lean. Another is to cook it properly. There are different low-fat cooking styles for different cuts of meat. For example:

- Broiling. This involves putting meat in the oven directly under the flame or electric element—preferably no more than 3 to 5 inches away—and is recommended for relatively thin cuts. Put the meat on a broiling rack with a drip pan underneath to catch the fat.
- Roasting. This is usually recommended for larger cuts of meat such as a roast. The meat is placed on a rack and cooked in a medium-temperature (350°F) oven.
- Stove-top grilling. Using a ridged cast-iron pan or one of the newer stove-top grills, this is a fast technique for cooking meat that is an inch thick or less. The fat flows down into the ridges and away from the meat.

Baste wisely. Traditional basting calls for sopping the beast with buttery, oily concoctions. Forget that. To keep your meat moist and flavorful, baste with defatted stock, a low-fat marinade, flavored vinegar, or even fruit juice.

Skip the skin. About one-half the fat in chicken is found in the skin or directly beneath it, so always peel the bird before you eat. It's a good idea to cook chicken before removing the skin, however, since this helps lock in flavor and moisture and doesn't add too much fat to the meat.

Go fish. Fresh fish and shellfish are always good choices because they're delicious, easy to cook, and low in fat. But it's better to bake or broil fish without added fat

than to fry it, which adds extra fat and calories to the meal, says Lisa Litin, R.D., a research dietitian at Harvard School of Public Health.

And once you get your fish to the table, "watch the cream sauces, tartar sauce, and additions of margarine or butter," Litin adds. One tablespoon of tartar sauce has 8 grams of fat—only slightly less heart-stopping than the 11 grams found in butter.

Exercise control. If you're eating humongous quantities, even the leanest meat is going to give you fat overload. Limit your meat serving to about 6 ounces, experts say. That's about the size of two decks of playing cards. Then, round out the meal with the other good stuff you've put on the table.

WOK ON THE WILD SIDE

A stir-fry meal may look and taste exotic, but it's really an easy, anything-goes, fantastically quick style of cooking. It requires little if any oil. And unlike traditional menus that feature meat, wok cookery gives vegetables star billing: They come out crisp, intensely colored, and packed with their original nutrients because the cooking process is so fast.

"The nice thing about stir-frying is that you can be creative. You can add whatever is on hand, using different types of vegetables, meats, and liquids, and they all give different flavors," says Pat Harper, R.D., a Pittsburgh nutritionist and spokesperson for the American Dietetic Association. "It's more like you're creating a meal rather than just cooking it." So if you, too, would like to be a da Vinci of da kitchen, here are some stir-fry basics.

Create a stir. The first thing you need in order to stir-fry is a wok, although a large frying pan will do in a pinch. "I use an electric wok. I find that's really handy to use," says Dr. Rosenbloom.

Begin with marinades. For extra flavor with no added fat, try soaking some of your ingredients in a marinade. An easy one to begin with is a mixture of garlic, ginger, and soy sauce. This works great when cooking seafood, tofu, tempeh, and eggplant.

Synchronize your stir-fry. You want all of your stir-fry ingredients to finish cooking at the same time, so it's a good idea to chop all the vegetables into pieces of roughly the same size. Meat takes the longest to cook, so toss that in first. Delicate items such as snow peas should go in last.

Get ready for spaghetti. Rice may be the traditional accompaniment for stir-fry, but switching to an alternative will give your meal a new look. "You can put stir-fry over noodles, you can put it over rice, you can put it over spaghetti or different shapes of pasta, so every time it's like a different meal," says Harper.

Let the oil slide. The great thing about wok cooking is that you can often prepare an entire meal without adding any fat beyond a spritz of no-stick spray. Contrast that to a recipe that calls for frying vegetables—broccoli, carrots, or onions, for example—in 3 teaspoons of vegetable oil, which could add 15 grams of fat to the meal.

Tuan Lam often forgoes the fat entirely. "A lot of our customers now don't want us to use a lot of oil," he says. "So we're using broth when we're cooking with vegetables."

Meats

Fred Flintstone was a lucky guy. Sure, he had to settle for Wilma instead of Betty, but when he pedaled home from his job at the quarry each night, he knew that he had a steaming, 10-pound slab of brontosaurus steak waiting on his plate for dinner.

And just think: None of those doctors who beef about how too much red meat clogs your arteries was even born yet.

Americans eat an average of around 235 pounds of meat a year. "That's an all-time high," says Jens Knutson, director of regulatory and industrial affairs at the American Meat Institute. More than half of the meat we consume is red meat. Poultry is next, at about 40 percent; and fish lags far behind, at roughly 6 percent.

That old mastodon masticator Fred Flintstone probably wouldn't see anything wrong with those figures, but most doctors would. And while there has been a slow shift from red meat to poultry in recent years, it appears that some weight- and health-conscious men may be counting their chickens for the wrong reasons.

OUR BEEF IS WITH FAT

Thanks to advances in food technology, red meat has grown increasingly lean. And researchers have found that our weight and cholesterol levels couldn't care less whether we eat chicken or beef. The meat just has to be lean.

Two studies have pointed to the fat content of beef—and not necessarily beef itself—as the problem. One study looked at 38 men with high blood cholesterol levels. (Foods that are high in saturated fat raise cholesterol as well as contribute to weight gain.) The researchers found that it didn't matter whether the men ate lean beef or lean chicken. Blood cholesterol levels decreased by the same amount.

Another study looked at whether beef protein or beef fat was the cholesterol-raising culprit. The answer was the fat.

So as long as it's lean, we can eat as much as we want? Not so fast. There's still cholesterol in the meat to worry about, and most of the cholesterol is in the meat's lean parts. Also, there's the iron factor. One 3-ounce serving gives you 20 to 30 percent of your Recommended Dietary Allowance of iron. High doses of iron have been linked to heart disease.

High red-meat consumption also has been linked to colon cancer, the second leading cause of death from malignancies in the United States.

Still, you don't have to deny yourself the

meat you love. You can eat it and still be healthy—and lean—if you follow some basic advice, says Lynne W. Scott, R.D, director of the diet modification clinic at Baylor College of Medicine in Houston. Eat small portions. Eat lean cuts. And eat them along with other low-fat foods.

THE KINDEST CUT

There are really two big things to look for if you want to continue eating red meat and still maintain your weight: portion size and fat content. Here are some ways to enjoy meat and good health.

Don't gamble with big portions. You can eat up to 6 ounces of lean meat a day and still be healthy, says Scott. How much is that? Next time you're playing poker with the boys, check out the deck of cards before you deal. That's about the size of 3 ounces of meat. About 15 percent of the calories in your diet should be protein, and 3 ounces will more than satisfy that.

Select wisely. Many companies pay the government to grade their meat. Grades are based on the animal's age and the amount of fat in its meat. Beef is graded prime, choice, select, standard, commercial, utility, cutter, and canner. You really only need to worry about choice and select.

Prime, which contains more marbling of fat in the meat than most of us wish to buy, is usually sold only to restaurants.

Choice and select are the grades most frequently found at supermarket meat counters. The others are so tough that you'd never eat them as a steak. They are used either in ground beef or in processed meats.

Prime tenderloin gets 48 percent of its calories from fat. The same steak rated choice gets 44 percent, and select checks in at 39 percent.

Buy lean cuts. In any animal, the leanest meat is located where the animal has larger, more active and powerful muscles. This makes sense. Think about your own body. Your biceps are probably much leaner than your rump. We could give you an anatomy lesson for each farm animal, but instead, we'll make it simple. Just look for round, ham, and leg cuts, suggests the USDA Agricultural Marketing Service.

When we're talking birds, light meat is lower in fat than dark meat. Backs and legs have the highest amount of fat.

Read the labels. In general, chicken and turkey are leaner than beef, but you really need to compare the fat content. Some ground beef is leaner than ground turkey. That's mainly because ground turkey can contain skin and fat that drives up the fat content. The same goes for hot dogs. (To be fair, there are some brands of low-fat and fat-free wieners out there, too.) Look at the grams of fat per ounce.

LEARNING TO LOVE LEAN

You know what happens when you cook lean meat. It tastes like lean meat—dry and chewy. It robs your mouth of saliva. It's the ultimate letdown. You smell steak. You see steak. But you don't really taste steak. When you get done eating, you're still craving steak.

It doesn't have to be that way. Stanley Lobel, a fourth-generation butcher at Lobel's

Meats on Madison Avenue in New York City, knows how you feel. And he says there's a really easy solution to the lean-steak problem: Marinate it.

Don't worry. You don't have to be Julia Child to pull this off. All you need is a bottle of fat-free Italian dressing, says Lobel, who runs the butcher shop with his brother Leon, son Mark, and nephew Evan. Pour it over the steak, then put the steak in the fridge for anywhere from a couple of hours to overnight. When you cook it, it will almost taste like that oozy, fatty, a-butter-knife-will-cut-it prime meat.

Remember, we said *almost*.

"In marinating, you not only build in the flavor but also make it more tender," says Lobel, who along with his brother has authored *Meat, All about Meat, How to Be Your Own Butcher,* and *The Lobel Brothers Meat Cookbook.*

"The only thing you might have to add to the dressing is lots of garlic if that's what you like. That would definitely do the trick. And it would be quite good. Of course, you're still going to miss the flavor of a real prime piece of meat. It's a give-and-take situation."

If you want to be daring, you can mix up your own marinade. Make it one-quarter acid and three-quarters oil, Lobel suggests. The acid softens the meat and the oil carries the flavors into the meat once the acid has softened it. For your acid, you can use anything from wine to vinegar to lemon juice. Any cooking oil will do, although some people prefer olive oil.

BE A HAMBURGER HELPER

Hamburgers are as American as, well, apple pie. They're also just as fattening. A typical burger or slice of apple pie packs more than 13 grams of fat.

We're not about to advise you to go burgerless on the Fourth of July—or any other time, for that matter, provided that you're keeping your meat consumption within recommended guidelines. (Remember, two card decks a day.) But there are some simple steps you can take to significantly cut the fat in your burger.

Blot and drain. After browning ground beef, place it in a dish covered with a double thickness of paper towel. Then, stick another paper towel on top and blot up the grease. If you want to remove even more fat, dump the ground meat into a colander and rinse with hot, but not boiling, water. Squeeze out the excess water. The water will wash away fat and cholesterol while leaving the protein, iron, zinc, and B_{12} behind. Using both of these methods can cut 50 percent of the fat from the beef.

Chill it. Once you've blotted and rinsed the meat, stick it in the refrigerator overnight. Whatever fat is left will harden. Then, you can scrape it off the next day, says Nancy D. Berkoff of the Los Angeles Trade Technical College. Obviously, if you're the type of person who figures out what you're having for dinner $1/2$ hour before you plan on eating it, this won't work for you.

Extend it. Remember Hamburger Helper? It will make your ground beef go a lot farther on a lot less fat. But the commercial product is also high in salt, so make your own. Mixing in bread crumbs, oatmeal, matzo meal, diced carrots, and other vegetables will add bulk and cut down on the amount of meat you're eating.

Pay the price. Now that you know how to defat your ground beef, don't think that you can buy the cheaper, higher-fat kind and make it healthy at home. You're wasting your money. The bulk in the cheaper beef will be from fat. Once you defat it, you'll have a lot less meat. It actu-

ally makes more sense to your wallet to purchase the more expensive, lower-fat meat, says Berkoff.

Order that burger well-done. Bacteria grows on the surface of beef, so grilling a steak on both sides will probably kill all of it regardless of how red it is on the inside. Hamburgers, though, are a different story. The surfaces of the ground beef that were exposed to air during the grinding process were spread throughout the burger when you made it, so you need to cook a burger until the center is gray.

Seafood

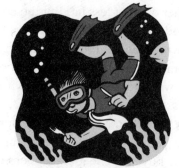

It's dinnertime, and Mr. and Mrs. Blandmouth find themselves in a large East Coast metropolis. They're in town from Nebraska as conventioneers at the Regis Philbin Charisma Conference, and now they need to eat. They're in a daring mood, so they decide to try out the city's famed seafood restaurant.

As the waiter talks about the sweet pompano, the juicy shad, and the rich bluefish, their eyes widen, a slight haze forming over their pupils. Mr. Blandmouth's right pupil wanders to the corner of his eye and catches Mrs. Blandmouth's left pupil in the corner of her eye—a small but inescapable signal that daring is now kaput. "I'll have the baked flounder without the sauce," says Mr. Blandmouth. "I'll have what he's having," follows Mrs. Blandmouth.

The Blandmouths have just ordered a bland meal. "Those who aren't fish eaters, they order plain flounder. I always think that it won't have any taste. I guess they have it to say that they ate fish," says Richard Bookbinder, owner of Bookbinder's Seafood House 15th Street, a well-known Philadelphia seafood establishment that occasionally entertains visitors like Mr. and Mrs. Blandmouth.

FISHING FOR GOOD HEALTH

Fish restaurant and market owners know only too well that seafood can be a hard thing to get to know, but there are many reasons why you should acquaint yourself.

For one, it's a healthy way to get the nutrients found in beef without also getting the fat. You need to eat only 3 ounces of fish every other day to satisfy your protein needs. Fish also is a good source of certain B vitamins that you can't always get from plants.

Seafood usually contains only 5 to 10 percent fat, compared with red meat, which is 30 to 40 percent fat. The leanest of beef— broiled top round—has 4.9 grams of fat per 3.5-ounce serving, compared to the leanest of fish—cod or flounder—which has no more than 2 grams of fat per 3.5-ounce serving. This makes fish a superb choice for keeping your weight under control.

"Even when you eat what is called a fatty fish, like salmon, it only runs between 6 and 10 percent fat. When you consider that a Big Mac is 45 percent fat and french fries are about the same percentage of fat, you're really eating a low-fat diet no matter how much fish you consume," says Gary J. Nelson, Ph.D., a research chemist with the USDA's Western Human Nutrition Research Center in San Francisco.

Even seafood that's considered to be high in cholesterol is better than eating meat, Dr. Nelson says. Crab, shrimp, and lobster may be higher in cholesterol than other seafood, but their total fat is only between 1 and 2 percent. "As long as you're not eating it in hollandaise sauce or pan-fried in gobs of butter, as long as you're just eating the boiled shrimp, it's so low in fat that you're probably better off than eating something else, like cheese or beef or pork."

Also, the cholesterol in shellfish doesn't come close to what you'll get from eggs. Two eggs at breakfast give you more than 400 milligrams of cholesterol—100 milligrams more than your daily recommended maximum amount. A 3.5-ounce serving of shrimp (about nine small shrimp) has just 166 milligrams of cholesterol.

Another reason to eat fish perhaps isn't as important as we once thought. For years, doctors pushed fish consumption because of an oil called omega-3 fatty acids that was thought to prevent heart disease, arthritis, stroke, and diabetes. But researchers have found that fish oil has fewer healthy powers than was formerly believed. It's not a reason to forgo fish, although you can save some money by skipping the fish-oil pills (unless they are prescribed by your physician for high triglyceride levels). It's just that fish doesn't seem to do anything magical for our hearts.

One study found that increasing your fish consumption from one time a week to every day will not significantly reduce your risk of heart disease. Another found that increased fish consumption didn't decrease the risk of heart disease or stroke. However, some research does suggest that moderate fish consumption may reduce your risk of dying from a heart attack, even if it doesn't prevent the heart attack in the first place.

"It seems like fish oil is not the panacea that was hoped for, although eating fish is a healthy alternative to red meat," says Walter C. Willett, M.D., Dr.P.H., professor of epidemiology and nutrition and chairman of the department of nutrition at the Harvard School of Public Health and a coauthor of both studies. "It's important to remember that you can get omega-3's from plant sources as well. And there is evidence that getting them from plants might be beneficial from the standpoint of heart disease. Some plant sources of omega-3's are canola oil, soybean oil, flaxseed, and walnuts. So I don't think the final answer is in on all forms of omega-3's."

SHELLFISH SAFETY

There is truly no bad seafood when it comes to fat and protein, Dr. Nelson says. But you may need to be wary of particular kinds for pollution reasons, and if you're allergic.

Shellfish often live amidst the garbage dumps of the sea. Oysters and clams feed by filtering 15 to 20 gallons of water per day, soaking up food particles as well as harmful bacteria and pollutants. Crabs, if they can't find any fresh food, are likely to be scavengers, eating dead material on the ocean's floor. Both eating habits make the creatures more susceptible to picking up people-sickening germs. It's more an issue with mollusks, such as clams, mussels, and oysters, because you're eating the entire body—including the stomach. When you eat crabs, you tend to pick out the white meat and stay away from the entrails.

That said, you don't have to give up shellfish. You just need to ask questions when you buy it.

Find out where it came from and whether those waters are clean or polluted, says Doris Hicks, a seafood technology specialist with the University of Delaware Sea Grant Program in Lewes. Each bushel of oysters, clams, or mussels must have a tag that is dated and that lists where it came from.

Here are two other safe shellfish strategies to keep in mind.

Make sure that they open. If the clamshell doesn't open when you cook it, you should throw the creature away. The closed shell means that the clam inside wasn't subjected to enough heat to kill the bacteria that are naturally present.

Don't get a raw deal. Think of downing raw oysters as bungee jumping. It can be a great experience, and it can be a dangerous one. You can prevent raw-oyster problems by not taking a chance and avoiding raw seafood altogether, says Hicks. Also, if you don't know where your oysters came from, not eating them during the months of May through August may help you avoid a rare type of food poisoning caused by red plankton.

If you have a chronic disease (for instance, any chronic form of liver, kidney, or gastrointestinal disease), you should never eat raw oysters or any raw shellfish, because you are more susceptible to its bacteria. The same rule applies to those suffering from immune-suppressing diseases such as AIDS or tuberculosis.

WHAT YOU NEED TO KNOW

Back to Mr. and Mrs. Blandmouth. Had they been a tiny bit more daring, they could have ordered grilled swordfish or tuna—both good starter fish. Neither have bones. They come in thick steaks, and they have more flavor than flounder. At least they could have gone home to Nebraska boasting about their dinner as well as their autographed photo of Regis.

Because there are so many varieties of seafood, it takes longer to become familiar with it than it would for, say, a slab of beef. But you don't have to spend your life wearing waders to understand it. All you have to do is divide it into the main types.

- The bonehead variety. Most restaurants debone your fish, so you usually won't have to worry about taking little bites and then using your tongue to smush the meat around in search of throat-scratching bones. But some fish are really bony. And if you don't like pulling food from your mouth every once in a while, they are best eaten carefully. These include trout, shad, sea bass, and catfish. "You would almost have to be a brain surgeon to get all the bones out," Bookbinder says.
- The robust variety. If you wake up in the morning and your dog is still licking your fingers, you had a robust fish. We're talking about the ones with the strong flavor and smell. They are oily, ranging in color from pink to red to blue or gray.

They include salmon, shad, tuna, mackerel, mahimahi, bluefish, and pompano.

- The "almost like meat" variety. These come in steaks and can be grilled. They are white-fleshed, so they aren't fishy-tasting. These include cod, halibut, mako, shark, skate, monkfish (cut into medallions), and swordfish.
- The pale, flaky variety. These come in fillets and are soft-fleshed and mild-tasting. They include orange roughy, perch, pollack, catfish, hake, sea trout, tilapia, fluke, flounder, and sole.

When you order fish at a fish store, be less concerned about the actual name of the fish than about the type. Let's say you're looking for something to grill. Don't go in and just look at the tuna. Consider swordfish and shark as well, says Hicks. For one, the store might not have tuna that day. Also, allowing yourself to substitute one fish for another can save you money. For instance, though swordfish is available year-round, it's much less prevalent on the East Coast in October and November, when fishing is a little tougher because of rough seas and

A BURGER TO GO

We know in our hearts—and in our guts—that we can't have all-beef patties, even if we hold the special sauce and cheese, as often as we may want.

But what's the alternative?

Try ground fish.

Fish burgers come in several varieties, including salmon, tuna, and, in the summer, Louisiana or Black Drum redfish. A betting man would lay down $100 that fish burgers would flop. And a betting man would lose.

"It caught on right away," says Robert Perose of Perose Seafood in Allentown, Pennsylvania, one of a growing number of stores where fish burgers are sold. "We make it into sausage. We make it into a veal Parmesan. Anything you would use ground beef for, this can be substituted. It's the closest thing to meat you can get."

Whether you have a salmon burger or a redfish burger, you're doing your weight some good. Both are low in fat. Salmon has less than a gram, and redfish contains less fat than boneless, skinless white chicken meat.

Because they are low in fat, the fish cook much faster than a regular beef burger. They take about 4 minutes per side on the grill.

We would never recommend that you eat something we haven't at least sampled ourselves, so we had lunch at Perose Seafood one day and tried the Cajun redfish burger. Now, we wouldn't exactly say that it tastes like a hamburger. It actually tastes *better* than most burgers. Light and spicy. Juicy. It was a lip-licking meal.

The ground salmon has a stronger fish taste. If you like salmon, you'll like a salmon burger. If you don't like salmon, you won't like a salmon burger.

stormy weather. So the price will probably be higher.

Here are some other pointers for buying and ordering fish.

Ask for directions. Let the store owner explain the best way to cook the fish. Many fish-store owners don't mind helping you out. Richard and Robert Perose of Perose Seafood in Allentown, Pennsylvania, will even do the work for you. On some nights, they sell already prepared fish. For instance, they'll have salmon with honey mustard already smeared on top. A sticker on the box explains how long to bake it. The brothers also have premade, microwaveable fish dinners. A chunk of seasoned fish comes with some vegetables and potatoes. Cooking time is only a couple of minutes.

Look for quick turnaround. You want to buy fish from a store that handles a lot of fish. That means that the fish will come and go quickly. It won't lie around.

Get fresh. You want to get the freshest fish possible. A fresh whole fish will have bright, clear eyes, shiny skin with a metallic luster, bright red gills, and smooth, well-attached scales, says Hicks. Also, the flesh should be firm and elastic. It should spring back after you press it.

Fillets should be moist and firm with no dried-out edges or gaping holes. And mollusks—oysters, clams, and mussels—should have tightly closed shells. If the shell is slightly open, tap it. If it closes, the creature is alive and edible. If it doesn't move, throw it away.

Keep it cold. When picking out fish at the store, make sure that it's cold to the touch. Fish is kind of like ice cream. You want to get it home before it melts, so make your trip to the fish store your last errand. And if you know that the drive home in 90°F heat will last more than ½ hour, take a cooler or pack the fish with a bag of ice. At home, put the wrapped fish in a bowl, cover it with a bag of crushed ice, and store it in the coldest part of your refrigerator—preferably in the middle drawer since it's protected from temperature fluctuations when you open and close the refrigerator door. Uncooked fish should be used within 1 to 2 days of purchase and kept between 33° and 34°F, says Hicks.

"You want to keep your fish cold, but not frozen," adds Perose.

Suffocate and freeze. When freezing fish, you don't want air to get to it. Make sure that the plastic wrap is skintight, then put the fish in a freezer storage bag or plastic container. This will prevent any damage to the fish from shuffling or rough handling, says Hicks. Fish will keep for 3 to 6 months in the freezer, depending on the type. Low-fat fish keeps longer than fattier fish.

Listen to old Ben. In *Poor Richard's Almanac*, Ben Franklin said that fish and guests smell after 3 days. That's how long your cooked leftovers will keep in the fridge, says Hicks.

Cereals

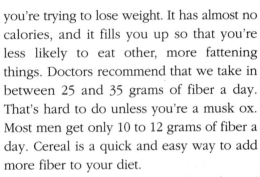

A sk most men why they don't eat breakfast and they'll probably say that they don't have time. What they really mean is that they hit the snooze button instead of getting up when the alarm goes off. And when it comes to breakfast, if you snooze, you lose.

But you don't have to roll out of bed an hour early and make pancakes from scratch. Just reach for a box of cereal, the lazy man's grub.

"Cereal, to me, is one of the easiest things in the world, not just in terms of making it but also in terms of cleaning up before I leave the house," says John Stanton, Ph.D., food-marketing professor at St. Joseph's University in Philadelphia. "It's one bowl. I don't even need to turn the stove on."

Actually, it's so easy, it doesn't seem possible that it's allowed to be good for you. But it is. Of all the things you can eat in the morning, Dr. Stanton says, cereal is one of the best choices.

Hot cereal has most of the same benefits as cold, but there's one hitch. It involves using either your stove or your microwave. "They just take longer. That's the only problem. I could eat oatmeal every day if someone would get up and make it for me," Dr. Stanton says.

BULK IN A BOWL

Men need fiber. It's good for your heart and digestive tract, and it's very good when you're trying to lose weight. It has almost no calories, and it fills you up so that you're less likely to eat other, more fattening things. Doctors recommend that we take in between 25 and 35 grams of fiber a day. That's hard to do unless you're a musk ox. Most men get only 10 to 12 grams of fiber a day. Cereal is a quick and easy way to add more fiber to your diet.

Elizabeth Somer, R.D., author of *Food and Mood*, recommends picking a cereal that has at least 2 grams of fiber per serving. Cereals made primarily from corn, wheat, oats, or rice—particularly bran cereals such as Kellogg's All-Bran—have as much as 14 grams of fiber per serving. Then again, some, like General Mills's Boo Berry, have none. So you have to check nutrition information on the box. Remember, that's what it's there for.

Just because some cereals will fill half of your daily fiber requirement doesn't mean that you need to eat twice as much. A lot of fiber comes from other foods as well.

"People know that they are supposed to eat more fiber, but they think that eating a bran cereal is the answer to their fiber

EAT EARLY, EAT LESS

John Stanton, Ph.D., food-marketing professor at St. Joseph's University in Philadelphia, knows a lot about nutrition. But even he admits that if he didn't eat a decent breakfast, he'd spend the morning scooping high-fat peanut butter into his mouth. That's his vice.

Everyone has similar pitfalls. It might be jelly doughnuts, chocolate chip cookies, or potato chips. Fat. Fat. And more fat.

This may explain the results of one of Dr. Stanton's studies. He found that those who eat breakfast—regardless of the kind of breakfast—have lower cholesterol levels than those who rush off to work hungry. "By skipping breakfast, people obviously are hungry during the day," Dr. Stanton says. "They seek to make up the missing calories in their day by picking high-calorie choices. And those high-calorie choices are usually high-fat choices."

needs. What they need to do is eat a high-fiber diet," Somer says. "A high-fiber diet that contains lots of fruits, vegetables, whole grains, and legumes provides a blend of different fibers."

Eating at least 2 grams of fiber a day will help lower your cholesterol, and eating 25 grams a day will lower your risk of colon cancer by 31 percent. Colon cancer is the third most prevalent and fatal cancer in men in the United States. A high-fiber diet lowers your risk of getting it by decreasing the time that waste sits around in your colon.

Many cereals also are crammed with vitamins. Most provide at least 10 percent of some of your vitamin and mineral needs. Some, such as Total, offer 100 percent of the recommended Daily Value for nine vitamins, iron, and zinc.

Not only do they have good stuff, many cereals also are lacking the bad stuff—fat. Most have only 2 grams or less per serving, although oat-based cereals and granolas usually have more. As a rule, look for cereals that have 2 grams of fat or less, says Somer.

Here are other key things to look for when picking out cereal.

Sugar. Keep it to 4 grams or less per serving, suggests Somer. If the cereal has fruit in it, you can allow for more. Just remember what fruit is. Froot Loops do not contain fruit. Raisin Bran does.

Protein. Try for at least 3 grams per serving, says Somer. The protein will perk up your brain, giving you peak mental performance all morning. It also will quiet your stomach through those morning meetings. No one wants to be the guy whose "grrring" tummy gets everyone's attention.

Dairy

The cow looks like a real slacker. It stands around in the pasture. It eats some grass. It chews. Stares into space. Chews. Maybe takes a nap. Chews some more. Stares into space again. Chews.

But its production abilities are awesome. Because of its four-compartment stomach, the cow can eat vitamin-packed, non-human-digestible grass, spit it up, chew on it, choke it back down, and eventually make milk we can drink. That milk is turned into an array of foods, from cheese to butter to yogurt.

Though eggs are not technically a dairy food—they're not made from milk—we'll be talking about them later in this chapter because you usually find them next to the milk cartons in the grocery store.

IT DOES A BODY GOOD

Though buffalo and goats supply milk and related products for various parts of the world, the cow has the U.S. market cornered.

How does it get from the farm to you? The thin, white liquid is pumped from the cow; cooled; processed; analyzed for bacterial count; heated to destroy bacteria, yeast, and molds (this is called pasteurizing); and then cooled again.

Though not required by law, most milk is also homogenized by being forced through very small pressurized tubes that break up the fat and disperse it evenly. If milk were not homogenized, cream would rise to the top. Low-fat and fat-free milk are not always homogenized, however, because much of the cream has been removed.

Packed with more than 40 nutrients, milk products provide a huge amount of essential vitamins and protein, including 75 percent of the calcium in the average American diet.

Calcium is what makes milk such a great food. That and the fact that you can guzzle it straight out of the carton. Three cups of milk, 3 cups of yogurt, or 3 to 5 ounces of cheese will cover your Daily Value of calcium. That means strong bones and teeth. Adequate calcium intake also may help prevent colon cancer and high blood pressure.

If you don't like milk, though, don't feel like you have to drink it. Broccoli, kale, turnip greens, seeds, and nuts are also considered good sources of calcium, but keep in mind that you'd have to eat a lot of them. You'd need 2½ cups of broccoli, 6 cups of pinto beans, or 30 cups of soy milk in order to get the same amount of calcium that you would from an 8-ounce glass of milk.

Obviously, milk is the easier alternative. To get the most from your milk, you'll want to keep it cold and in the dark. Strong sunlight and fluorescent light will destroy vitamins.

SKIM THE FAT

The problem with milk and milk products is that many are high in fat. Whole milk gets nearly 50 percent of its calories from fat, and Cheddar cheese packs a whopping 74 percent of its calories from fat.

When you're trying to lose weight, you don't have to give up milk products. You just need to give up the ones high in fat. One of the simplest ways to do that is to switch to fat-free or low-fat milk and low-fat cheese.

What's the difference between low-fat and fat-free? The low-fat, or 1%, variety sounds pretty good, doesn't it? But it still gets 20 percent of its calories from fat.

Fat-free milk has as much fat removed as is technologically possible. It gets 6 percent or less of its calories from fat, and all of the good stuff is left in.

"When the fat changes, nothing else does," says Robin Bagby, R.D., program-development specialist for the College of Health and Human Development at Pennsylvania State University in University Park. "Fat-free milk is still a good source of protein. That hasn't changed. It's a good source of calcium. That hasn't changed. It's only less fat."

Switching to fat-free milk may be more palatable if you do it in small steps. If you're used to drinking whole milk, first try 2%. Then, go down to 1% and work your way down to fat-free. Try different brands of fat-free. You might find one brand more palatable than another, says Bagby.

MARGARINE VERSUS BUTTER

First, they told you that butter is loaded with artery-clogging saturated fat. So you switched to margarine. Then, they said that margarine is loaded with artery-clogging trans fatty acids. So you decided that you may as well eat whatever you damn well please because the doctors can't make up their minds.

But the butter-versus-margarine debate really isn't all that complicated. The bottom line is that they're both bad for you.

There's no disagreement over the evils of butter's saturated fat. It's loaded with calories and it clogs your arteries. The consensus of the health world is to limit saturated fat to no more than 10 percent of your daily calories.

Margarine may be lower in calories, but it often contains trans fatty acids. Studies have shown that both saturated fat and trans fats increase your risk of coronary heart disease because they lower high-density lipoprotein (HDL), the good cholesterol, and raise low-density lipoprotein (LDL), the bad cholesterol. Nutritionists can't tell you to keep your intake to a particular amount because you have no way to gauge how much of the stuff you're eating. Unlike saturated fat, trans fats aren't listed on food labels. If you see partially hydrogenated vegetable oil on the list of ingredients, you know that the food has trans fatty acids lurking inside. But you have no way of knowing how much.

What's a health-conscious guy to do?

Jump in the tub. If you have to choose, go for a lower-fat margarine alternative. In a 1-tablespoon serving, most margarines have 2 grams of saturated fat compared to butter's 7, and the margarine has no cholesterol. Go for the tub versions or liquid "squeeze" versions of reduced-fat or fat-free margarines. The softer the margarine, the fewer trans fatty acids.

Spread out. When cooking or baking, try to use oil instead of butter or margarine. For spreads, think of other things to smear on top: jam, honey, hot peppers, relish. "It's experimenting with what tastes good to you and slowly weaning yourself back," says Bagby. "It's small steps over time."

Cut your hydrogenated fat. Hydrogenated fat is the main source of trans fats, so cutting down on your intake of products that list hydrogenated or partially hydrogenated fat high on their list of ingredients should help reduce your trans fat intake as well.

SAY CHEESE

According to legend, cheese was discovered by accident. Several thousand years ago, a guy stuck some milk in a sheep's-stomach pouch and set out on a daylong journey. The heat and the stomach enzymes turned the milk into a snowy white cheese curd and a liquid called whey.

Sounds kind of unappetizing, doesn't it? But we know that the next time you see some Swiss cubes on a party tray, the memory of that story won't keep you from stuffing cube after cube into your mouth.

Men like cheese. With most cheeses averaging 66 percent of their calories from fat, cheese is one of the most common fat boosters in our diets. Just one small, 1½-inch cube of hard cheese takes care of one-third of our day's maximum intake of saturated fat.

It's a good thing that food scientists have figured out how to defat cheese by adding more milk protein and taking away milk's cream. But if you're used to eating regular cheese, don't expect reduced-fat or fat-free versions to meet your taste standards, even though these versions are improving. To get the most out of them, substitute part of the regular cheese you're putting in a casserole or a pasta salad or on a pizza with a fat-free or reduced-fat version. That way, you'll still get the flavor of the regular cheese, but with less of the fat. Another good reason to blend a regular cheese with its fat-free counterpart in a hot dish is that some of the fat-free cheeses don't melt very well.

Here are a few other ways to enjoy cheese without getting all the fat.

Stay light, eat white. White cheeses such as mozzarella, Swiss, ricotta, and Parmesan are generally lower in fat than yellow cheeses such as Cheddar and American because they are often made with low-fat or reduced-fat milk instead of whole. Be aware, though, that food coloring can be used to make higher-fat cheeses white, so if you buy white American or white Cheddar cheese, you'll get just as much fat as you would in the yellow versions.

In general, white cheeses are good choices to buy in the reduced-fat variety. You won't miss the taste as much because white cheeses tend to have a milder flavor than yellow cheeses, says Gregory D. Miller, Ph.D., vice president of nutrition research and technology transfer for the National Dairy Council in Rosemont, Illinois.

Make it old and hard. If you're going to eat the real heart-clogging stuff, then at least do your teeth some good. Have it for dessert. A few studies indicate that hard, aged cheeses such as Monterey Jack and Cheddar may reduce cavity-causing bacteria.

Melt it and hide it. Fat-free cheese tends to look like plastic when melted. So if you hide it in a casserole, you won't notice it as much.

YOGURT:
THE WONDER DAIRY FOOD

It might reduce colon cancer. It might boost immunity. It might aid digestion. A cup a day just might make you live to be 100.

Thing is, these are all "mights."

"There's some interesting data that suggest that the bacteria in yogurt can change the bacteria in the colon. It's certainly exciting data. I don't think it's proven. It's somewhat speculative, but it is consistent," says Dennis A. Savaiano, Ph.D., professor and dean of the School of Consumer and Family Sciences at Purdue University in West Lafayette, Indiana. "I think we're in the same stage with yogurt and immunity. The data look promising, but this is a hard issue to prove."

Even with all the magical, life-enhancing qualities aside, yogurt is a nutritional powerhouse. A cup provides 300 to 450 milligrams of calcium, more than milk. It also supplies more B vitamins, phosphorus, and potassium than milk. And a cup of low-fat yogurt gives you one-fifth of your recommended daily protein intake.

Plain, fat-free yogurt can be used as a substitute for just about any fat-laden condiment, but some yogurts are better than others. Here's how to pick the best.

Get cultured. If your package of yogurt includes the statement "meets the National Yogurt Association criteria for live and active culture yogurt," it means that the yogurt has at least 10 million cultures per gram. And doctors think that those bacteria are what give yogurt its health-promoting qualities. An easy way to be sure that your yogurt contains significant amounts of these cultures is to look for the National Yogurt Association "LAC" seal on yogurt containers, says Timothy Morck, Ph.D., director of nutrition, regulatory, and consumer affairs for the Dannon Company in Tarrytown, New York.

Check the fat content. Yogurt can get almost half of its calories from fat. Read the labels and choose the low-fat and fat-free varieties.

Consider the calcium. If you're lactose intolerant, you may want to consider using yogurt as your primary dairy product because the cultures aid in digestion. Just make sure to choose yogurt that supplies 20 to 40 percent of your Daily Value for calcium in an 8-ounce serving, recommends Dr. Morck.

Check the date. As yogurts with live cultures age, they continue to produce lactic acid, which causes them to have more of a "bite" or tart taste. You won't get sick eating them, but you may not like the way they taste, especially if you prefer a mild, sweet flavor, Dr. Morck says. Unless you or the supplier had the yogurt sitting in the hot sun, it will last at least until the date on the cup. That date is generally the last day that the product should be sold in stores, he says, but you can feel confident eating most yogurts up to a week after the date. If you are concerned about eating it after that date, call the manufacturer's phone number, located on the product's container.

Keep the whey. When you open yogurt and there's some runny liquid floating on top, don't pour it out. It's whey. It contains protein and calcium. Stir it in, says Dr. Morck.

THE UPS AND DOWNS OF EGGS

For a while, eggs were portrayed as the ultimate evil in the food world. We're not going to tell you to start making omelettes every morning. But we are going to remove some of the stigma.

The reason that eggs got such a bad rap is because of the high amount of cholesterol they pack. Two eggs will put you well over your recommended limit. But it seems that we don't have to worry as much about dietary cholesterol as we once thought. High levels of cholesterol in the blood are a problem, but the cholesterol in food plays only a limited role.

Still, no one is going to tell you to eat more than four eggs a week.

"When you have two eggs for breakfast, that's 400 milligrams of cholesterol. Even if you go to a strict no-cholesterol diet for the rest of the day, you've already taken in more than the recommended amount, which is 300 milligrams. So a person who eats two eggs for breakfast plus bacon, which has cholesterol, and then goes on to eat regular meals will end up with probably 500, maybe 600 or 700, milligrams of cholesterol," says Gary J. Nelson, Ph.D., a research chemist with the USDA's Western Human Nutrition Research Center in San Francisco. "Even though cholesterol is less critical in raising your blood cholesterol level than dietary saturated fat, when you get up into 700 or 800 milligrams per day, it does have a significant effect."

Point is, you don't have to feel guilty every time you eat an egg. Just keep them to less than four a week and don't cook them in butter.

You can cut some of the cholesterol from your omelette by not putting in as many yolks. If you don't want to pick out the yolk yourself, buy egg substitutes.

Pastas and Grains

In ancient Rome, white bread was revered as the food of the gods. The concept was so ingrained that the politically powerful members of society mixed chalk in with their flour to ensure that their loaves were as pasty as possible.

Lots of things have changed since then. Rome fell. (For lack of Wonder Bread? You be the judge.) And the idea that white bread is the ultimate nutritional powerhouse has been relegated to the dung heap of history, somewhere between that wacky old flat-Earth theory and the even more frightening notion from the 1970s that men could look fetching in lime green leisure suits.

Why is dark bread better? For the same reason that whole wheat pasta is better than pasta made from white flour. It's the same reason that brown rice is better than white. And it's the same reason that oatmeal is better than Cream of Wheat. It all depends on what part of the grain is used to make the food.

PLANTING THE SEED OF GOOD HEALTH

Grains are seeds that come from grasses. You can think of them pretty much as anything you've seen waving in the wind while you've been driving along some desolate country road: wheat, corn, oats, barley, millet, rice, and rye.

To understand why some parts of the grain are better than others, you first need to know the parts of the grain.

Endosperm. This is the largest part of the grain, but the least nutritional. It contains starch, some protein, and a few B vitamins.

Germ. The smallest part of the grain and the most nutritionally concentrated, it contains protein, oils, and the B vitamins thiamin, riboflavin, niacin, and pyridoxine. It also has vitamin E and the minerals magnesium, zinc, potassium, and iron.

Bran. The grain's fiber powerhouse, this coating around the endosperm contains B vitamins, zinc, calcium, potassium, phosphorus, magnesium, and some other minerals. A bowl of high-bran cereal with milk has as much potassium as a medium-size banana.

Though the endosperm has barely any nutritional value, it's refined (processed by removing the bran and germ) and ground up to make the white flour that is a key component in white bread and pale pasta. The government requires manufacturers to enrich such refined products with thiamin, riboflavin, niacin, and iron.

But products that are made with the other parts of the grain—oat bran muffins, whole wheat bread, wheat germ, brown rice—are naturally more nutritious.

About now, you're probably wondering whether you're ever allowed to eat white bread and pale pasta again. The answer is yes. You just want to eat more of the dark stuff, too, says Jane Folkman, R.D., spokesperson for the Massachusetts Dietetic Association in Boston.

The most important reason to eat a lot of whole grains is fiber. Fiber helps you lose weight. It lowers cholesterol. And it keeps your digestive tract running smoothly. But fiber grams do not add up easily. One bagel has about 0.5 gram, a slice of whole wheat bread has 1.5 grams, and a cup of enriched spaghetti has 2.2 grams. So you can see why nutritionists want you to eat 6 to 11 servings of grains and cereals a day.

"If you eat more foods such as brown rice and whole wheat pasta, it's a lot easier to meet that recommendation," says Neva Cochran of the American Dietetic Association. Grains are also low in fat and high in complex carbohydrates.

WEIGHING IN

But can't too many grain products such as pasta and bread make you fat?

No. It's true that starchy foods can raise insulin to abnormally high levels in about 10 to 20 percent of the population. That makes them more susceptible to heart disease, but it doesn't make them fat. Many such people have insulin problems because they are already overweight, because they don't exercise, or because their genes made them that way.

Going strictly by the numbers, it would seem that eating more pasta and other grain products would help with weight loss. Grains are carbohydrates, which have 4 calories per gram. Fat has 9 calories per gram. If we ate the same amount of food but cut the fat and increased the carbohydrates, it would make sense that we would lose weight.

The problem is that we haven't done that. Between 1978 and 1990, Americans cut their average intake of dietary fat from 36 percent to 34 percent of total calories. Basically, that's 1 fewer teaspoon of butter a day. But we gained weight.

Why? It wasn't the switch from fatty meats to nonfatty pastas and grains. We got fatter because we ate more during the same time period, increasing our daily calories. And we began exercising less, says Gerald Reaven, M.D., professor emeritus of medicine at Stanford University School of Medicine.

Pasta is not fattening unless you eat six bowls of spaghetti when you usually would eat only one. Try to follow the Food Guide Pyramid. Six to 11 servings of pastas and grains really isn't that much when you consider what counts as a serving—one slice of bread, ½ cup of cooked cereal, or ½ cup of rice. Some specialty-shop bagels are so large that they equal 4 servings. And a typical serving of spaghetti will count as 3 servings.

THE BREAD OF LIFE

Different breads have different amounts of fiber, varying from 1 gram to more than 3 grams per slice. Read the label to find high-fiber breads.

Also, as we said before, look for breads made from whole grains. That means that the bread should have the word "whole" somewhere in its name. For instance, whole wheat bread has more zinc, magnesium, fiber, and other nutrients than refined white bread. The refining process strips those nutrients. Wheat bread usually has twice the fiber of white bread.

If you're looking to buy wheat bread, be careful to read the labels. Some breads have wheat-sounding names but are really made with refined flour. To make sure that you're getting whole wheat, look for "whole wheat" or another whole grain as the first ingredient on the label, says Cochran.

It's okay to eat other stuff like French bread, rye, pumpernickel, sourdough, and English muffins, because they are packed with healthy complex carbohydrates, says Cochran. But don't fool yourself into thinking that you're getting whole grains. You might get a pinch of the whole rye seed with your bread, but most of it is made from refined flour. And the dark

BAGEL BLUNDERS

All you wanted was a quick breakfast. Instead, you got a quick trip to the emergency room to have your finger stitched up.

"People are often embarrassed to tell you," says Mark Smith, M.D., chairman of the department of emergency medicine at Washington Hospital Center and clinical professor of emergency medicine at the George Washington University School of Medicine and Health Sciences, both in Washington, D.C. "We noticed that it was sufficiently common that we identified it as a syndrome. You usually get one or two people a weekend."

George Washington University hospital doctors were seeing so many bagel injuries that they did some research. They called some bagel stores, and they came up with some cutting-edge advice.

Get a grip. Some bagel shops or kitchen supply stores sell devices that will hold your bagel steady as you slice. They keep your fingers out of the knife's way.

Make a lateral move. Put the bagel flat on the table and slice parallel to the table. Though your hand should be out of harm's way, not too many experts are fond of this method. This is no time to get cocky.

Stay above the fray. With your thumb and index finger, hold the bagel perpendicular to the table. Your thumb and index finger should be shaped like an upside-down U. If you're holding the bagel in your left hand, for instance, your thumb should be toward you, to the left. Put the knife edge in the space between your thumb and index finger and cut down. "This way, your fingers are above the knife and it's hard to cut yourself," Dr. Smith says.

color of pumpernickel usually comes from coloring.

USING YOUR NOODLE

They are proud of their pasta over there in Europe. So proud, in fact, that they openly bicker about who invented it. One crowd argues that Marco Polo brought it back to Europe after he visited Kubla Khan. But Italians don't buy it. A few years back, they decided that pasta was so important that it should have its very own museum. At this National Museum of Pasta Foods, they argue that Italians served noodles at least 100 years before Marco Polo even thought about China. It just seemed new because the Chinese were serving pasta differently.

Another thing they tell you at this museum: Whatever you do, don't overcook the noodles. With that in mind, here's what you need to know in order to eat pasta like an Italian.

Experiment with shapes. There are more than 300 different shapes that fall into five basic categories. There are long, round noodles such as spaghetti and angel hair, and long, flat ones such as linguine and lasagna. There's the tube variety such as ziti, macaroni, and penne, and the corkscrew type such as fusilli and rotini. Finally, there's the potluck category that includes everything that doesn't fit into the above. That includes those wagon wheels, the ABCs in alphabet soup, and specialty pastas shaped like chile peppers, bicycles, and even sex organs.

Consider the flour. You want to buy pasta that's made from a good flour. In most cases, you want something made from 100 percent semolina (ground durum wheat). It's what's known as a hard flour. It won't absorb much water when cooked, so it will always turn out firm. It's good with a variety of sauces, from light sauces made with olive oil to heavy, chunky sauces. Some refrigerated pastas are made from regular bread flour (ground up endosperm), which is known as a soft flour. If you like limp pasta, that's fine. But be forewarned: No matter what you do, it will never turn out firm. Asian noodles offer an expanded selection in taste because they are made with so many varied sources: buckwheat, rice, mung beans, potato starch, and sweet potatoes.

Know your dough. The pasta you buy at the grocery store is usually what's known as dry pasta. It's fine for almost all occasions, but if you want to treat yourself, try refrigerated fresh or soft pasta, available at specialty shops and some supermarkets. It cooks faster, tastes doughier, and usually costs more dough. It also is usually made with egg, which means that it has more cholesterol. It will keep in the refrigerator for only a day or two, so plan to cook it up quickly. It freezes well, however.

Eat Popeye pasta. Some pastas have ingredients other than flour, and that's what makes some nutritionally different from others. Some types contain egg, which means as much as 145 milligrams of cholesterol per serving. Others have some spinach, and almost all semolina products are enriched with extra nutrients. Spinach and wheat pastas can be a good way to boost your nutrient intake. For example, a cup of cooked spinach spaghetti has 42 milligrams of calcium, 87 milligrams of magnesium, 81 milligrams of potassium, and 151 milligrams of phosphorus. One cup of regular, cooked spaghetti, in comparison, has 10 milligrams of calcium, 25 milligrams of magnesium, 44 milligrams of potassium, and 76 milligrams of phosphorus.

Keep it in the dark. You can keep dried, uncooked pasta in a cool, dry cupboard for up to a year. You can refrigerate cooked pasta for 3 to 5 days. The cooked pasta will continue to absorb flavor from the sauce unless you store it separately.

Follow directions. To avoid clumpy pasta, make sure you give it enough water. Boil 4 to 6 quarts of water per pound of pasta. Also, stir often. In terms of cooking time, there's really no magical advice. Follow the package directions, according to Donna Chowning Reid, director of communications for the National Pasta Association in Arlington, Virginia. Each manufacturer has tested its pasta to determine the optimum cooking time, and each pasta is different. If you're not the clock-watching type, you can nibble a piece every so often. Pasta is done when it's firm yet cooked all the way through.

CONVERTING TO RICE

It's been around since 2800 B.C., and next to spaghetti, rice is probably one of the easiest things to cook.

It comes in three different sizes. Long-grain rice is four times as long as it is wide. Short-grain rice is round. Long-grain rice comes out fluffy and easy to separate. Medium-grain is more moist and tender, and short-grain sticks together after cooking—good for rolling sushi.

Rice comes in many varieties, but the most familiar are brown and white. Brown rice provides more fiber, vitamin E, phosphorus, and calcium than white rice. But most white rice is enriched and provides more thiamin and iron than brown rice. Here are some ways to spice it up.

Try something new. Other varieties of rice include converted, aromatic, and wild. Converted rice is Uncle Ben's. It has been steamed under pressure before milling, which returns some of the bran's nutrients without keeping the bran intact. The rice turns out firm and fluffy. Aromatic rice is the term used to describe any variety of rice that has a strong, nutty aroma. Wild rice is not really a member of the rice family; it's the seed of an aquatic grass. It has more protein than white rice and has a nutty flavor.

Keep a lid on it. Once opened, uncooked rice should be stored in a tightly sealed container in a cool, dry place. The shelf life for brown rice is shorter than for white. The bran layers of brown rice have oil that can go rancid, so the U.S.A. Rice Council suggests storing it in the refrigerator. It will keep in the fridge for about 6 months.

Go slow. When cooking rice, slowly add it to boiling water. Make sure there's enough water for the rice to float freely. And of course, follow the package directions.

Produce

It's a nightmare, that childhood memory. Your mom sticks a plate of mushy, overcooked, sulphury-stinking green balls down on the table and bellows, "Eat." Yes, the dreaded brussels sprouts—the name alone can make a grown man gag.

So imagine the stomach pains Ann Parker must have suffered when she started her new job promoting the Santa Cruz Beach Boardwalk's annual Brussels Sprouts Festival.

Parker hated those tiny green balls. Hated them.

And here the public relations director had to convince people to come to a place that served brussels sprouts pizza, brussels sprouts ice cream, brussels sprouts cookies, and brussels sprouts shish kebab for 2 days straight. Know what she did? She learned to like brussels sprouts.

Just goes to show that you can learn to like anything if you set your mind to it.

Fortunately, it doesn't have to be only brussels sprouts. But to boost your odds of taking weight off and keeping it off and of preventing a host of serious illnesses, you should eat five to nine servings of fruits and vegetables a day, says Jerianne Heimendinger, R.D., Ph.D., former director of the National Cancer Institute's Five-a-Day-for-Better-Health! program and currently acting director of the Lifestyle Research Center at the AMC Cancer Research Center in Denver.

A serving is any of the following: ¾ cup of 100 percent fruit juice, a medium-size piece of whole fruit, ½ cup of chopped vegetables, 1 cup of salad greens, ¼ cup of dried fruit, or ½ cup of cut fruits or vegetables.

HELP YOURSELF

At the buffet table of life, the sign over the salad bar always reads, "All you can eat."

In general, produce contains only small amounts of those things that doctors and nutritionists have been trying to get us to consume less of, namely, fat and calories. Plus, it's loaded with most of the stuff that doctors say we need more of: fiber, vitamins A and C, and an assortment of antioxidants.

Fruits and vegetables contain hundreds of hard-to-pronounce and harder-to-spell cancer-fighting compounds known collectively as phytochemicals. About 35 percent of cancer deaths are thought to be related to diet. And in many studies, people who ate a lot of vegetables and fruits cut their risks of cancer in half compared with people who hardly touched the stuff.

Thing is, no one fruit or vegetable has all the phytochemicals. Tomatoes and watermelon have a particular kind of compound that's different from the compounds in carrots and sweet potatoes. Broccoli and brussels sprouts have anticancer compounds that are different from the cancer-fighting sulfurous compounds in garlic and onions.

Doctors believe that those substances and a host of unknown others work in conjunction with one another to prevent many of the leading forms of cancer, so you can't just eat tons of the one fruit or one vegetable that you like and say that you've had your five servings that day. You need a variety.

To get what are believed to be the essential phytochemicals in your diet, you need to eat something in these food categories every day.

Red fruits: tomatoes, watermelon, guavas, pink grapefruit

Cruciferous vegetables: broccoli, cauliflower, brussels sprouts, cabbage

Citrus fruits: oranges, grapefruit, and tangerines

Tearjerkers: garlic and onions

Orange vegetables: carrots, pumpkins, and sweet potatoes

If you're not that crazy about fruits and vegetables, you'll want to concentrate on those that produce the most nutritional bang for your buck with each serving. Here's a breakdown of the nutrients provided by some produce powerhouses that are recommended by the National Cancer Institute's Five-a-Day-for-Better-Health! program.

- 50 percent of the recommended Daily Value for vitamin A: apricots, bok choy, cantaloupes, carrots, chile peppers, spinach, winter squash, and sweet potatoes
- 50 percent of the recommended Daily Value for vitamin C: broccoli, brussels sprouts, cauliflower, chili peppers, green peppers, grapefruit, kiwis, oranges, cantaloupes, papayas, and strawberries
- 4 or more grams of fiber (most fruits and vegetables have between 1 and 3 grams): figs, pears, prunes, dried peas, and beans

LEARNING TO LIKE IT

Okay, you're convinced. You *should* eat more vegetables. But you've known that for years. The problem is that you still don't *want* to eat them.

Most of us have no problem eating vitamin-vacant iceberg lettuce. But cruciferous vegetables, such as bok choy, broccoli, brussels sprouts, cabbage, and cauliflower, present a greater challenge. Some guys hate just about every vegetable imaginable except lettuce and carrots.

What makes one guy a vegetable lover and another a vegetable hater?

It might all come down to another hard-to-pronounce and harder-to-spell compound called 6-n-propyl-thiouracil. It seems that people who are really sensitive to that compound are also pretty sensitive to both bitter and sweet tastes, says Ann Ferris, R.D., Ph.D., professor and head of the department of nutritional sciences at the University of Connecticut in Storrs.

Researchers assume that there is a link between tasting that compound and dislike of bitter-tasting foods, but they've never established a definite link. And women seem to be more sensitive to 6-n-propyl-thiouracil than men, Dr. Ferris says.

Possibly, vegetable hating is partly socialization, Dr. Ferris says. "When you're a child, there's an assumption that you're not going to like brussels sprouts. There's an assumption that nobody's going to like brussels sprouts," she says. "A lot of it is that we're socialized as children not to like them."

That's why some doctors feel that you can make yourself like or at least tolerate your most despised vegetable simply by eating it a lot.

That's how Ann Parker learned to like brussels sprouts. As a part of the Santa Cruz Brussels Sprouts Festival, she tried them in pizza. She had them stir-fried. She had them spun into saltwater taffy.

"The big surprise was, I think I only had two dishes I didn't like during the 5 years that I promoted it," Parker says. "It's like any food. You have to prepare it correctly. People would come to the festival thinking that they hated them, then they would taste some of the recipes and they would change their minds."

PRODUCE MORE

If you want to increase your produce consumption, you have to think produce. All the time.

"Try and incorporate it into every meal," says Clare Hasler, Ph.D., director of Functional Foods for Health, a joint program of the University of Illinois at Urbana-Champaign and Chicago. "Just really try to make it a part of your diet. It's a major behavior and dietary change. If you're eating three meals a day and two or three snacks, you should have your five servings right there."

Meal by meal, here are some easy ways to get more produce into your diet.

Breakfast

- Drink 6 ounces of orange juice.
- Put ½ cup of fruit (sliced bananas, strawberries, blueberries) on your cereal or pancakes.
- Eat a bowl of fruit.

Snacks

- Instead of coffee or soda, have 6 ounces of 100 percent fruit juice such as pineapple, grapefruit, or orange. Drinking a blend of different fruits and vegetables is great because it provides more than one type of phytochemical.
- Try fat-free fruit bars, whole fruit (apples, bananas), or cut vegetables for snacks instead of candy.

Lunch

- Have a salad. To cut down on preparation time, make it at the grocery store salad bar or buy presliced, bagged lettuce and vegetables. A large salad with 2 cups of leafy greens can count for two or more servings. Try to mix in lots of different-colored vegetables. Besides making your salad prettier, they increase the number of phytochemicals.

THE FORBIDDEN FRUIT

We know that, nutritionally, apples are good for us. But for centuries, we've looked to apples to provide us with other benefits. Here are just a few less common ways we can use them.

To win races. In Greek mythology, the huntress Atalanta offered to marry any chap who could beat her in a race. The losers—and there were many—lost their lives. She speared them. But that didn't deter her suitors, one of whom was Milanion. Not relishing the idea of being speared to death, Milanion tricked her into losing. He dropped three golden apples as he raced. Atalanta stopped to pick them up and lost.

To make body parts. We all know about how Eve fed Adam that apple. But what a lot of us don't know is exactly what happened once Adam ate it. Yeah, yeah, they got their eviction notice from paradise; Eve was cursed with painful childbirth. But some people believe that yet another thing happened that fateful day: Adam got a new body part. He never could manage to swallow that apple. It got stuck in his throat, and the Adam's apple was created.

To tell the future. So you've been seeing this woman for a while. It's a promising relationship. You like her. Your friends like her. Heck, your dog likes her. But, well, you're still a little wary about tying the knot. What to do? Cut an apple in half. An even number of seeds means that marriage is the way to go. But if you cut open a seed while slicing the apple, it means that there's trouble ahead.

- Eat vegetables such as carrots or celery sticks on the side, or eat a piece of fruit.
- Add lettuce, tomato, sprouts, and other vegetables to your sandwiches.

Dinner

- Make vegetables a part of the main dish. Stir-fry chicken with broccoli or snow peas.
- Have a salad.
- Garnish the main dish with sliced fruit.

Dessert

- Stick fruit on top of cake or ice cream.

MAKING TIME

Probably the biggest reason that men don't eat enough produce is the time factor. You may have time to buy a head of broccoli. Then, it sits in the fridge. Sits in the fridge. Sits in the fridge. Then, you notice a gooey, slimy growth. It's time to chuck it.

Don't be so traditional. There are lots of ways to get produce into your diet besides cooking it as a side dish.

Shake it. Instead of letting the stuff sit in the fridge, shove it in the blender and make a shake out of it. One example is fresh strawberries with orange juice. Or make grapefruit-juice ice cubes and stick them in pineapple juice.

Buy them ready to go. Buy prepackaged, already-sliced items to snack on at home. These can include canned pears, sliced watermelon, and baby carrots. Make sure that canned fruits are packed in 100 percent fruit juice.

You may think that you're getting fewer vitamins when someone else does the cutting. Not true. Research shows that bagged vegetables don't breathe as much as unbagged vegetables. That means that they use up fewer nutrients.

Cut them in advance. Wash and cut up vegetables such as carrots, celery, and zucchini for easy access. Wrap them in plastic or keep them in water to keep them fresh.

Have drinks available. Keep small bottles or cans of 100 percent fruit juice in the fridge. That way, you can grab one to drink on the way to work.

Keep them ready. Always try to have a piece of fruit such as a banana or apple handy. Take easy-to-eat fruits and vegetables to eat in the car. Top choices include apples, bananas, carrots, grapes, and pears. Keep dried fruits—prunes, raisins, peaches, figs—in the glove compartment.

Freeze them. Put bagged vegetables you're not going to eat soon in the freezer to make them last.

KEEPING PRODUCE FRESH

If no self-respecting man would stop to ask for directions to someplace he really wants to go, he's sure not going to ask some supermarket produce manager for directions on how to store fruits and vegetables. We understand that. So to make your life simpler, Kathy Means, vice president of membership and public affairs for the Produce Marketing Association in Newark, Delaware,

has provided a list of handling tips for 20 commonly used fruits and vegetables. All of these are available year-round.

Bananas. Store them at room temperature to ripen. Refrigerate ripe ones (yellow with black specks). It will turn the skins black, but the insides will be fine. They will keep a few days, depending on the stage of ripeness.

Apples. Store them either at room temperature or in the fridge. They will keep for weeks if refrigerated.

Oranges. Their peak season is October through May. You can store them at room temperature if you plan to eat them within 2 weeks. Otherwise, store them in the refrigerator. They'll keep for weeks there. To get juicier oranges, pick out those that seem heavy for their size.

Cantaloupes. Store ripe ones in the fridge, where they will last a few days. You cannot judge ripeness by thumping. Ripe ones have a cantaloupe smell and will be slightly soft at the blossom end.

Grapes. Store them in a plastic bag in the fridge. They'll keep there for a few days. Wash them before serving, not before storing.

Avocados. Store ripe ones in the warmest part of the refrigerator for up to 3 days. You can ripen them at home by putting them in a loosely closed paper bag at room temperature. Keep checking them because there is a fine line between ripeness and overripeness. When they yield to gentle pressure, they're ready to eat. You can get them to ripen faster by sticking a ripe banana or tomato in the bag. The fruit will give off a natural gas that will heat up the bag and help them ripen.

Lemons. You can store them at room temperature for a few days or, for longer storage, keep whole lemons in the fridge for up to a month. To release more juice, stick the fruit in the microwave for 10 sec-onds, then roll it on a countertop before squeezing.

Strawberries. Their peak season is April through August. Store them unwashed in the refrigerator. They'll keep for a few days. Wash before eating.

Peaches. Their peak season is April

BETTER BRUSSELS SPROUTS

No one can force you to eat brussels sprouts. But we're going to let you in on a few secrets that might help you make those little green balls go down easier. Here's the reasoning: If you can learn to like brussels sprouts, you can learn to like anything.

First, you should know that until the mid-1960s, sprouts were handpicked. Then came a revolution. By crossbreeding different kinds of sprouts, scientists created a variety that could be machine-harvested.

"A lot of the characteristics were fine for farming, but the one characteristic that they didn't pay a lot of attention to was taste," says Steve Bontadelli, a brussels sprouts grower in Santa Cruz, California, the sprouts capital of the United States. "So they were real bitter, and that's what a lot of people in our generation were raised on. They never tried them again."

Today, however, brussels sprouts science has far surpassed what it was in the 1960s. Today's hybrids are better tasting and milder. Some are even, shall we go so far as to say, sweet.

There's one bad characteristic that has not been bred out of today's sprouts. They still stink. Not to worry. You can do something about that smell. Cook them with a few celery stalks. That goes for any stinky vegetable.

Also, you want to flavor them. Garlic is a great complement. Or if you have a roast in the oven, toss in some frozen sprouts during the last ½ hour to let them soak up the meat juices.

Here are some other sprout strategies.

Avoid the middle. Buy sprouts in either the late season (December to January) or the early season (July to September). Those varieties are milder than ones grown during other times of the year.

Buy them young. Buy younger, smaller sprouts. They're milder.

Let X mark the spot. When preparing them, cut an X in the butt of each one to make them cook evenly. And whatever you do—and this goes for all vegetables—don't overcook them. Mushy brussels sprouts rank as one of the ultimate gross-out foods. "That's another thing our moms used to do a lot, cook the heck out of them. Then there's this yucky, mushy thing you eat," says Bontadelli. "They are much better al dente. You can put a fork in them, but you don't want them to mush out."

through October. Ripen them at room temperature and refrigerate them when ripe. They'll keep for a few days in the refrigerator. Buy firm but slightly soft peaches with yellow between the red parts. Ripe ones smell peachy.

Grapefruit. Their peak season is January through June. You can store them for a few days at room temperature and for a week or more in the refrigerator. Choose heavy fruit.

Potatoes. Store them in a cool, dry, dark place for up to 2 months. Refrigeration will alter the taste.

Head lettuce. To make it last longer, core it by slamming it against something (some guys use the wall, others the counter) and then ripping off the stem. Rinse, drain, and stick it in a tightly closed bag or container in the crisper section of the refrigerator. Whole lettuce will last about a week.

Tomatoes. Store at room temperature until ripe, then eat immediately. Once a tomato is sliced, it should be refrigerated or it will quickly go bad. But be forewarned: Tomatoes lose their taste in the fridge.

Onions. Store in a cool, dry, dark place with good air circulation in a loosely woven bag, basket, or crate. They'll keep for weeks. Refrigerate cut onions in a covered container.

Carrots. Remove the green tops and store unwashed in a plastic bag in the refrigerator. They store well for 2 weeks.

Broccoli. Put it unwashed in a plastic bag in the crisper. It will last 3 days or more.

Cucumbers. Refrigerate, either cut or whole, in a plastic bag. An unpeeled cucumber will last for a week.

Bell peppers. Store in a plastic bag in the fridge for up to 5 days.

Cauliflower. Store it unwashed in a plastic bag in the crisper. It can keep for a week, but eat it as soon as possible to avoid a strong taste and smell.

Mushrooms. Refrigerate them in a paper bag. They will last about 2 days. Wash them before eating, not before storing.

Jim Palmer, Hall of Fame Pitcher

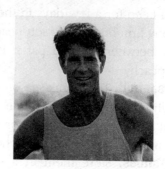

The first time that Hall of Fame pitcher Jim Palmer really ate healthy, it wasn't by choice.

"In 1968, I'd hurt my arm and I was down in Puerto Rico (for rehab)," the former Baltimore Orioles great recalls. "I went from about 210 or 212 pounds to 190 just because I didn't eat as much junk food.

"Down there, I was eating more rice and bananas and things like that. More native-type food. And I lost 20 pounds."

Today, almost 30 years later, Palmer still tips the scales in the low 190s. "But I know that, within a matter of moments, I could be at 210 by going back to my old eating habits," he says. "Pie à la mode, eating all the things you know are bad for you but that make you feel good for the moment. I think that's where the discipline comes in."

And that discipline has clearly paid off. Jim Palmer, now in his fifties, is the Dick Clark of the sporting world. He has maintained his trim, athletic build and boyish good looks long after the end of his remarkable 21-year baseball career. Between broadcasting stints for network television and local Orioles games, and his commercial campaigns for such high-profile clients as The Money Store and Jockey

underwear, Palmer is probably on the tube more now than he was in his playing days.

But Palmer didn't cut any Dorian Gray deals or discover the magic fountain of youth, although he does spend part of the year at his winter home in Juno Beach, Florida. "You make lifestyle decisions," he says. "I don't want to live a boring life. But I want to make conscious decisions that are going to be healthier."

A MAJOR-LEAGUE CHANGE-UP

Growing up as a three-sport schoolboy star, Palmer never worried much about what he ate. As an all-state football, basketball, and baseball player in Arizona in the early 1960s, Palmer's basic diet consisted of the same staples as any other all-American boy's: hamburgers and hot dogs.

"I just felt that whatever I ate would be superseded by going to basketball practice, doing my homework, and then going for a 2-mile run," Palmer says. "I never worried about the nutritional value. I just felt that I would be in good shape, regardless of what I ate. That's how naïve I was."

Coming out of high school, Palmer rejected a scholarship offer to play basketball for UCLA. (If he had said yes, he would have played with another pretty fair player, a kid named Lew Alcindor—known around the world today as Kareem Abdul-Jabbar.) The 18-year-old Palmer, meanwhile, got a then-whopping $50,000 bonus to sign with the Orioles.

When he was in the minor leagues, it was tough to eat well. Players got $3 a day in meal money, and it didn't go very far. "You'd have grilled cheese sandwiches," Palmer recalls. "Then, everybody said you ought to eat wheat bread. So you'd try to eat healthy by having a grilled cheese sandwich that was fried in butter on whole wheat bread."

When he hit the majors, Palmer quickly learned that if he didn't take responsibility for his own health and fitness, nobody else would. In the minors, he had played for the hard-driving Cal Ripken Sr., father of future Hall of Famer and Orioles ironman Cal Ripken Jr. "Everybody ran hard who played for Cal, because he made you," Palmer says. "Then, when you got to the big leagues, you were on your own. They thought that since you were in the big leagues, you ought to be able to make conscious decisions that were going to be the right ones.

Well, a guy would stay out late drinking or have a headache or didn't feel like running or was a little overweight, and he wouldn't run. And then it would reflect in his performance."

Postgame spreads in major-league locker rooms back then usually featured meat and potatoes, and there were always plenty of candy bars on hand for a quick energy boost. Today, you'll find healthier foods—fruits and vegetables—mixed in with the candy bars, but Palmer says that many athletes still have the naïve notion that nutrition doesn't matter.

"There's a certain imperviousness to health when you're young and vibrant and full of life," says Palmer, a three-time Cy Young Award winner who chalked up 268 victories en route to being the only pitcher ever to win World Series games in 3 decades. "You look around, and how many guys shortened their careers because they didn't take care of themselves? An unbelievably great amount of them."

EATING FOR LIFE

Palmer took great care of himself throughout his playing days, but he pinpoints a West Coast visit to Hollywood stuntman Ted Grossman's home in 1978 as a real turning point in terms of nutrition. When he checked the food supply there, Palmer recalls, all he saw were fruits, vegetables, nuts, and rice. "And I'm going, 'What am I going to eat? This is all healthy stuff.'"

Palmer had eliminated many of the really high-fat items from his diet following his Puerto Rico trip in 1968, but he credits his friendship with Grossman with truly opening his eyes to the full benefits of eating for health and nutrition.

He may be a true believer, but he doesn't consider himself to be a fanatic. "Life's too short not to have a Mrs. Field's cookie or some Häagen-Dazs ice cream or whatever," says Palmer, who still lives in Baltimore most of the year with his wife, Joni. "Moderation—that is the key. There are people who are overly zealous about everything, whether it's religion or diet or just work, work, work. It's nice to have a happy, pleasant mix where you can eat health-consciously, but you don't have to overdo it."

Conscious decisions are what it all comes down to for Jim Palmer. And all of those little daily decisions add up to one big one: to lead a longer and healthier life.

"I want to live as long as I possibly can. I don't want to know what's after life. That's going to happen soon enough. It's inevitable that that's going to happen. So you make conscious lifestyle decisions."

Index

Underscored page references indicate boxed text. **Boldface** references indicate photographs.

Calf muscles, 251
Calf raise, 272–73
Calorie Control Council, 12
Calories
  in alcohol, 13–14, 14, 83
  in cheeseburger, 49
  counting, 16–19
  exercise for burning, 23
    aerobic dance, 113
    chores and yardwork,
      128
    cycling, 113
    jumping rope, 137
    pro baseball, 153
    running, 49, 113, 153, 157
    skiing, 166
    tennis, 49
    Tour de France cycling,
      153
    walking, 53, 113, 125
  in frozen food, 301–2
  time of consumption of, 64
Campbell, Wayne W., 58–59,
    107–8, 196–97
Cancer
  colon, 11, 291, 338
  colorectal, 291
  diet and, 11
  dietary fat and, 291–93
  fiber and, 338
  fruits for preventing, 302–3,
    349–50
  lung, 11, 291
  pancreatic, 291
  prostate, 11, 291
  vegetables for preventing,
    302–3, 349–50
Candy, 77
Canned food, 304–7, 323
Canned Food Information
    Council, 305, 307
Cantaloupes, 353
Capilene, 166
Cappaert, Jane, 170

Carbohydrates, 11, 18, 66,
    90–91
Carrera, Richard, 174, 176
Carrots, 355
Cauliflower, 355
CDB Research and Consulting,
    10
Centers for Disease Control
    and Prevention, 56, 152
Cereals, 77, 337–38, 338
Chang, Michael, 28–30, 28, 29
Changes in lifestyle and
  clothing, 95-97, 96
  diet, 64–68, 65, 67
  dining out, 79–83, 80, 81,
    87
  holidays, 89–94, 90, 92
  snacks, 74–78, 76, 77
  socializing, 79–83, 80, 81,
    93–94
  traveling, 84–88, 87
  work, 69–73, 70, 71
Cheese, 341–42
Cheeseburger, 49
Chest exercises. See Upper-
    body workout
Chicken, 300, 326
Chinning bars, 136, **136**
Cholesterol
  dietary fat and, 290–91, 343
  fiber and, 290, 338
  heart disease and, 5
  high-density lipoprotein,
    14–15, 290–91, 297, 340
  lipids and, 4–6, 5
  low-density lipoprotein, 15,
    289–91, 297, 340
  olive oil and, 292, 297
  overweight and, 290–91
  shellfish and, 333
  sources of, 5, 290
  vitamin C and, 290
Chores, 127–29, 128
Cinnamon, 297

Circadian rhythm, 258–59,
    260–61, 262
Clams, 333–34
Cleaning plate, avoiding, 65, 92
Climbing stairs, 72–73, 270–71
Clothing. See also Shoes
  Capilene, 166
  changes in lifestyle and,
    95–97, 96
  cotton, 192
  cycling, 154–56
  dancing, 133
  Lycra, 191–92
  martial arts, 175–76
  running, 160
  skiing, 166–68
  spandex, 155–56
  Thermax, 166
  tips for dressing lean and,
    95–97, 96
  weight-lifting, 191–92
Coates, Budd, 157–58, 160,
    191–92
Cochran, Neva, 345–46
Cocktails, 83
Coffee, 297
Colbeth, Doug, 278–80, **278**
Coleman, Douglas L., 22
Colon cancer, 11, 291, 338
Colorectal cancer, 291
Commuting, exercise and,
    263–66, 265
Competition, athletic, 52, 173
Complex carbohydrates, 18
Concentration curl, 241, **241**
Concentric phase, 187
Connelly, A. Scott, 293
Convenience food
  canned food, 304 –7, 323
  in convenince stores, 300
  fast food, 88, 295, 298–300,
    299
  frozen food, 301 –3, 323, 336
Converted rice, 348

American intakes of, 345
body weight and, _292_
cancer and, 291–93
cholesterol and, 290–91, 343
corn oil and, 291
evolutionary perspective on,
    288–89
food labels and, 293, 297
heart disease and, 289–90,
    297
hydrogenated, _21_, 341
in
    common foods, _291_
    dairy products, 340–41, 343
    fish, 332–33
    frozen food, 302
    margarine vs. butter,
        340–41
    meat, 328–29
    milk, 340
    red meat, 300, 325, 332
    shellfish, 333
    snacks, _77_
lipids and, 4–6, _5_
monounsaturated, _21_, 289,
    297
omega-6 fatty acids, 291
omega-3 fatty acids, 305–6,
    333
polyunsaturated, _21_, 289–90
pros and cons of, 288
reducing, 17, 19, 23–24,
    40–42
saturated, 11, _21_, 289, 302,
    341
serving sizes and, 23–24
skimming, when cooking,
    321
taste and, 23
3-gram rule and, 23
trans fatty acids, 340–41
triglycerides, _5_, 333
weight and, _292_
weight gain and, 17, 22–23

Dieting, 16–19, 49
Digging with shovel, _128_, 129
Dining out
    changes in lifestyle and,
        79–83, _80_, _81_, _87_
    ethnic food and, _87_
    fast food and, 88, 295,
        298–300, _299_
    salads and, 80
    vegetables and, 82
Dinner, 68, 352
Dip, 235, **235**
Discipline, _29_, 48–49
Dishman, Rod K., _110_
Donkin, Scott, 129
Dough, pasta, 347
Doughnuts, 71–72
Downhill skiing, 166–67
Downing, Dan, 132
Dressings, 80–82
Dried fruits, 295
Drugs, circadian rhythm and,
    258
Dumbbell curl, seated, 202,
    202
Dumbbell fly, 237, **237**
Dumbbell kickback, 242, **242**
Dumbbell row, one-arm, 238,
    238
Dumbbells, 190, 269
Dumbbell sidebend, 225, **225**
Duncan, John, 124–26, 130,
    149, 151–52

E

Eating habits, _22_, _65_
Eating schedules, 23, 64–65,
    75, 294–95
Eccentric phase, _187_
Eccrine glands, 115
Ectomorph, 106–8, _107_
Egg noodles, 296
Eggs, 343

Endomorph, 106–8, _107_
Endosperm, 344–45, 347
Endurance, _154_, 170
Equipment for
    cooking, 320–22
    cycling, 153–54, 155
    exercise at work, 269
    pullups, 136
    rowing, 173
    skiing, 167
    swimming, 170
    weight lifting, 187, 189–94,
        _192_
Erdman, John, 7–8
Erector spinae, 234
Ethnic food, _87_
Exercise. *See also* Aerobic
        exercise; *specific types*;
        Stretching; Time for
        exercise; Workouts
    in afternoon, 259
    body clock and, 259, 262
    calories burned by, 23
        aerobic dance, _113_
        chores and yardwork, _128_
        cycling, _113_
        jumping rope, 137
        pro baseball, 153
        running, 49, _113_, 153, 157
        skiing, 166
        tennis, 49
        Tour de France cycling,
            153
        walking, 53, _113_, _125_
    commuting and, 263–66, _265_
    competitive, 52
    elderly and, 57–59, _58_
    energy-boosting, 66
    in evening, 23, 259, 262
    everyday
        chores, 127–29, _128_
        dancing, _113_, 132–34, _133_
        golf, 130–31
        jumping jacks, 135, **135**

holidays and, 89–94, _90_, _92_
labels on
    canned food and, 306
    dietary fat and, 293, 297
    FDA definitions and, 312
    frozen food and, 302
    meat and, 329
    reading, 297
    sodium and, 306
low-fat, 24, _43_, 77–78, _77_,
    295–97, 322–25, _322_
multicourse meals and, _65_
preferences, _11_
raw, 334
roles of, 42, _43_
second helpings of, _65_
spicy, 23, 93–94
substitutions, _43_, 77
toppings, 24, 80–82, 91–92,
    296
24-hour plan for, 64–68, _65_,
    _67_
Food diary, _37_
Food Guide Pyramid, 12,
    308–10, _309_, _310_, 345
Foreman, Doug, 144–45, **144**
Foreman, George, 57, 127, 129
Foreyt, John P., 4–5, 8–9,
    13–14, 20, 36, _37_
Franklin, Barry, 268
Franklin, Ben, 336
Free weights, 187, 189–90
French fries, 300
Frog-leg crunch, 218, **218**
Front lat pulldown, 201, **201**,
    238, **238**
Front lunge, 210, **210**
Froot Loops, 338
Frozen food, 301–3, 323, 336
Fruits. _See also specific types_
    cancer prevention and,
        302–3, 349–50
    canned, 306
    citrus, 350

cooking, 349–55, _352_, _354_
dried, 295
fiber in, 93
fresh, 352–55
meal plans including, 351–52
red, 350
Furman, Ashrita, 25–27, **25**, _26_,
    57

G

Gallagher, Drury, 168–69
Galloway, Jeff, 159
Gardner, Christopher, 289–90
Garlic, 330
Gear. _See_ Equipment for
Genetics
    fat cells and, 4
    metabolism and, 21, 39
    weight gain and, 20–24, 39
Germ, 344
_Gi_, 175–76
Ginger, 325
Gloves, weight-lifting, 192
Glucose levels, 6
Gluteus maximus, 251
Gluteus medius, 251
Gluteus minimus, 251
Goals
    fitness, 111
    Men's Health Weight-Loss
        Formula and
        maintaining, 39–41, _40_
    setting, 34–38, _37_, 46–47
    weight-lifting, 187–88
Goggles, swimming, 170
Goldman, Bob, 46
Golf, 130–31
González, Michael J., 289,
    291–92, 309, _309_
Grains, 344–48, _346_
Grapefruits, 290, 355
Grapes, 353
Graves, James E., 234, 245

Grazing, 75, 295
Greens, 80, 92, 295, 325
Grilling, _324_, 326
Ground beef, 49, 299–300,
    330–31
Ground fish, _335_
Guista, Antoine, 168
Gut. _See_ Abdominal fat
Gyms, 52, 186–87, _268_

H

Hagerman, Frederick C.,
    171–73
Halberg, Franz, 64
Hamburger, 49, 299–300,
    330–31
Hamburger Helper, 330–31
Hamstrings, 251, _265_
    flexibility of, _196_
Hanging knee-raise crossover,
    224, **224**
Hanging leg-raise crossover,
    224, **224**
Hanging single-knee raise, 223,
    223
Hansell, John, 83
Harper, Pat, 294–95, 326
Harrison, Chip, 128, 135
Harville, Susan, 320, 325
Hasler, Clare, 351
HDL. _See_ High-density
    lipoprotein
Health clubs, 52, 186–87, _268_
Heart disease
    alcohol and, 15
    cholesterol and, _5_
    dietary fat and, 289–90, 297
    fish for preventing, 333
    insulin levels and, 345
Heat exhaustion, 117
Heatstroke, 117
Heel raise, 255, **255**, 265–66
    one-leg, 210, **210**

National Academy of Sports Medicine, <u>48</u>

National Cancer Institute, 302, 350

National Museum of Pasta Foods, 347

National Safety Council, 58

National Strength and Conditioning Association, <u>48</u>

National Yogurt Association, 342

Neck exercises. *See* Shoulders-and-neck workout

Nelson, Gary J., 332–33, 343

Newman, Steven M., 124, 126

Nieman, David, <u>150</u>

Noodles, 296, 327, 347

NordicTrack, 167

No-stick cookware and spray, 321, 323, 327

Nutmeg, 297

Nutrition, 294–97. *See also* Diet; Food(s)

Nutrition Facts panel, 308, 310

Nuts, 83

O

Ob gene, 21

Oblique crunch, 222, **222**, 229, **229**

Obliques, 216

Oblique twist, 223, **223**, 231, **231**

Oils, 291–92, 296–97

Oleo, 340–41

Olive oil, 292, 297

Olympic power bench, 190

Olympic weights, 189–90

Omega-6 fatty acids, 291

Omega-3 fatty acids, 305–6, 333

One-arm dumbbell row, 238, **238**

One-legged squat, 73

One-leg heel raise, 210, **210**

Onions, 355

Oranges, 353

Otter Bar Lodge, 55

Oven roasting, 321, 326

Overload principle, <u>187</u>

Overweight, <u>71</u>, 290–91. *See also* Body fat; Weight gain

Oysters, 333–34

P

Pace, Adele, 259, 267, 269, <u>270</u>

Palmer, Jim, 356–58, **356**

Pancreatic cancer, 291

Parker, Ann, 349, 351

Parties, lifestyle changes and, 93–94

Pastas, 327, 344–48, <u>346</u>

Peaches, 354–55

Pear type of body-fat distribution, 7–8

Pectoralis major, 234

Pectoralis minor, 234

Pedals, clipless bike, 155

Peikin, Steven, <u>65</u>, 80, 82, 91

Pelchat, Marcia Levin, <u>22</u>, 74, 76, <u>76</u>

Pelvic lift, 251, **251**

Pépin, Jacques, 313–15, **313**

Peppers, 355

Perose, Richard, 336

Perose, Robert, <u>335</u>, 336

Personal trainers, <u>48</u>

Perspiration, 115–17, <u>116</u>

Peters, Tom, 138–40, **138**

Phospholipids, <u>5</u>

Physical activity. *See* Exercise; *specific types*

Phytochemicals, 349–50

Pizza, 300

Polyunsaturated fat, <u>21</u>, 289–90

Popcorn, 77, <u>81</u>

Portions of food. *See* Serving sizes

Posture, <u>58</u>, 131

Potatoes, 82, 293, 300, 355

President's Council on Physical Fitness and Sports, 8, <u>35</u>, 38

Pressure cooker, 321

Prevention Index, 10

Price, Joan, 46, 51–52

Produce. *See* Fruits; Vegetables

Progress, recording, 52

Prostate cancer, 11, 291

Protein, 11, 19, 66, 338

Pulldowns
  front lat, 201, **201**, 238, **238**
  triceps, 241, **241**

Pullups, 136, **136**

Pushups
  between chairs, 206, **206**
  decline, 206, **206**
  desk, 207, **207**, 275, **275**

Q

Quadriceps, 251

R

Radicchio, 325

Raglin, Jack, <u>150</u>

Raised-leg exercises
  crunch, 220, **220**
  curl, 252, **252**
  knee-in, 221, **221**

Raisin Bran, 338

Rappelfeld, Joe, 161–63, <u>162</u>

Reaven, Gerald, 345

Recommended Dietary Allowance, 328